Pathology of Tumours
of the Oral Tissues

Pathology of Tumours of the Oral Tissues

R. B. Lucas
M.D., F.R.C.P., F.R.C.Path.

Professor of Oral Pathology in the University of London
Pathologist, Royal Dental Hospital of London

THIRD EDITION

CHURCHILL LIVINGSTONE
Edinburgh London and New York 1976

Churchill Livingstone
Medical Division of Longman Group Limited

Distributed in the United States of America by
Longman Inc., 19 West 44th Street, New York, N.Y. 10036
and by associated companies, branches and
representatives throughout the world.

© Longman Group Limited 1976

First Edition 1964
Second Edition 1972
Third Edition 1976

ISBN 0 443 01397 7

Library of Congress Cataloging in Publication Data

Lucas, Raleigh Barclay.
    Pathology of tumours of the oral tissues.

    Includes index.
    1. Mouth—Tumors. 2. Histology, Pathological.
I. Title. DNLM: 1. Mandibular neoplasms—
Pathology. 2. Maxillary neoplasms—Pathology.
3. Mouth neoplasms—Pathology. WU280 L933pj
RC280.M6L8   1976   616.9′92′31   75-43545

Printed in Great Britain

Preface to the Third Edition

THE rate of advance of knowledge in these times, and the rapidity with which factual information accumulates, ensure that even if textbooks can be said to be fully up to date when their authors have written the last word, they will certainly have fallen behind by the time they have gone through all the time-consuming processes of production and have finally become available to their readership. Nevertheless, in this edition, an endeavour has been made to incorporate the significant advances of recent years and to revise the subject matter where necessary. In this task I have had much help and assistance from Professor A. C. Thackray, and Professor Ivor R. H. Kramer has also made valuable suggestions. It is a pleasure to express my thanks to these colleagues. I should also like to thank my colleagues of the Royal Dental Hospital for permission to use their clinical records, and particularly to Dr. B. K. Wignall for radiographs. Mr. Keith Taylor, Miss Usha Desai and the photographic department of the hospital have been of great assistance, and Mr. John Mercer of my own department has again devoted his expertise to the illustrations. Miss Jill Waight has dealt with the typing with skill and patience.

London, 1976   R. B. Lucas

Preface to the First Edition

THIS account of tumours of the oral tissues has been written from the point of view of the diagnostic pathologist whose principal interest lies in the histological evaluation of biopsy and operation material. Naturally, the full assessment of the patient and his disability depends on the integration of all the available information, and of this morbid anatomy and histology represents only one fraction, though frequently a decisive one. The inclusion of remarks on the clinical and radiological features of the various lesions dealt with here is not, however, an attempt to provide a full description of all aspects that have to be taken into account in arriving at a diagnosis. These remarks are, rather, intended only to give the pathologist who may not be especially familiar with lesions in the oral region some idea of the general aspect and behaviour of these lesions, and a comprehension of what is likely to be in the clinician's mind when he sends material to the laboratory. Detailed accounts of these aspects of the subject are available in a number of excellent texts, for those who require fuller information.

Again for the benefit of those who may not have any specialised knowledge of the oral tissues, a short account of the normal histology and development of these tissues has been included. This feature likewise is not intended to replace the full descriptions provided in the special works on the subject. It is intended for those whose interests are primarily in pathological interpretation and who require only a sufficient background of embryology and histology, which for this purpose they may find it convenient to have at hand.

With regard to the principal subject matter, a wide view has been taken, for the pathologist will be interested not only in neoplasms but also in those non-neoplastic lesions that require to be considered in the differential histological diagnosis of tumours, in those that present clinically in such a manner that the clinician may regard them as possible neoplasms pending pathological examination, or in those that, though as yet non-neoplastic, may constitute possible premalignant conditions. For these reasons, a number of lesions that are not neoplastic have been included.

I have much pleasure in acknowledging the help I have received from many sources. My colleagues of the Royal Dental Hospital have generously placed at my disposal their clinical records, and have also furnished me with data and material from their cases elsewhere. In this regard I would wish particularly to thank the following for material from which the indicated figures have been prepared and for radiographs and clinical data: Mr. H. P. Cook (Figs. 19c, d; 64); Mr. B. W. Fickling (Figs. 15b; 16e; 51c, d); Mr. J. H. Hovell (Figs. 16d; 50) and Dr. D. Greer Walker (Figs. 16c; 28). Colleagues from other hospitals have been no less generous, and I should like to thank Mr. K. G. Boobyer and Dr. H. Miller for clinical data, radiographs and sections (Fig. 58); Dr. N. C. Gowing for clinical data and sections (Figs. 24c, d; 62c, d); Mr. G. T. Hankey, Professor A. E. W. Miles and Dr. J. P. Waterhouse for clinical data, radiographs and sections (Fig. 27); Professor A. B. MacGregor for clinical data, radiographs and sections (Fig. 52); Professor H. A. Magnus and Dr. B. C. Cardell for sections (Figs. 24a, b; 84); Mr. R. W. Raven and Mr. J. N. W. McCagie for clinical data and radiographs (Fig. 69); Mr. M. Tempest for specimens and clinical data (Figs. 65a, b; 73; 101c, d; 102b, c, d); Dr. A. C. Thackray for sections (Figs. 40; 63; 75d, e; 86) and Mr. P. A. Toller for specimens and sections (Figs. 16a, b; 38a; 49; 109a).

I owe a special debt of gratitude to Dr. S. Blackman and the Department of Radiology of the Royal Dental Hospital for the radiographs of our own hospital cases and for much helpful

vii

guidance, and to the Photographic Department for making the reproductions. I am also greatly indebted to Mr. K. R. Ray for much follow-up data.

My thanks are due to the following authors, editors and publishers for permission to reproduce their copyright material: Mr. H. P. Cook and the editor of *Oral Surgery, Oral Medicine, Oral Pathology* (Fig. 64a); Professor W. J. Hamilton and Messrs. Heffer (Figs. 1, 2, 4); Mr. Rainsford Mowlem, Mr. G. L. Fordyce and the editor of the *Proceedings of the Royal Society of Medicine* (Fig. 54d); and to the editors of the following journals for permission to reproduce figures from my own publications: *Journal of Clinical Pathology* (Fig. 109b); *Journal of the Royal College of Surgeons of Edinburgh* (Figs. 104c, d); *Oral Surgery, Oral Medicine, Oral Pathology* (Fig. 25a); *Proceedings of the Royal Society of Medicine* (Fig. 30a, with B. W. Fickling; Fig. 61a, with H. J. J. Blackwood). I am also indebted to Dr. S. Blackman and Messrs. John Wright and Sons Ltd for permission to reproduce from *An Atlas of Dental and Oral Radiology* the radiographs in Figs. 52, 53, 57, 72, 107 and 108.

I am particularly glad to acknowledge my indebtedness to Professor Ivor R. H. Kramer, who read the manuscript, made many useful suggestions and gave me the benefit of his wide experience. The views expressed, however, are not necessarily his.

Finally, I wish to express my thanks to my laboratory staff for their unfailing help and assistance. In particular, Mr. John Mercer, F.I.M.L.T., spent much time and effort on the preparation of the photomicrographs. Miss J. Middleton, Medical Artist to the Hospital, made the line illustrations (Figs. 3, 33, 34, 89). The great burden of secretarial work was cheerfully carried by my secretary Mrs. Brenda Coode. Miss Gillian Bayliss prepared the index.

Messrs. J. & A. Churchill were as courteous and helpful as ever to their authors, and I wish to thank in particular Mr. A. S. Knightley for unfailing patience and assistance.

London, 1964   R. B. LUCAS

Contents

I
EMBRYOLOGY AND HISTOLOGY
OF THE ORAL TISSUES

1. Embryology and Histology of the Oral Tissues

DEVELOPMENT OF THE ORAL CAVITY AND FACE

The Oral Cavity. The stomatodaeum is present in the 3-week embryo as a shallow cavity in the head region, with the brain above it and the pericardial sac below (Fig. 1). Dorsally the stomatodaeum is separated from the pharynx by the buccopharyngeal membrane, though this structure soon disintegrates to establish the continuity of the cavity with the foregut. At the back of the cavity, where it is bounded by the buccopharyngeal membrane, there is a cranial prolongation of the stomatodaeum, Rathke's pouch, from which the anterior part of the pituitary gland develops.

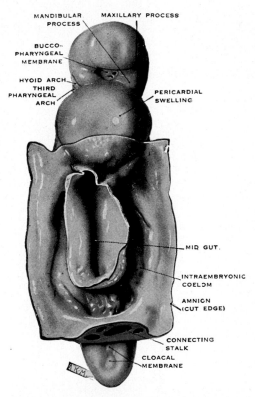

Fig. 1 The ventral aspect of a reconstruction of a 20-somite human embryo of about 26 days. Modified from Davis. × c. 32. (From Hamilton, Boyd and Mossman's "Human Embryology," Heffer, Cambridge.)

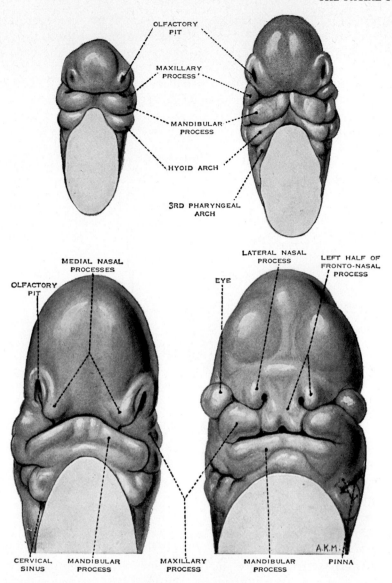

Fig. 2   Drawings of the ventral aspect of the head region of human embryos to show the development of the face. A—5·7 mm; B—6·7 mm; C—11·8 mm; D—14 mm (based on Streeter). (From Hamilton, Boyd and Mossman's "Human Embryology," Heffer, Cambridge.)

The Facial Processes. The mandibular processes arise at the sides of the primitive mouth cavity (Fig. 2). Each process grows forward to meet its fellow from the opposite side in the midline, thus forming the mandibular or first branchial arch. This arch constitutes the lower border of the oral cavity and separates it from the heart. Above the oral cavity the appearance of two depressions, the olfactory pits, divides the face into a central and two lateral areas. The central area forms the frontonasal process and the lateral areas are the lateral nasal processes. The portions of the frontonasal process in the region of the nasal pits constitute the medial nasal processes, and the inferolateral portion of each medial nasal process forms the globular process.

The maxillary processes develop as outgrowths from the dorsal part of the mandibular processes on each side and grow forward, beneath the developing eye, to form part of the upper boundary of the opening of the oral cavity. When each maxillary process reaches the region of the nasal pit it comes into close relationship with the other processes. At first, the various processes are demarcated from each other by grooves, but by the seventh week the grooves have been obliterated by fusion of the processes, due to proliferation of the mesoderm and disintegration of the covering ectoderm in the area of union (Fig. 3).

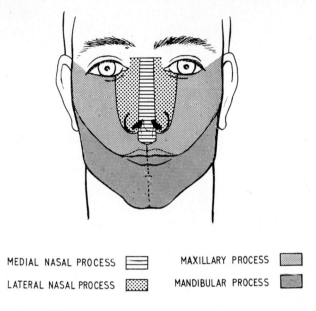

MEDIAL NASAL PROCESS

LATERAL NASAL PROCESS

MAXILLARY PROCESS

MANDIBULAR PROCESS

Fig. 3 Diagram of the adult face to show the areas derived from the various embryonic processes.

The Palate. At the same time as the maxillary processes are uniting with the other processes of the face they are also sending shelf-like extensions into the oral cavity. These extensions are the palatal processes, which eventually meet in the midline to form the posterior portion of the palate. The anterior portion is formed by similar shelf-like processes that extend backwards from the frontonasal process to fuse with each other and with the extensions from the maxillary processes. This fusion is incomplete, so that there remains a small gap in the midline, the incisive foramen. Another process also arises from the maxillary process where it forms the lateral wall of the oral cavity. This is the tectoseptal process, which grows towards the roof of the mouth to unite in the midline with its fellow from the opposite side, thus separating the brain capsule from the oral cavity. The united processes then turn downwards to form the posterior part of the nasal septum. The anterior part of the septum is formed by an extension from the frontonasal process. When the downward-growing nasal septum reaches the level of the palate, the palatal processes have not yet reached the midline. This follows, and the palatal processes and the lower border of the nasal septum then unite. The primitive oro-nasal cavity is now divided into right and left nasal cavities on each side of the septum above the palate, and the oral cavity below the palate (Figs. 4 and 5).

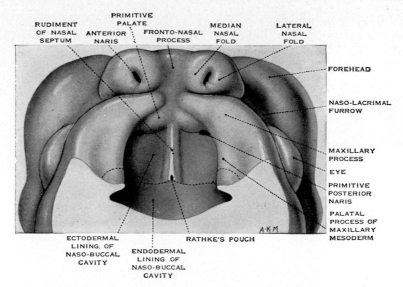

RUDIMENT OF NASAL SEPTUM — ANTERIOR NARIS — PRIMITIVE PALATE — FRONTO-NASAL PROCESS — MEDIAN NASAL FOLD — LATERAL NASAL FOLD

FOREHEAD

NASO-LACRIMAL FURROW

MAXILLARY PROCESS

EYE

PRIMITIVE POSTERIOR NARIS

PALATAL PROCESS OF MAXILLARY MESODERM

ECTODERMAL LINING OF NASO-BUCCAL CAVITY — ENDODERMAL LINING OF NASO-BUCCAL CAVITY — RATHKE'S POUCH

A·K·M

Fig. 4   A drawing of the roof of the stomatodaeum of a 13·5 mm human embryo. A distinct palatal process from the maxillary mesoderm is now present. This will later meet its fellow of the opposite side and fuse with it and with the down-growing nasal septum. The latter is now seen as a ridge in the roof of the primitive nasal cavity portion of the stomatodaeum. The previous site of attachment of the buccopharyngeal membrane is shown by the interrupted line. (From Hamilton, Boyd and Mossman's "Human Embryology," Heffer, Cambridge.)

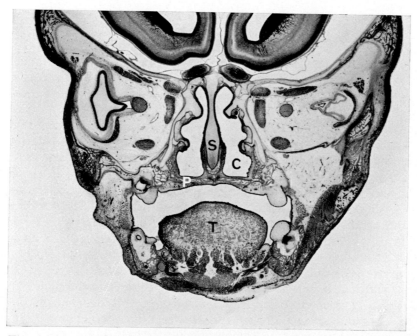

Fig. 5   Frontal section through the head of an approximately 12-week embryo. The palatine processes and nasal septum have united. ×4.
S Nasal septum   P Palate   C Nasal cavity   T Tongue

The nasopalatine duct, traversing the incisive foramen, provides a communication between the oral and nasal cavities in many animals but in man only the upper end remains patent, the lower end terminating blindly in the palatine papilla. Jacobson's organ is a small detached portion of the olfactory plate that lies in the nasal septum above the nasopalatine duct. It is vestigial in man.

The Tongue. A series of eminences similar in shape to the mandibular or first branchial arch develop parallel to the arch and below it. These are the second, third, fourth and fifth branchial arches. The first, second and third arches give rise to the tongue, the posterior part developing from the third arch and the anterior part from the first and second arches. Two eminences develop within the oral cavity on the first arch, one on each side, and a third eminence develops in the midline, somewhat dorsally to these two. This is the tuberculum impar. These three swellings form the body of the tongue, while an outgrowth from the third arch forms the base. The base grows to meet the body, the junction between the two parts being marked by the sulcus terminalis, which persists throughout life. The thyroid gland develops from a down-growth of epithelium from the floor of the mouth, at the same time as the tongue is developing. The point of origin of this downgrowth, which becomes the thyroglossal duct, is marked on the dorsum of the tongue by the foramen caecum, situated between the anterior and posterior parts.

The epithelium of the tongue is at first of simple cuboidal type. From this there develop first the vallate and later the fungiform and filiform papillae.

For full accounts of the development of the oral tissues, see Keith (1948), Sicher (1972) and Hamilton, Boyd and Mossman (1974).

DEVELOPMENT OF THE JAWS AND THE TEETH

The mandible develops in the mandibular arch, Meckel's cartilage appearing before ossification occurs. This cartilaginous rod extends from the otic capsule, where it gives rise to the incus and malleus, through the mandibular arch to the midline to meet its fellow of the opposite side. At the sixth week of embryonic life a thin plate of bone appears in the arch, immediately ventral to Meckel's cartilage, and ossification then proceeds rapidly. Most of Meckel's cartilage disappears, but near the middle line the extreme end of the cartilage is at first enclosed in a bony tunnel. Later, this portion of the cartilage also disappears.

The maxilla develops in the maxillary process. Ossification commences about the seventh week, from a centre or centres close to the nasal capsule. The maxillary sinus develops as an outgrowth from the lateral wall of the nasal capsule, first appearing at about the fourth month.

The teeth commence development in the sixth week of embryonic life. At this stage, proliferation of the oral ectoderm along the whole length of the jaw results in a ridge of epithelium growing down from its deep surface into the underlying mesoderm. This ridge is the primary epithelial band which divides, a little later, into outer and inner processes. The outer process is the vestibular lamina, which subsequently takes part in the separation of the lip and cheek from the jaw. The inner process is the dental lamina, from which the teeth develop. The first sign of the development of the individual teeth is the appearance of separate bud-like swellings at intervals along the dental lamina in each jaw. These are the enamel organs of the deciduous teeth. At this early stage each enamel organ consists simply of an aggregation of epithelial cells, but the cells proliferate rapidly and in such a manner that the growing organ assumes a cap-like shape. At the same time the mesoderm immediately adjacent to the developing enamel organ proliferates, forming a condensation termed the dental papilla. This structure will later give rise to dentine formation and will itself ultimately become the pulp of the tooth (Figs. 6 and 7).

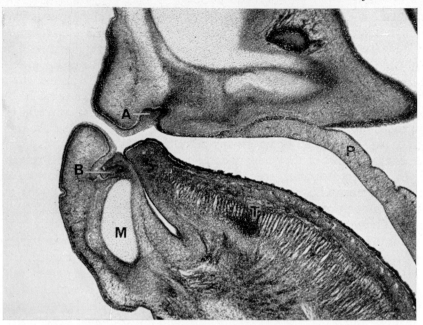

Fig. 6 Sagittal section through oral region of a 12-week embryo, showing tooth germs in both jaws. × 30.

A Tooth germ in maxilla   T Tongue   P Palate
B Tooth germ in mandible   M Meckel's cartilage

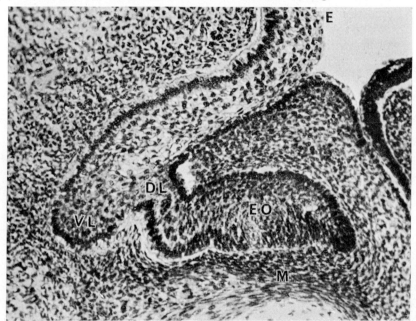

Fig. 7 Higher magnification of the mandibular tooth germ in Fig. 6. The oral epithelium has grown into the jaw to give rise to the dental lamina and tooth germ and the vestibular lamina. The tooth germ is at the cap stage and just deep to the cap can be seen the commencing condensation of the mesenchyme to form the dental papilla. × 200.

E Oral epithelium   DL Dental lamina   EO Enamel organ
VL Vestibular lamina   M Condensing mesenchyme

The cap-shaped enamel organ continues its growth, becoming elongated as it extends more deeply into the mesoderm of the jaw. Since the cells of its deep surface proliferate least rapidly it becomes bell-shaped rather than cap-shaped, with the dental papilla remaining within the cavity of the bell. While the enamel organ is thus enlarging, the free end of the dental lamina proliferates. This proliferation gives rise to the enamel organ of the permanent tooth, and it will go through the same changes as the enamel organ of the deciduous tooth. Subsequently, the dental lamina is penetrated by ingrowth of the surrounding mesoderm, which breaks it up into isolated groups of cells. The tooth germ now lies free in the jaw, and the remnants of the dental lamina mostly disappear. Some groups of cells persist, however, and may cornify to form small epithelial pearls, or they may undergo cystic change. Epithelial cells or microcysts originating in this way are frequently seen in the jaws of infants, and in sections of fetal material, but they mostly disappear with eruption of the teeth. Similar rests are often seen in the follicles of teeth that remain unerupted.

The Enamel Organ. As the aggregate of epithelial cells that buds off the dental lamina grows into the cap stage the cells differentiate to form a peripheral layer that is continuous with the basal layer of the oral epithelium and that encloses a central area of polyhedral cells. The peripheral cells are of low columnar type while the central cells are polyhedral, but changes take place in both these cell groups as growth proceeds. When the enamel organ reaches the cap stage those cells of the peripheral layer that line the deep surface of the organ become taller, while the cells lining the rest of the enamel organ remain low columnar in type. By the time the bell stage is reached four distinct layers or zones can be seen. These are (1) the external enamel epithelium, (2) the internal enamel epithelium, (3) the stellate reticulum, (4) the stratum intermedium (Fig. 8). The external enamel epithelium is that portion of the peripheral layer of cells that covers the convex surface of the enamel organ. These cells are of low cubical type. The internal enamel epithelium is the zone of the peripheral cells that lines the deep surface of the enamel organ, that is to say, the concavity of the cap or the hollow of the bell. These cells are tall columnar and will presently become ameloblasts and form enamel. The mass of cells that is enclosed within the external and internal enamel epithelium, and that forms the greater part of the enamel organ, is the stellate reticulum. To begin with, these cells are much the same in appearance as are the cells of the oral mucosa, but following the differentiation of the outermost cells to form the enamel epithelium the internal cells become star-shaped and separated to some extent from one another by the accumulation of intercellular fluid, though they still remain in contact by means of intercellular processes. Those cells of the stellate reticulum immediately adjacent to the internal enamel epithelium are flattened, and constitute the stratum intermedium. The area where the cells of the internal and external enamel epithelium meet is the cervical loop. It is here that most of the further growth of the enamel organ takes place, and in due course the loop will become the root sheath of Hertwig.

Fig. 8   Consecutive stages in the development of the tooth germ. **a** and **b,** bell stage. × 30. **c,** dentine and enamel are forming. × 30. **d,** higher magnification of enamel organ to show the cellular layers. × 75.

OE	Oral epithelium		Ex	External enamel epithelium
DL	Dental lamina		SI	Stratum intermedium
B	Bud for permanent tooth		CL	Cervical loop
SR	Stellate reticulum		DE	Dentine and enamel formation
In	Internal enamel epithelium		DP	Dental papilla

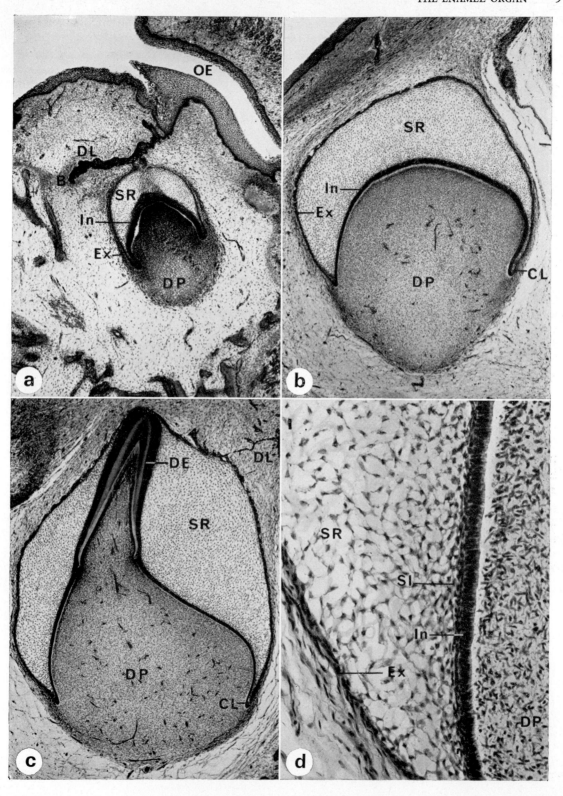

Dentinogenesis. By the time the internal enamel epithelium has differentiated, the meso-dermal cells of the dental papilla have laid down fine argyrophil fibres and those cells of the papilla nearest to the enamel epithelium have become columnar and arranged side by side in a single layer. These are the odontoblasts, their differentiation resulting from the organising effect of the internal enamel epithelium upon the mesodermal cells of the dental papilla. Thus there are now two rows of cells facing each other, the cells of the internal enamel epithelium and the odontoblasts, separated only by a basement membrane.

Dentine appears in the region of the basement membrane, between the two rows of cells. To begin with it is in the form of an organic matrix, but as deposition continues calcification takes place in those areas first laid down. The zone of dentine most recently deposited—that next to the odontoblasts—always remains uncalcified so long as dentinogenesis continues, and is termed the predentine zone. Dentinogenesis begins first at the crown area of the tooth and the process spreads till dentine is being laid down all round the dental papilla, except its base. As the dentine is deposited tubules appear in it, each one containing a process from an odontoblast (Fig. 9).

Amelogenesis. Soon after the cells of the internal enamel epithelium have assumed a tall columnar appearance the nuclei become regularly arranged at the inner ends of the cells. Following this, the odontoblasts differentiate and dentine is laid down as just described. It is only after dentine formation has commenced that amelogenesis can take place, and this is heralded by the cells of the internal enamel epithelium becoming shorter again. These cells are now known as ameloblasts. At the end of each ameloblast, next to the dentine, an area of the cytoplasm becomes granular and demarcated from the rest of the cell by a condensation, the terminal bar. From this area of the cell, the Tomes' process, enamel matrix is secreted and after a certain amount of the matrix has been laid down mineralisation commences. The mineral is in the form of crystallites of hydroxyapatite and these have a preferred orientation within the matrix, probably dictated by the ameloblasts. This gives the enamel a prismatic structure. Mineralisation con-tinues, and to such an extent that when it has been completed the enamel consists almost entirely (96 per cent) of inorganic material. From this stage onwards enamel cannot be demonstrated in decalcified sections, for the small amount of organic material that remains after decalcification is insufficient to maintain the general structure of the tissues. In such sections, therefore, the enamel is represented by an empty space. Where organic enamel matrix is still present, however, it can be readily examined, as it resists decalcification and stains well by routine methods. In cross-section its prismatic structure is well seen (Fig. 9). As the zone of enamel matrix increases in thickness the ameloblasts retreat towards the periphery of the enamel organ. That is to say, the stellate reticulum of the enamel organ becomes progressively reduced in size till eventually it disappears completely and the ameloblasts come into contact with the external enamel epi-thelium. When this occurs the formation of enamel is complete and the ameloblasts, as a last function, deposit a thin layer, or enamel cuticle, on the surface of the enamel. After this they become smaller and similar to the cells of the external enamel epithelium. Thus, what was once the enamel organ now consists merely of the former ameloblasts and the external enamel epi-thelium without any intervening stellate reticulum. This remnant is now termed the reduced enamel epithelium, and together with the enamel cuticle forms Nasmyth's membrane.

Formation of the Root. Though at first all the layers of the enamel organ are present in the cervical loop, as this structure continues to elongate the stellate reticulum and stratum inter-medium disappear so that the internal and external enamel epithelium come into contact. This double layer is then known as the root sheath of Hertwig. No enamel is formed in this region, but dentine is laid down to constitute the root of the tooth. Much of this process takes place after the tooth has entered the oral cavity, for at the time of eruption the roots are still largely unformed. When the root dentine has been completely laid down, a process that takes up to two to three

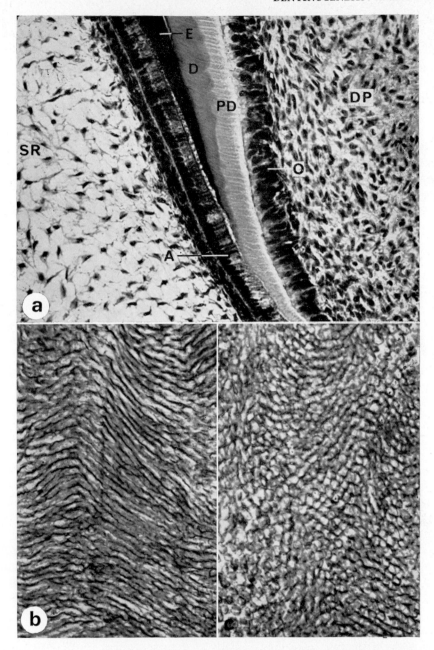

Fig. 9 **a,** developing dentine and enamel, laid down in juxtaposition. × 200. **b** and **c,** longitudinal and transverse sections of developing enamel. The longitudinal section shows the rod structure and the transverse section the roughly hexagonal appearance of the rods. × 480.

DP	Dental papilla	PD	Predentine	E	Enamel
O	Odontoblasts	D	Dentine	A	Ameloblasts
		SR	Stellate reticulum		

years for the permanent teeth and less for the deciduous teeth, the root sheath disintegrates. Its remnants, however, persist around the roots of the teeth as the epithelial rests of Malassez. In cross-sections of the teeth the rests appear as small groups of epithelial cells lying in the connective tissue of the periodontal membrane, close to the root of the tooth. In tangential and longitudinal sections the rests are seen to form chains of cells of varying length, sometimes in an intercommunicating network.

Cementogenesis. When the epithelial root sheath breaks up, the surrounding connective tissue comes into contact with the dentine of the root. This induces those cells close to the dentine to differentiate into cementoblasts, which then deposit cementum upon the root.

The Dental Follicle. At an early stage in the development of the tooth, the cells of the mesoderm condense around the tooth germ and in due course become fibroblasts. They then lay down fibrous tissue to form a sac or follicle within which the tooth continues to develop. Later, when ossification commences in the jaw, bone will grow around the follicle to form a cavity or crypt enclosing it.

Eruption of the Teeth. When formation of the dentine and enamel of the crown have been completed the tooth commences to move towards the oral mucosa. The crown is covered by the reduced enamel epithelium and when this reaches the oral mucosa the two layers of epithelium fuse. Continued movement of the tooth leads to the crown proceeding through the fused layers and thus entering the oral cavity.

STRUCTURE OF THE MATURE TOOTH

The greater part of the mature tooth consists of dentine. The root dentine is covered by a thin layer of cementum and the dentine of the crown is covered by enamel. Internally, the dentine contains the dental pulp in the pulp chamber. The root of the tooth occupies a socket in the alveolar bone, to which it is attached by the connective tissue fibres of the periodontal ligament (Fig. 10).

The Pulp. The pulp consists of loose connective tissue and carries the blood, lymphatic and nerve supply to the tooth. Where it meets the dentine, the surface of the pulp is covered by a layer of odontoblasts. These are columnar cells with oval nuclei, and each cell has a process that lies within a corresponding tubule in the dentine. Immediately internal to the odontoblast layer there is a narrow cell-free zone (Fig. 11).

Dentine. Physically and chemically dentine is very similar to bone, consisting of 30 per cent organic material and water, and 70 per cent inorganic material. As in bone, the organic fraction consists of collagen fibrils embedded in a mucopolysaccharide cementing substance, and the inorganic fraction consists mainly of calcium phosphates in the form of apatite crystals. Unlike bone, however, dentine contains no cell bodies but only cell processes, those of the odontoblasts, in the dentinal tubules. The dentinal tubules are 2 to 3μ in diameter and each runs through the whole thickness of the dentine from the cell body of the odontoblast to the outer surface of the dentine. There are cross-communications between the tubules, containing anastomosing branches of the odontoblast processes (Fig. 11). Calcification of the dentine occurs in spherical or globular masses or calcospherites, which coalesce to give a uniformly mineralised tissue. Where calcification is incomplete the separate globules can be seen, with the uncalcified or hypocalcified ground substance in between them. Such areas are referred to as interglobular dentine.

Enamel. As previously mentioned, mature enamel can be studied only in ground sections unless special methods are employed, since it is completely removed by routine histological decalcification. The inorganic fraction of enamel is hydroxyapatite and the small organic fraction

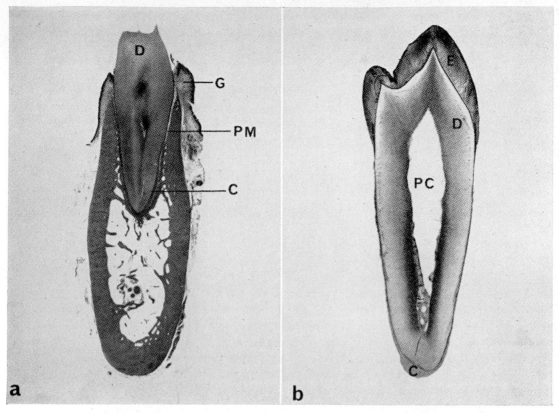

Fig. 10 **a,** decalcified section of tooth in situ in the mandible. × 2·5. **b,** ground section of tooth. × 4

E	Enamel	C	Cementum
D	Dentine	PM	Periodontal ligament
PC	Pulp chamber	G	Gingiva

is a complex of proteins. Proline is present but there is little if any cystine, so that this organic fraction of enamel differs in character both from keratin and collagen.

Enamel consists of rods or prisms in an interprismatic substance that is slightly less mineralised than the rods themselves. Each rod runs from the enamel-dentine junction through the whole thickness of the enamel to its surface, following a slightly wavy course. The rods are roughly hexagonal in cross-section, with an average diameter of 4 μ.

Cementum. Cementum is a modified type of bone that covers the dentine of the tooth root in a thin layer (Fig. 11). Two varieties of cementum occur normally, acellular and cellular. Acellular or primary cementum, the type first formed, covers the root from the enamel-cementum junction to close to the apex. As the name implies, this thin layer of cementum is homogeneous and contains no cells. Cellular or secondary cementum covers the apical portion of the root, and in a thicker layer than the acellular cementum covers the coronal end of the root. Lacunae containing the cementocytes are present, corresponding to the lacunae for osteocytes in bone. The cementocytes are very similar morphologically to osteocytes, though they are usually somewhat larger. The processes of the cementocytes do not radiate in all directions like those of osteocytes, but tend to be directed away from the dentine towards the periodontal ligament. Well-marked incremental lines running parallel with the root surface are seen in the cementum and it is quite normal to find successive increments of both acellular and cellular cementum occurring in any order or distribution, though that mentioned above is the usual finding. Cementum is continuously deposited throughout life. The principal function of cementum is to give attachment to the fibres of the periodontal ligament.

Periodontal Ligament. The connective tissue fibres generally termed the periodontal ligament or membrane constitute a suspensory ligament that attaches the tooth to the bony alveolus. The fibres are attached to the cementum, and for the most part run in bundles to the alveolar bone. Those from the cementum nearest to the crown, however, run across the alveolar crest to the cementum of the adjacent tooth, and some also run into the gingiva (Fig. 11).

HISTOLOGY OF THE ORAL CAVITY AND FACE

No special description of the normal structure of these tissues is necessary, though some remarks on the oral mucosa may be useful.

The mucous membrane surrounding the necks of the teeth is the gingiva or gum (Fig. 12). The gingiva is firmly attached to the tooth in a cuff-shaped manner, but the arrangement of the tissues is such that a shallow sulcus is formed. This gingival sulcus tends to collect food and debris, particularly in the absence of adequate oral hygiene, and this provides a favourable situation for bacterial growth. Even in gingivae that appear completely normal clinically, at least a sparse infiltration of macrophages and lymphocytes can be noted in the subepithelial connective tissue in the region of the gingival sulcus. The epithelium is usually keratinised, though often in otherwise normal tissues keratinisation is lacking, or there may be parakeratosis. The epithelial pegs and dermal papillae are long and slender. The mucous membrane covering the jaws farther away from the gingiva constitutes the alveolar mucosa. Here the epithelium lacks a stratum corneum and epithelial pegs are poorly developed or absent.

The mucous membrane elsewhere in the mouth shows some variations in the different areas (Fig. 13). The epithelium of the hard palate is well keratinised and has numerous long pegs. Mucous glands are present in the subepithelial connective tissue posteriorly. The palatine papilla contains the blind endings of the nasopalatine ducts, which are lined by columnar epithelium with numerous goblet cells. Small islets of cartilage are sometimes found in this area, derived from the paraseptal cartilages. Islets of epithelium may be present, usually close to the papilla but also elsewhere in the midline of the palate. These may show cornification. They are the remnants of the epithelium that covered the line of fusion of the palatal processes. The oral aspect of the soft palate is covered by non-keratinised squamous epithelium. The free borders of the nasal surface are also covered by squamous epithelium but the remainder of this surface

---

Fig. 11   **a,** longitudinal section of tooth, showing pulp, odontoblasts, predentine zone and dentine. × 200. **b,** longitudinal section of root of tooth, showing attachment to the alveolar bone by the periodontal membrane. × 12. **c,** longitudinal section of tooth. A relatively thin layer of acellular cementum lines the dentine. Epithelial rests are present in the periodontal ligament. × 75. **d,** transverse section of tooth, showing a thin layer of acellular cementum covering the dentine, then several increments of cellular cementum and finally another layer of acellular cementum. × 85.

P	Pulp	CC	Cellular cementum
O	Odontoblasts	PM	Periodontal ligament
PD	Predentine	E	Epithelial rests
D	Dentine	A	Alveolar bone
AC	Acellular cementum	C	Cementum

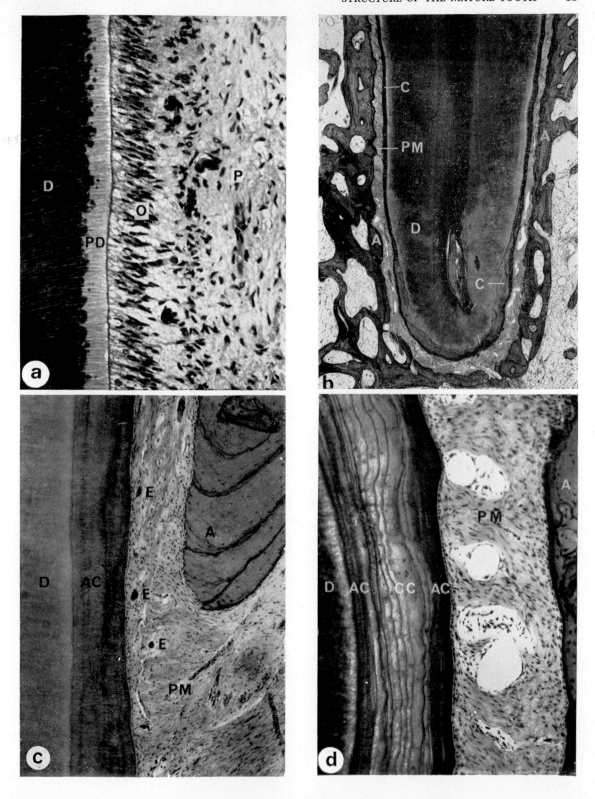

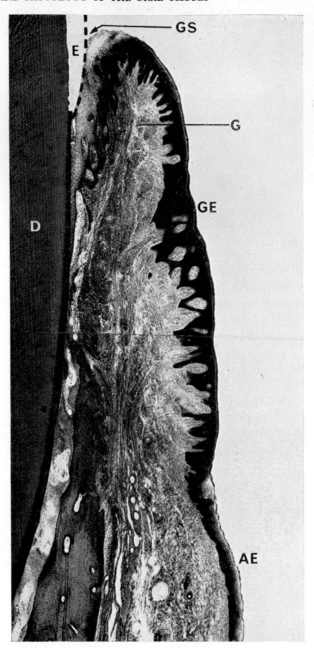

Fig. 12   Longitudinal section of tooth and gingiva. The gingiva forms a shallow sulcus at its free extremity. The epithelium is keratinised and has numerous pegs and the connective tissue shows chronic inflammatory infiltration. The epithelium of the alveolar mucosa lacks pegs and is not keratinised. × 35.

D	Dentine	GS	Gingival sulcus
E	Indicates position of	G	Gingiva
	enamel in undecalcified	AE	Alveolar epithelium
	tooth	GE	Gingival epithelium

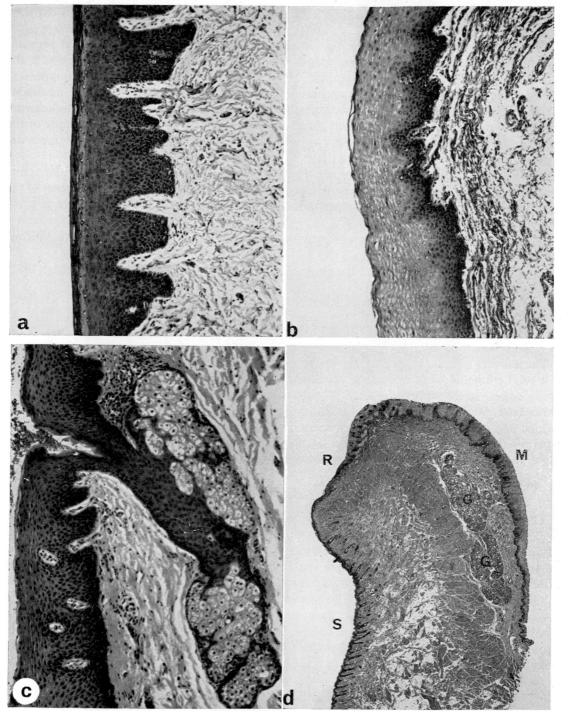

Fig. 13 Variations in the mucosa in different areas of the mouth. **a,** hard palate, showing keratinisation and numerous epithelial pegs. × 75. **b,** floor of mouth. The epithelium is not keratinised and the epithelial pegs are short. × 75. **c,** check. A sebaceous gland ("Fordyce spot") opens on to the mucosal surface. × 75. **d,** lip. The character of the different zones is seen in this low power view. × 7·5. R Red zone S Skin M Mucosa G Mucous glands.

cytoplasm and numerous long thin processes lie between the bases of the secretory cells and the basement membrane. The tentacle-like processes embrace the secretory cells and are thought to be concerned, by virtue of their contractility, in the flow of secretion from the secretory cells.

The alveoli discharge into the intercalated ducts, which are lined by low columnar or cubical cells and surrounded by myoepithelial cells. These ducts join to form the striated ducts, lined by a single row of columnar cells that show perpendicular striations in the cytoplasm of the basal area, near the basal membrane. The striated ducts are intralobular; the lobules are then connected by the junction of the striated ducts to form the excretory ducts, lined by pseudo-stratified epithelium.

Lymphatic tissue is often associated with the parotid gland. Small lymph nodes are frequently to be found within the capsule and sometimes the nodes themselves contain salivary tissue. Lymph nodes adjacent to the gland, outside the capsule, have also been shown to contain salivary tissue. Lymphatic tissue may also be present around the duct of the submandibular gland, but only as rather diffuse deposits and not in the form of definite nodes. Similarly, lymphatic tissue is infrequently found in connection with the sublingual gland.

Sebaceous glands normally occur in the parotid gland, arising from those intercalated and striated ducts that end blindly.

Distribution

MAJOR GLANDS

1. Parotid gland. The parotid gland is situated below and in front of the external ear. Accessory glands are often present as small masses along the course of the parotid duct. The duct opens into the vestibule of the mouth opposite the second upper molar tooth.

2. Submandibular gland. This gland lies beneath the mandible, with its duct opening at the side of the frenulum of the tongue close to the floor of the mouth. Accessory glands may be present along the course of the duct.

3. Sublingual gland. There is one major sublingual gland situated beneath the mucous membrane at the side of the frenulum of the tongue, and several lesser sublingual glands. The duct of the major gland opens near, or into, the duct of the submandibular gland. The minor glands open along a fold of mucous membrane beneath the tongue.

MINOR GLANDS

1. Labial glands. These are the numerous glands situated in the submucosa of the inner surface of the lips.

2. Buccal glands. These glands are situated in the mucous membrane of the cheek.

3. Retromolar glands. Glands situated in the retromolar fossa behind the lower third molar tooth.

4. Glands of floor of mouth. These are the lesser sublingual glands, described above.

5. Glossopalatine glands. A group of glands extending posteriorly from the lesser sublingual glands, to ascend in the mucosa of the glossopalatine fold.

6. Palatine glands. These are some 400 glands distributed over the hard palate and soft palate. There are a few glands in the uvula.

7. Tonsillar glands. Many small glands are found outside the capsule of the palatine tonsil. Glands are also present over the pharyngeal tonsil.

8. Lingual glands. On each side, a collection of glands situated close to the inferior surface of the tongue near the tip, is referred to as the anterior lingual gland. Other glands are found at the base and borders of the tongue.

ABERRANT SALIVARY TISSUE

Rarely, salivary tissue may be found lying in an indentation on the lingual surface of the mandible. Probably it is derived from the sublingual or submandibular glands. Harvey and Noble (1968) give a good account of mandibular bony indentations or defects, citing the literature.

REFERENCES

Hamilton, W. J., Boyd, J. D., and Mossman, H. W. (1974) *Human Embryology*. 4th Edition. Cambridge. Heffer.

Harvey, W., and Noble, H. W. (1968) Defects on the lingual surface of the mandible near the angle. *Brit. J. oral Surg.*, **6,** 75.

Keith, A. (1948) *Human Embryology and Morphology*. 6th Edition. London. Edwin Arnold & Co.

Scott, J. H., and Symons, N. B. B. (1974) *Introduction to Dental Anatomy*. 7th Edition. Edinburgh and London. Churchill Livingstone.

Sicher, H. (1972). *Orban's Oral Histology and Embryology*. 7th Edition. St. Louis. The C. V. Mosby Company.

II
TAXONOMY OF ORAL TUMOURS

2. Nomenclature and Classification of Oral Tumours

Many of the lesions of the oral tissues that present clinically as tumours are not neoplasms but are non-neoplastic developmental anomalies or overgrowths of inflammatory or other causation. From the point of view of pathological diagnosis it is of course important to bear all these conditions in mind. Accordingly, the term "tumour" is used here in its broader sense and is not restricted to lesions that are definitely neoplastic.

In the oral region both neoplasms and non-neoplastic tumefactions arise from the tissues specially concerned with the teeth as well as from the non-dental tissues such as nerve, bone, vascular tissue, salivary tissue and others. Those arising from the dental tissues are commonly referred to as odontogenic tumours and those from the non-dental tissues as non-odontogenic tumours.

TUMOURS OF THE DENTAL TISSUES

The term "odontome" or "odontoma," which continues to be used, though now in a more restricted way, was originally employed as a general designation for any tumour arising from the dental formative tissues. Broca's (1866) classification subdivided the odontomes according to the stage of development of the tooth at the inception of the tumour, but Malassez (1885) and Bland-Sutton (1888) laid the foundations of modern taxonomy by basing classification on the tissue from which the tumour arose. Gabell, James and Payne (1914) modified Bland-Sutton's classification but still included, as had previous authors, non-neoplastic cysts of dental origin. This classification recognised three main groups of odontomes:

EPITHELIAL ODONTOMES, arising from the dental epithelium.
COMPOSITE ODONTOMES, arising from both dental epithelium and dental mesenchyme.
CONNECTIVE TISSUE ODONTOMES, arising from dental mesenchyme only.

The epithelial odontomes included the neoplasm then known as multilocular cyst and now as ameloblastoma, and also non-neoplastic epithelial cysts. The composite odontomes were those lesions in which the abnormal tissues derived from both epithelium and mesenchyme and formed either irregular calcified masses or recognisable tooth-like structures, and the connective tissue odontomes included fibrous and other connective tissue tumours that were thought to arise from dental mesenchyme. In the following years more detailed study of the odontomes led to a gradual replacement of this terminology by one more compatible with general pathological usage, with the different lesions designated so far as possible in accordance with the parent cell type. Thus the multilocular cyst became the adamantinoma or ameloblastoma and the connective tissue odontomes became fibromas or cementomas, according to their structure. The composite lesions, consisting of both epithelial and mesenchymal dental elements, however, retained their original designation as odontomes. Thoma and Goldman (1946) systematised the more recent terminology in their classification of odontogenic tumours, omitting the non-neoplastic cysts.

The classification, later somewhat amplified by the American Academy of Oral Pathology (Robinson, 1952), ran as follows:—

I. EPITHELIAL TUMOURS.
Adamantoblastoma.
Enameloma.

II. MESENCHYMAL TUMOURS.
Odontogenic fibroma.
Dentinoma.
Cementoma.

III. ODONTOGENIC MIXED TUMOURS (ODONTOMAS).
Soft odontoma—epithelium and mesoderm.
Soft and calcified odontoma—adamantoblastoma arising in conjunction with a forming or completely formed odontoma; all sorts of histologic variations due to the inductive effects of one tissue on another.
Completely formed odontoma with enamel, dentine, pulp, cementum, periodontal membrane.

(*a*) Compound (many small teeth).
(*b*) Complex (irregular tooth structure).

It will be observed that the term "odontome" has now been narrowed to designate only those lesions that consist of both epithelial and mesenchymal elements. More recently, it has been further restricted to include only those mixed lesions that contain fully formed dental tissues of both epithelial and mesenchymal origin, that is to say, both enamel and dentine. Thus, Thoma and Goldman's soft odontoma, which consists of ameloblast-like epithelial cells and fibroblastic cells but no enamel or dentine, is now known as ameloblastic fibroma, and the odontomes are now represented only by the lesions that contain the calcified dental tissues. It is in this sense that the term odontome is in current use.

Recent classifications by Pindborg and Clausen (1958) and Gorlin, Chaudhry and Pindborg (1961), based on the inductive changes exerted by dental tissues on each other, have brought up to date the older classifications by omitting some lesions and including others that have been more recently described. It is clear, however, that much work remains to be done on the classification of the odontogenic tumours, and that new schemes will appear, for some of the lesions concerned are of infrequent occurrence and their life history is not fully known at present. The following list of odontogenic tumours groups the various lesions according to their structural characteristics, as this is a convenient and logical subdivision for use by the diagnostic pathologist and the morphologist. It should be noted that very occasionally there are encountered lesions that appear to occupy intermediate positions between the main groups, or that appear not to fit into any of the groups. However, such lesions are the exception rather than the rule. The nomenclature used here is based on that recommended by the World Health Organization (Pindborg and Kramer, 1971).

1. LESIONS CONSISTING OF ODONTOGENIC EPITHELIUM.
Ameloblastoma.
Adenomatoid odontogenic tumour.
Calcifying epithelial odontogenic tumour.
Calcifying odontogenic cyst.

Calcification may occur in these lesions but only in the form of amorphous deposits and not usually as fully developed enamel or dentine. Calcification is rare in ameloblastoma but is a very distinctive feature of the calcifying epithelial odontogenic tumour. Small scattered deposits are usually seen in the adenomatoid odontogenic tumour and may represent a type of enamel. Tubular dentine may, exceptionally, occur in the adenomatoid odontogenic tumour. Dentine, and enamel, may occur in the calcifying odontogenic cyst.

2. LESIONS CONSISTING OF ODONTOGENIC EPITHELIUM AND MESENCHYME.

Ameloblastic fibroma.
Ameloblastic sarcoma.

These tumours are "mixed," consisting of neoplastic odontogenic epithelium similar to that seen in ameloblastoma, and a mesenchymal element that is also neoplastic. This is usually fibroblastic in type but may, rarely, be sarcomatous.

3. LESIONS CONSISTING OF ODONTOGENIC EPITHELIUM AND CALCIFIED DENTAL TISSUES.

Odontoameloblastoma

The epithelial component of the tumour consists of odontogenic epithelium, but mature enamel and dentine are also present.

4. LESIONS CONSISTING OF CALCIFIED DENTAL TISSUES, BUT WITHOUT ODONTOGENIC EPITHELIUM

(except that directly associated with the formation of the calcified tissues).

Complex odontome
This lesion consists of a tumour-like mass of enamel, dentine and cementum, deposited in an irregular manner.

Compound odontome
This odontome is more highly organised, the enamel and dentine forming recognisable tooth-like structures. Many such teeth may be present, in a fibrous capsule.

Dens invaginatus (dilated odontome)
A developmental malformation in which an invagination of enamel is formed in a tooth.

Enameloma
A developmental malformation consisting of small ectopic deposits of enamel on a tooth.

Dentinoma
A tumour-like lesion in which the only calcified tissue is dentine.

Cementoma
A basically fibrous lesion in which cementum or cementum-like tissue is also present.

5. LESIONS CONSISTING OF ODONTOGENIC MESENCHYME.

Fibroma.
Myxoma.

Apart from the occasional presence of small groups of odontogenic epithelial cells, these lesions are histologically similar to fibroma and myxoma elsewhere in the body.

TUMOURS OF DEBATABLE ODONTOGENIC ORIGIN

Pigmented tumour of the jaws of infants.
Congenital epulis.

The pigmented tumour of the jaws occurs only in infants and has often been described as a pigmented ameloblastoma in the belief that it is basically an odontogenic tumour. The congenital epulis closely resembles the granular cell myoblastoma found in adults.

TUMOURS OF THE NON-DENTAL TISSUES

The primary non-odontogenic tumours and tumour-like lesions of the oral tissues include many that are familiar in other parts of the body. Again, it is not proposed to classify these lesions in a rigid manner, but to group them in such a way—mainly on a structural basis—that pathological comparisons will be facilitated.

Primary tumours of the non-dental tissues

EPIDERMAL

Leukoplakia; other white lesions of the oral mucosa.
Squamous cell papilloma.
Keratoacanthoma.
Squamous cell carcinoma and its variants; verrucous carcinoma; intraepidermal carcinoma; basal cell carcinoma.

FIBROUS CONNECTIVE TISSUE

Fibroma; myxoma; fibrosarcoma.
Fibrous epulis; denture fibrosis; pyogenic granuloma.
Fibromatosis.

ADIPOSE TISSUE

Lipoma.

CARTILAGE

Chondroma, chondrosarcoma.
Chondroblastoma; chondromyxoid fibroma.

BONE

Osteoma, osteomatosis.
Osteoid osteoma and osteoblastoma.
Torus palatinus and torus mandibularis.
Osteosarcoma.

VASCULAR TISSUE

Haemangioma; angiosarcoma.
Haemangiopericytoma.
Glomus tumour.

NEURAL TISSUE

Neurilemmoma and neurofibroma; neurofibromatosis; neurosarcoma; traumatic neuroma.
Neuroblastoma, ganglioneuroma.

MUSCLE

Leiomyoma; leiomyosarcoma; rhabdomyoma; rhabdomyosarcoma.
Myoblastoma.

LYMPHOID TISSUE

Lymphomas; lymphosarcoma, reticulum cell sarcoma, Hodgkin's disease, Burkitt's tumour.
Leukaemia.

GIANT CELL LESIONS

Giant cell tumour of bone.
Giant cell granuloma.
Giant cell lesions in hyperparathyroidism.
Giant cell epulis.

EWING'S TUMOUR

MYELOMATOSIS

MELANOMA

TUMOURS OF THE SALIVARY GLANDS

Secondary tumours

Metastatic deposits from a wide variety of primary growths may occur in the oral tissues.

REFERENCES

Bland-Sutton, J. (1888) Odontomes. *Trans. odont. Soc., Lond.*, **20**, 32.

Broca, P. (1866) *Traité des Tumeurs*. Paris. Asselin.

Gabell, D. P., James, W. W., and Payne, J. L. (1914) *The Report on Odontomes*. London. The British Dental Association.

Gorlin, R. J., Chaudhry, A. P., and Pindborg, J. J. (1961) Odontogenic tumors. Classification histopathology, and clinical behavior in man and domesticated animals. *Cancer*, **14**, 73.

Malassez, L. (1885) Sur le rôle des débris épithéliaux paradentaires. *Arch. physiol. norm. et path.*, **5**, 309; **6**, 379.

Pindborg, J. J., and Clausen, F. (1958) Classification of odontogenic tumors. A suggestion. *Acta odont. scand.*, **16**, 293.

Pindborg, J. J., and Kramer, I. R. H. (1971) *International Histological Classification of Tumours, No. 5. Histological Typing of Odontogenic Tumours, Jaw Cysts and Allied Lesions*. Geneva. World Health Organization.

Robinson, H. B. G. (Ed.) (1952) Proceedings of the fifth annual meeting of the American Academy of Oral Pathology. *Oral Surg.*, **5**, 177.

Thoma, K. H., and Goldman, H. M. (1946) Odontogenic tumors. A classification based on observations of the epithelial, mesenchymal, and mixed varieties. *Amer. J. Path.*, **22**, 433.

III
TUMOURS OF THE DENTAL TISSUES

3. Ameloblastoma

The first detailed description of ameloblastoma was given by Falkson (1879) although earlier authors, including Broca (1868), were aware of the tumour. The term adamantine epithelioma was introduced by Malassez (1885) and subsequently many synonyms were used, including adamantinoblastoma, epithelial odontome and multilocular cyst. The now current ameloblastoma was introduced by Churchill (1929) and Ivy and Churchill (1930).

A very full account of the historical aspect of ameloblastoma is given by Baden (1965).

Incidence

Frequency. Ameloblastoma accounts for approximately 1 per cent of all oral tumours. The literature consists mainly of single case reports and small series, but extensive reviews with statistics of age, sex, race, site of growth and other details have been made by Robinson (1937) and Small and Waldron (1955). The last-named authors surveyed 1,036 cases, including the 379 of Robinson's earlier series. A more recent report from the Mayo Clinic reviews 126 cases, with a detailed analysis of clinical findings, pathology and results of treatment (Mehlisch, Dahlin and Masson, 1972).

Age and Sex. Small and Waldron found that the average age of patients at the time of reporting to hospital was 38·9 years, but the average age at the time of discovery of the tumour was 32·7 years. Most patients were between the ages of 20 and 50 years. The tumour can occur in young children (Young and Robinson, 1962; Topazian, 1964; Lewin, 1966). The oldest patients have been over 80 years of age. Because of the slow-growing nature of ameloblastoma, it is likely that very often the tumour has existed for an appreciable period before its discovery.

Rather more males than females are affected by ameloblastoma.

Race. The tumour is said to be more frequent in Africans than in the white races. In the United States, for example, ameloblastoma accounts for 0·07 per cent of all malignant tumours. In Denmark, tumours of the jaw account for 0·1 per cent of all tumours registered (Clemmessen, 1965). In Africa, on the other hand, tumours of the jaws represent 3·6 per cent of all tumours, and ameloblastoma accounts for 0·3 per cent of all tumours (Davies and Davies, 1960; Dodge, 1965; Kovi and Laing, 1966). Tumours of the jaws, including ameloblastoma, also appear to have a higher incidence in Korea (Chung and colleagues, 1969). However, it will be appreciated that in the less developed countries there may be special difficulties in the collection of data.

Location. About 80 per cent of tumours occur in the mandible, generally in the molar region or the ramus, though the premolar area and the symphysis may also be affected. Maxillary tumours occur more often in the molar area or the antrum and floor of the nose than in the anterior region.

An unusual feature of tumours in Nigerians, apart from the increased frequency mentioned above, is that most of the growths occur in the region of the mandibular symphysis and premolar area. Akinosi and Williams (1969) suggest that this might be due to the severe oral sepsis and calculus formation that is so frequently present in these patients.

Etiology

Very little is known about possible causal factors. New (1915) thought that irritation might be concerned since the tumour occurs so often in the posterior part of the mandible, where its occurrence might be connected with difficulty of eruption of the third molar. Robinson found that in about a third of the cases in his survey there was a history of previous oral infection, extraction of teeth, injury to the teeth or jaws or other abnormalities. Hertz (1951) and Forsberg (1954) have also considered that trauma or inflammation are etiologically significant. Of course, such lesions, as well as anomalous eruption of the third molar, are common in otherwise normal persons and little can thus be concluded from such observations.

Geschickter (1935) considered that rickets might be a factor. Pronounced defects in the development of the tooth germs occur in rickets in man, and in pigs maintained on a rachitogenic diet during the period of active dental development irregularity of the ameloblastic layer of the enamel organ occurs, with islands of cells budding off and becoming isolated to form ameloblastoma-like follicles. However, no unequivocal tumours have been produced in such dietary experiments. On the other hand, tumours that are quite comparable with ameloblastoma in man have been produced in mice by the injection of polyoma virus (Stanley and colleagues, 1964, 1965; Main and Dawe, 1966; Lucas, 1969). Csiba and colleagues (1970) have found particles with some of the characteristics of paramyxoviruses in an ameloblastoma.

Clinical Features

Ameloblastoma is a tumour that grows slowly and with few or no symptoms in the early stages. Not infrequently it is first noticed during routine dental examination. Later, there is gradually increasing facial deformity noted by the patient himself or by others, and teeth in the area of the tumour may become loosened. Pain is seldom a complaint, even in cases of quite long standing.

Examination in an early case, of the type, for instance, that comes to light as a result of oral X-ray examination, may show very little in the way of objective changes, perhaps an enlargement of the jaw that is just detectable. Later, the lesion becomes very obvious, with an ovoid or fusiform enlargement that is hard but not tender. In the maxilla, the sinus becomes involved and the tumour may extend into the orbit or nasopharynx. Because of the slow growth of the tumour it is probable that even in apparently early cases it has already been present for an appreciable period before detection. In the absence of treatment the tumour continues to enlarge and the surrounding bone becomes so thin that fluctuation or egg-shell crackling may be elicited. Perforation of the bone, however, is a late feature. In the past, tumours growing slowly but steadily in this way have reached enormous dimensions, but such cases are practically never seen now except in the less developed countries, where large growths are still encountered. It is also now uncommon to obtain what was formerly a not unusual history—that of a series of operations on the jaw for a "cyst" or an "abscess," carried out over a period of years, with recurrence after each one.

Radiological examination shows an area of bone destruction that is either polycystic or monocystic in appearance (Fig. 15). In the polycystic type the bone is replaced by a number of small well defined radiolucent areas giving the whole lesion a honeycomb or soap-bubble appearance, and at the same time the jaw itself is expanded. Although this radiographic picture is seen quite frequently it is not pathognomonic, for a similar picture may be found in giant cell lesions, fibromyxoma and some non-neoplastic cysts. In the monocystic type there is a well defined area of radiolucency forming a single compartment. If this is associated with an unerupted tooth, the appearances closely resemble those of a dentigerous cyst. If the roots of teeth are involved the picture may resemble that of a radicular cyst.

Pathology

Macroscopic Appearance. Apart from biopsy material, the specimen as received by the pathologist consists of the tumour with a surrounding margin of normal bone or of the completely

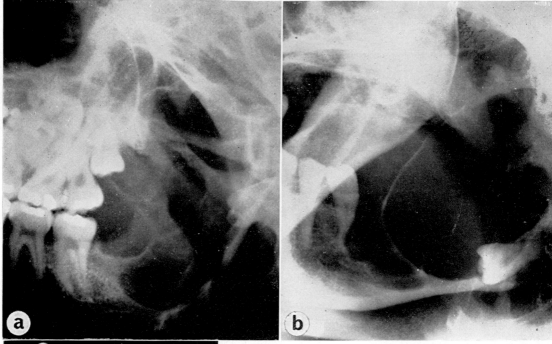

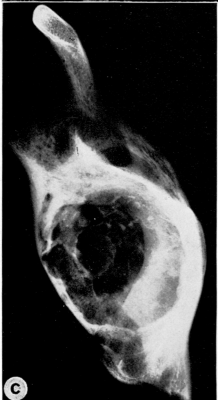

Fig. 15   Radiographic appearances of ameloblastoma. **a,** the typical picture, in which compartments in the bone separated by distinct septa produce a multiloculated or soap-bubble effect. **b,** the monocystic type of tumour. The monolocular cystic space in association with the unerupted and displaced third molar tooth produces an appearance identical to that of a dentigerous cyst. Gross specimen shown in Fig. 16**e,** and microscopic appearance in Fig. 22**c. c,** radiograph of the specimen shown in Fig. 16**d,** demonstrating the multiloculated appearance and expansion and destruction of the cortex.

Fig. 16   Gross specimens of ameloblastoma, showing variations from almost completely solid to entirely cystic growth. **a,** ameloblastoma replacing the whole of the left side of the body of the mandible. The tumour is almost entirely solid, except for a cyst at the anterior end and another at the posterior end. **b,** a tumour of the ascending ramus and body of the mandible, with solid and cystic areas. **c,** a tumour of the body of the mandible with some solid areas but with several large cysts. **d,** a tumour of the ramus of the mandible consisting mainly of two large cysts with some intervening solid areas. The lesion shows a multiloculated appearance in the radiograph (Fig. 15**c**). **e,** a unilocular ameloblastoma from the mandible. This thin-walled cyst, with some mural nodules, simulated a dentigerous cyst. Radiograph shown in Fig. 15**b,** and microscopic appearance in Fig. 22**c.**

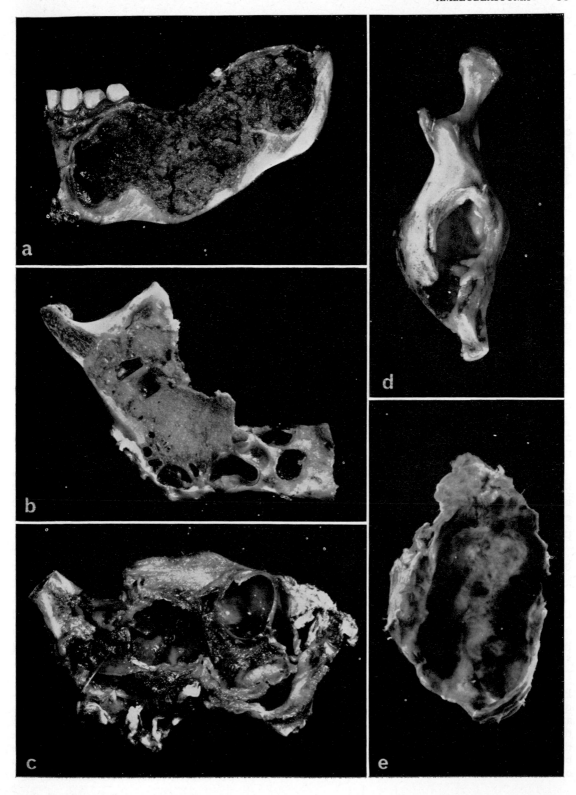

the outer layer are of variable size. Sometimes they are columnar or cubical, but they may be low cubical or flattened. When columnar they approach most closely in appearance to the normal ameloblast, or rather to the preameloblast, for they do not possess the Tomes' processes of the normal mature ameloblast and differ from it also in other details. These cells have well defined oval nuclei situated at the end of the cell nearest to the centre of the follicle. The cytoplasm may be finely granular or homogeneous and vacuoles are often present. Mitotic figures are rarely seen.

The central area of the tumour follicle consists of cells very similar to those of the stellate reticulum of the normal enamel organ and, as in that structure, they may be separated from the peripheral cells by a layer or two of flattened cells similar to those of the normal stratum intermedium. However, this feature is often lacking. The general resemblance of the ameloblastoma follicle to the normal enamel organ has also been emphasised by the histochemical and electron-microscopic studies of Clausen, Philipsen and Pindborg (1961) and Moe, Clausen and Philipsen (1961). The more recent ultrastructure studies of Lee, El-Labban and Kramer (1972) and Mincer and McGinnis (1972) confirm the resemblance. On the other hand, Mori and colleagues (1964, 1965) found that the enzyme activity distribution resembled that of squamous cell carcinoma and homologous non-neoplastic epithelium rather than that of tooth germ.

Microcyst formation within the tumour follicles is a common occurrence and the coalescence of small cysts to form larger ones is responsible in the course of time for macroscopic cyst formation (Kronfeld, 1930). In some cases the microcysts form by what appears to be a simple melting away of the central portions of the stellate areas of the epithelial follicles, leaving a clear space lined by a layer of flattened cells. In other cases cyst formation is accompanied by well marked cellular changes (Fig. 18). Thus there is swelling of the cells in the central area of the follicle and the cytoplasm becomes homogeneous and stains bright red with eosin. Neighbouring cells tend to coalesce and the centres of the follicles thus come to be occupied by masses of highly eosinophilic material which show the outlines of the individual cells composing them. This material is also strongly PAS positive. Cyst formation occurs within the eosinophilic masses and extends. Hodson (1957) has described the presence of mucin in the cysts and in the surrounding epithelium in some tumours. He has also found glycogen in the tumour epithelium in some cases. It is to be noted that cholesterol is almost never found in ameloblastoma, either in the cysts or as deposits in the stroma, although it is very common in radicular and dentigerous cysts.

Krompecher (1918) noted that instead of the development of eosinophilic masses within the follicles, cells with granular cytoplasm might be present (Fig. 18c, d). This is a rather uncommon feature of the tumour, which has also been noted by Frantz and Stix (1932), Aisenberg (1953), Shafer and Spivey (1954) and others. The granular cells, which occur singly or in large masses within the follicles, replace in whole or part the stellate reticulum. They are round or sometimes polyhedral with granular cytoplasm and small darkly-staining nuclei that are usually compressed against the cell wall. Distinct nucleoli are seen where there has been less compression and the nucleus remains central. The cytoplasmic granules are eosinophilic and PAS positive. Campbell (1956), McCallum and Cappell (1957) and Mallik (1957) have observed transition forms between

---

Fig. 18   **a,** a higher magnification of a field from the tumour shown in Fig. 17a. The structure of the tumour follicles is clearly shown, each consisting of a central area of stellate cells and a peripheral layer of cubical cells. Cyst formation occurs amongst the stellate cells. × 200. **b,** in this tumour the peripheral cells of the tumour follicles are columnar rather than cubical. The polarisation of the nuclei, which are situated towards the centres of the follicles, is clearly seen. × 500. **c,** granular cells in ameloblastoma. These cells occur mainly in the centres of the follicles, replacing the stellate cells. × 80. **d,** higher magnification, showing that the granular cells closely resemble those seen in myoblastoma. × 500.

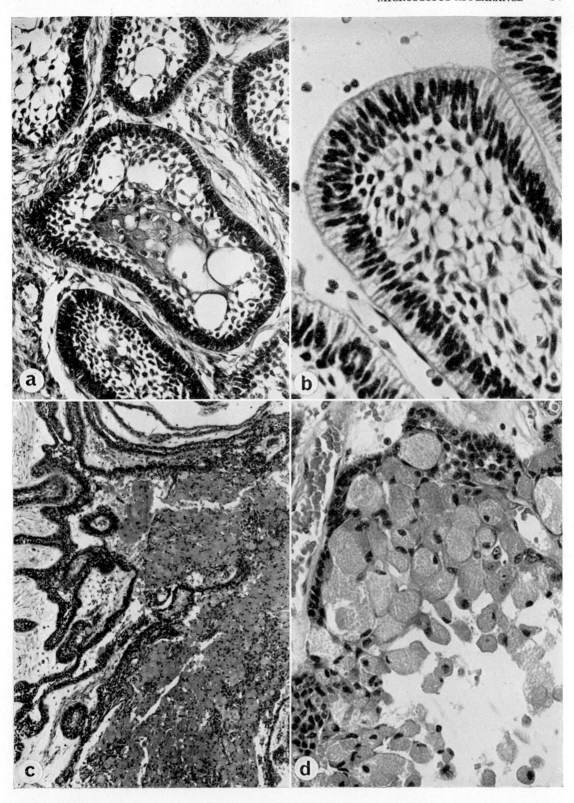

the stellate and columnar cells and the granular cells. They note that the granular cells are very similar to those of the congenital epulis and the myoblastoma but do not consider that there is sufficient evidence otherwise to relate these lesions to ameloblastoma. However, the fact that cells exactly like those of the congenital epulis are thus seen clearly to develop from epithelium suggested to Ardoin (1936) and Willis (1967) that that lesion, like the ameloblastoma, derives from dental epithelium. Hoke and Harrelson (1967) also subscribe to this view, pointing out that the cytoplasm of the normal ameloblasts undergoes granular change during amelogenesis, and there is also some ultrastructural evidence pointing to the epithelial origin of the granular cells (Navarette and Smith, 1971). Granular cells have also been reported in the fibrous element of ameloblastic fibroma (p. 78). Hartman (1974) has analysed a series of twenty cases of granular cell ameloblastoma, and gives the literature.

Squamous metaplasia is another variable feature in ameloblastoma. Small areas of squamous change, with the formation of intercellular bridges, are not infrequently noted, though extensive change of this type is uncommon and the formation of distinct epithelial pearls is rare. In the few cases in which squamous change is extensive the follicles may consist almost entirely of squamous epithelium, but some remaining traits of the original ameloblastomatous structure can usually be detected (Fig. 19). In cystic tumours the epithelium lining a cystic space may, occasionally, show well marked keratinisation, particularly after irradiation. Areas of calcification may be found, rarely, in the metaplastic squamous epithelium (Pindborg and Weinmann, 1958).

Apart from the case of the rare odontoameloblastoma, it is generally considered that enamel is not formed in the ameloblastoma. In the normal development of the teeth enamel is deposited only when dentine has first been laid down by the odontoblasts. In the tumour, odontoblasts and dentine are not found and the epithelial cells do not reach the stage of differentiation into ameloblasts. However, some workers have found small quantities of enamel or enameloid material in some tumours (Boyle and Kalnins, 1960), but this must be considered exceptional. Kalnins (1971) and Kalnins and Rossi (1965) have also found enamel-like deposits in craniopharyngiomas (p. 52). It is not certain whether the odontoameloblastoma should be considered as an entity in its own right, or simply as an ameloblastoma in which enamel and dentine have formed. The epithelial element of the tumour is identical to that of the usual type of ameloblastoma and in addition dentine and enamel are present. It should be noted that while odontogenic epithelium and dentine and enamel are present in immature odontomes, the epithelium in these lesions resembles normal odontogenic epithelium and not the epithelium of an ameloblastoma. Moreover, the behaviour of the odontoameloblastoma, so far as is known, for it is a very rare tumour, is similar to that of the ordinary ameloblastoma.

In the plexiform type of ameloblastoma the anastomosing strands of epithelium show the same layers as do the discrete cell islands of the follicular type (Fig. 20). Thus, the cell strands are bordered by a single layer of cubical or columnar cells, with an internal area of stellate cells. Cyst formation is also seen in this type of growth, but it occurs very frequently in the stroma as well as within the epithelium. Siegmund (1929) first noted the occurrence of stromal cysts in ameloblastoma. They have also been described by Lucas and Thackray (1952).

Cysts of the stromal type can be recognised by the fact that the cystic spaces occur on the side of the columnar epithelial layer opposite to that on which the stellate cells are situated. Various

---

Fig. 19   Squamous metaplasia in ameloblastoma. **a, b,** the stellate cells of the follicles are largely replaced by squamous cells showing intercellular bridges. × 300 and × 500. **c,** extensive squamous metaplasia, with the follicles consisting almost entirely of squamous cells, and in some epithelial pearls are present. × 80. **d,** higher magnification shows the squamification with keratinisation at K, and also at A evidence of the original ameloblastomatous structure. × 200.

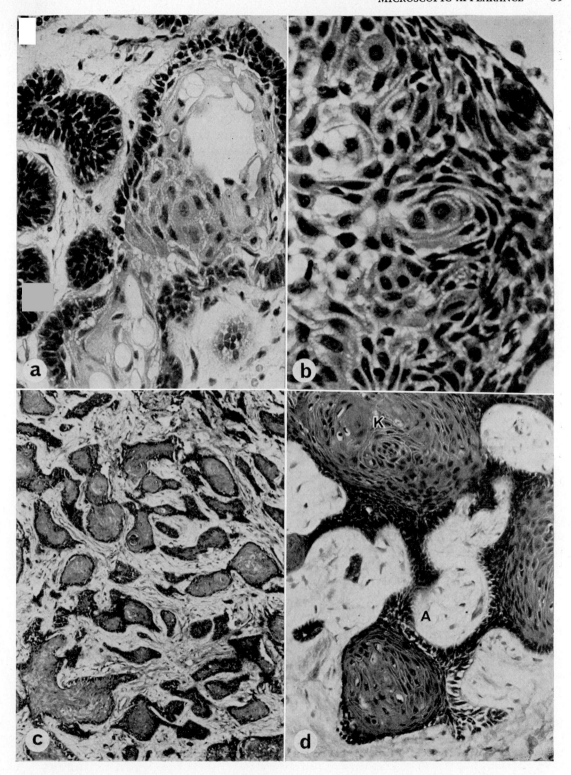

degrees of cystic change can often be seen in the same tumour. The earliest change appears to be loosening of the connective tissue, with a rather oedematous appearance. This is followed by progressive degeneration of the stromal cells and the appearance of microcysts containing homogeneous material that stains pale blue with haematoxylin. The process continues till no formed elements remain, a completely clear cyst being left. Blood vessels appear to be the most resistant elements to the degenerative process that produces the cysts, since capillaries may often be seen in cysts though destruction of connective tissue is practically complete. In some cases, stromal cyst formation is accompanied by the accumulation of large numbers of foam cells.

An unusual variation in the plexiform type of ameloblastoma is extreme vascularity of the stroma. Kühn (1932) reported a case of this type as a combination of ameloblastoma and haemangioma, and others have been reported by Oesterreich (1936), Aisenberg (1950, 1953), Lucas (1957), Thoma and Goldman (1960), Oliver, McKenna and Shafer (1961), Gardner and Spouge (1966) and Grover and colleagues (1971). The excessive vascularity occurs in connection with the stroma of the tumour, as shown in Fig. 21. There are greatly dilated capillaries in the stromal cysts, though sometimes only free blood is present and no endothelium can be detected. No blood or blood vessels are present within the epithelium. The reported tumours of this type have generally been referred to as adamantinohaemangioma, or by some similar designation, and are considered to be mixed tumours. There is no evidence, however, to indicate that the unusual vascularity in these cases is due to a neoplastic process. There is an entire absence of vasoformative activity on the one hand, while on the other the appearances suggest that the process is essentially degenerative, with the blood vessels dilating to occupy the spaces left by the disappearing stroma. It has already been noted that in the process of formation of stromal cysts in the ordinary type of plexiform ameloblastoma the blood vessels often persist when all other elements of the stroma have disappeared, though ultimately they too vanish and a completely cystic space is left. In the unusual vascular types of ameloblastoma probably the first change is also cystic degeneration in the stroma, but subsequently the vessels persist and dilate instead of disappearing. Thus appearances such as those seen in Fig. 21 are produced, in which the vessel is represented by a single layer of endothelium that is almost in apposition with the tumour epithelium. Such dilated vessels ultimately rupture and the stromal cyst then comes to contain free blood.

Thoma and Goldman (1960) describe the association of ameloblastoma and neurinoma in connection with a case reported by Braunstein (1949). The tumour was originally reported as an ameloblastoma occurring in the buccal mucosa and not attached to bone. In the recurrence there were characteristic ameloblastoma follicles in a connective tissue stroma with an extensive plexus of small irregularly disposed bundles of myelinated nerve fibres. This appearance in a recurrence has also been seen by Kramer (1961), who suggests that the neural element represents traumatic neuroma resulting from the previous operation. Another example of the association of a neural tumour and ameloblastoma is reported by Hodson (1961). In this case a neurilemmoma of the mandible was invaded by ameloblastoma.

Local Spread and Metastases. Generally speaking, ameloblastoma is a tumour that causes expansion of the bone more than destruction. At the same time, there is a certain amount of

---

Fig. 20 Plexiform ameloblastoma. **a,** the epithelial strands form an interlacing pattern. Cyst formation is prominent, most of the cysts being in the stroma. × 30. **b,** higher magnification showing the plexiform strands composed of stellate cells enclosed in an outer layer of columnar cells. An epithelial cyst is present at EC and stromal cysts at SC. Persisting capillaries are seen at Cap. × 200. **c,** a stromal cyst filled with foam cells. × 200. **d,** another common type of plexiform ameloblastoma, with minimal cyst formation × 30.

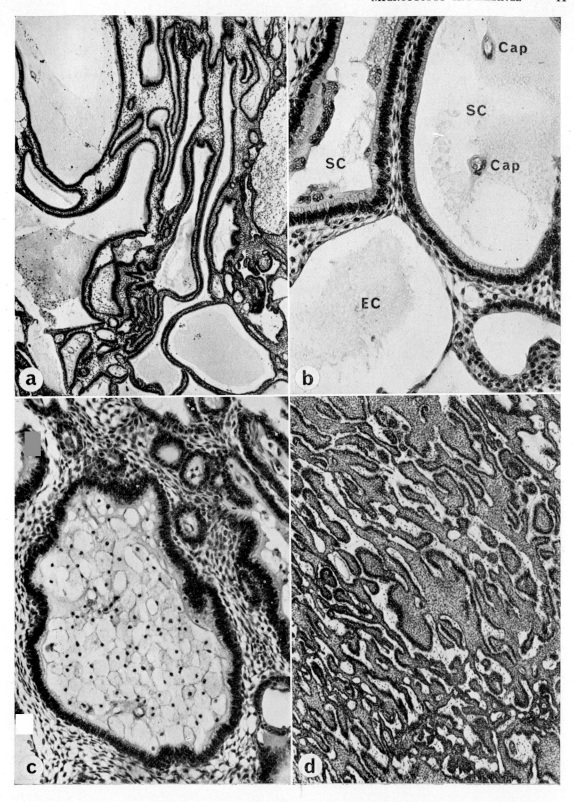

local invasion of the surrounding bone and though this is generally limited in extent it is quite sufficient to make it likely that tumour will remain after conservative treatment such as curettage. Recurrence of ameloblastoma after curettage is, therefore, common. Formerly a standard method of treatment it has now been abandoned, though the pathologist may still see specimens of recurrent growth from old patients who may have had several recurrences over the years. With the present-day treatment of complete excision of the growth together with an adequate margin of adjacent normal tissue, a permanent cure is much more likely.

In the absence of treatment ameloblastoma can grow to a great size, but still remains localised. Recurrences also may remain more or less localised, though involving a rather greater area of bone on each occasion. As already mentioned, many patients have continued for very long periods, with a curettage of the lesion perhaps every four or five years. However, this is not always what happens; unsuccessful interventions can be followed by extensive spread of the tumour. This is not due to accelerated growth but to the fact that the widening area to be dealt with at successive interventions, particularly in the case of maxillary growths, takes the operation into areas where a radical excision that will remove all growth becomes progressively more difficult to achieve. McWhirter (1952) has suggested radiotherapy as a possible alternative to surgery in some cases, and individual reports (Hair, 1963) have recorded success with this type of treatment, but it is generally agreed that ameloblastoma is radioresistant.

There appears to be no correlation between the histological pattern in ameloblastoma and its clinical course. A number of cases have been reported in which the tumour has pursued a more aggressive course than usual, but these are rare. Some of the earlier examples have been reported as carcinoma ameloblasticum or ameloblastic sarcoma, but it is difficult or impossible to judge from the records the real nature of these cases. McGregor (1935) and Wunderer (1953) give the earlier literature on cases of this type. Misdiagnosed squamous cell carcinoma or adenoid cystic carcinoma may well account for some examples, but there do seem to occur, although very rarely, tumours that have at least some of the characteristics of ameloblastoma and also the histological attributes of malignancy (Jones, 1966). But even such tumours may in fact be squamous cell carcinomas that have an ameloblastoma-like appearance—for example, one of Shear's (1969) cases of intra-alveolar squamous cell carcinoma would seem to be of this nature—so this question must remain open until more cases have been studied.

Regarding distant spread, the position is rather like that of basal cell carcinoma. That is to say, metastatic dissemination in ameloblastoma is very rare, but undoubted cases have occurred. Small and Waldron (1955) collected over 30 cases from the literature, up to the time of their report, in which metastatic deposits had occurred, but as they point out in their detailed analysis the great majority of these reports could not be regarded as offering acceptable evidence of metastasis from undoubted ameloblastoma. Here again, as in the case of many of the reports on tumours that have been particularly aggressive locally, misdiagnoses have been made in some cases and others are insufficiently documented or illustrated, or are otherwise equivocal. Carr and Halperin (1968) have collected and analysed the cases reported since Small and Waldron's review, and similar remarks apply.

In the few cases of ameloblastoma with metastases that can be accepted, the dominant feature is long-standing local disease, operated on a number of times over the course of years, with finally

Fig. 21 An unusually vascular ameloblastoma. **a,** essentially this is a tumour of plexiform pattern with dilated or ruptured capillaries in the stroma. EC, an epithelial cyst. SC, stromal cysts, × 80 **b,** higher magnification showing a dilated capillary in a stromal cyst. × 200. **c,** another stromal cyst with a rupturing capillary and escape of blood into the cyst space. × 200.

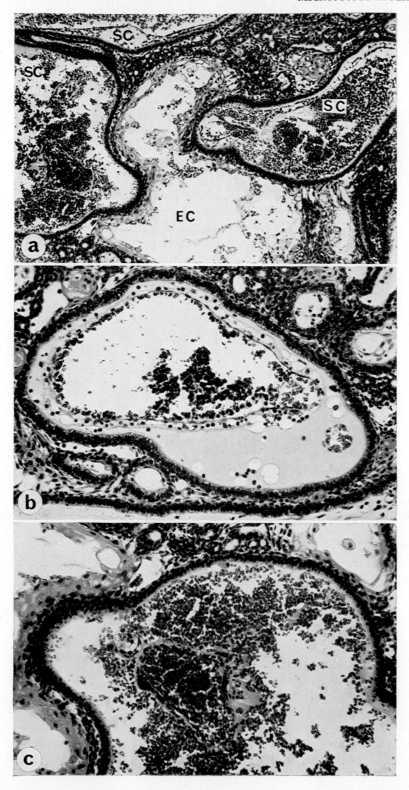

metastatic deposits in the lungs. For example, Vorzimer and Perla's (1932) patient had a mandibular tumour of over 20 years' duration. This was operated on several times and areas of infiltration developed in a lower lobe of the lung with tumour growing extensively in the related bronchial tree. The photomicrographs of the primary and secondary tumours show typical ameloblastoma. The localisation of tumour in one area of lung together with tumour in the related bronchi suggests that growth was aspirated in this case, rather than disseminated by the blood stream. Schweitzer and Barnfield (1943) also illustrate typical primary tumour and secondary deposits in the lungs in a patient who had 24 operations over 14 years for a mandibular tumour. There was also extensive invasion of the maxilla and base of the skull, illustrating the degree of local spread that can follow unsuccessful attempts at removal. In this case, the multiple nodules of growth in the lungs and pleura suggest haematogeneous dissemination rather than aspiration. Lee, White and Totten's (1959) case is similar, a mandibular tumour having been operated on many times in the course of 14 years and ultimately extending to the maxilla, antrum, orbit and cranial cavity. Six years before death multiple pulmonary metastases developed, which the authors think to be the result of blood spread, though aspiration dissemination in this as in the other cases cannot be excluded, in view of the numerous surgical operations. Other recent cases in which there were metastatic deposits in the lungs have been recorded by Tsukada, De La Pava and Pickren (1965), Harrer and Patchefsky (1970) and Sehdev and colleagues (1974).

Although pulmonary metastases, very probably deposited by aspiration, thus seem to be the usual form of dissemination, there are also cases where lymph node deposits have been noted (Simmons, 1928; Stoll, Marchetta and Shobinger, 1957). However, in the case reported by the last-named authors the tumour that was found in a cervical lymph node was squamous cell carcinoma. The patient had had an ameloblastoma for years, which finally recurred locally, together with squamous cell carcinoma. The authors think that squamous metaplasia in the ameloblastoma might have proceeded to the stage of carcinoma with, subsequently, metastasis to the regional nodes, but it might well be that two separate but coexisting lesions were concerned. Shatkin and Hoffmeister (1965) report a somewhat similar case in which there was a long history, many curettages, insertion of radium and subsequent excisions. Finally, the patient died with extensive local disease, the tumour having recurred as ameloblastoma and squamous cell carcinoma. There was a deposit of ameloblastoma in the lung and squamous cell carcinoma in a cervical lymph node. However, metastatic deposits of characteristic ameloblastoma can occur in lymph nodes, as in Dahlgren, Ekström and Mossberg's (1971) case.

Metastasis to bone has also been reported. In Hoke and Harrelson's (1967) case there was again a tumour of many years' standing, with several surgical interventions, and finally metastatic deposits in the cervical vertebrae. Sugimura and colleagues (1969) report a case with metastasis to a lumbar vertebra, but this case was exceptional in that the history was quite short, with only two operations. However, the primary tumour showed unusual features, including hyperchromatism and pleomorphism. The local recurrence was in the form of a spindle-cell growth, as was the metastatic deposit. These authors, and also Ikemura and colleagues (1972), list the cases of ameloblastoma with metastases that have been reported in the Japanese literature.

With regard to the remaining cases in the literature, either no histological examination of the supposed secondary lesion was carried out or no photographs are published, or the photographs do not offer convincing proof that the tumour in question is ameloblastoma. In the earlier cases it is often difficult to discern precisely what tumour is illustrated, while in the more recent examples it is obvious that the tumour shown is certainly not a typical ameloblastoma, being very probably squamous cell carcinoma or adenoid cystic carcinoma of salivary gland origin.

Histogenesis

The resemblance of the tumour epithelium to the normal enamel organ suggests that amelo-blastoma arises from the dental epithelium, or is at least very closely connected with it, but the precise point of origin is unknown. Possibilities include the enamel organ itself, the rests of Serre which represent the remains of the dental lamina, the rests of Malassez which are the remnants of Hertwig's root sheath, the oral mucosa and the epithelial lining of odontogenic cysts.

Enamel Organ. The early histologists thought that the enamel organ was a likely origin for the ameloblastoma on account of the obvious histological similarities. Such an origin, of course, implies that tumour growth starts at an early age, during the period of existence of the enamel organ as such. For this reason Bland-Sutton (1922) considered origin from the enamel organ to be unlikely. Most of his patients were middle-aged when their tumours first appeared, long after the regression of the enamel organs. On the other hand, more recent investigators have found the age of onset to be earlier than in Bland-Sutton's cases and the tumour does occur most often in the region of the mandible where supernumerary tooth germs are most frequently present. Also, as Robinson has pointed out, a tooth is quite often missing at the site of the lesion. Since the ameloblastoma is characteristically slowly growing and symptomless in its earlier stages, a tumour might well originate from a supernumerary tooth germ or from a germ of the normal series (hence the possibility of a missing tooth at the site of the lesion), appreciably prior to the time of the patient's first noticing it. The occasional occurrence of the tumour as a monolocular cystic lesion surrounding the crown of an unerupted tooth also suggests that in some cases the enamel organ may give rise to the neoplasm. Kegel (1932), Geschickter (1935), Zegarelli (1944) and Byars and Sarnat (1945) are amongst others who have also supported the enamel organ theory of origin.

Cell Rests. After the tooth buds have separated from the dental lamina that structure regresses and disappears, although isolated groups of epithelial cells remain unobtrusively in the connective tissue as the rests of Serre. Thoma and Goldman (1960) suggest that the dental lamina itself may give rise to ameloblastomas; such tumours would, of course, appear early in life. If tumours arose from the rests of Serre, as Manley (1954) thought possible, they could appear at any age. Spouge (1967) also suggests that the tumour arises from dental lamina or its derivatives.

When the enamel organ itself regresses epithelial rests are left around the roots of the teeth in the periodontal membrane. These cell rests were first demonstrated by Malassez (1885) and were suggested by him and others as the origin of ameloblastoma (Bump, 1927; McFarland and Patterson, 1931). The occurrence of small ameloblastomas between adjacent normal teeth is of interest, since in such cases epithelial rests would seem likely starting points. Such cases, however, are uncommon; examples have been reported by Kotanyi (1936), Thoma (1944), Quinn and Fullmer (1953) and England (1960).

A detailed account of epithelial rests in the jaws is given by Hodson (1962).

Oral Mucosa. A number of authors have observed that an ameloblastoma may show a connection with the oral mucosa. Siegmund and Weber (1926) illustrate some cases of this type, but they consider that the tumour might equally well have grown up to and established connection with the surface epithelium as have originated from it. Similar cases have been reported by Fish (1948), Champion, Moule and Wilkinson (1951), Wilkinson (1952) and others, and most authors have taken the view that the connection between mucosal and tumour epithelium could well be incidental. Most ameloblastomas are essentially intraosseous tumours, or at least present as such by the time they are seen, and even in those cases in which the mucosa is involved this would seem to be a secondary matter, occurring only after a comparatively long period of primarily intraosseous growth. Hertz (1951), Forsberg (1954) and Hodson (1957), however, raise the question of a mucosal origin for at least some tumours. Instances of extraosseous tumours such as that reported by Stanley and Krogh (1959) lend more support to the possibility of surface origin, but cases of this type are rare.

In line with the possible relationship between the ameloblastoma and the surface epithelium, some authors have considered the tumour to be a type of basal cell carcinoma. This is a view of some long standing (Krompecher, 1918; Sprawson and Keizer, 1933; Sprawson, 1937). Examples of ameloblastoma showing remarkable histological resemblances to basal cell carcinoma are encountered from time to time, and both tumours are related to derivatives of the covering ectoderm, if not arising directly therefrom. They resemble each other, too, in their natural history, for they are both neoplasms of slow growth and local malignancy only. There is, however, an important difference in response to radiation; the ameloblastoma is on the whole radio-resistant, in striking contrast to the radiosensitivity of the basal cell carcinoma.

Cysts of Dental Origin. A number of early reports (New, 1915; Bump, 1927; Schroff, 1931; and others) drew attention to lesions that appeared clinically and radiologically to be ordinary cysts of dental origin but which proved in fact to be ameloblastomas and Cahn (1933) advanced the view that all dentigerous cysts should be considered as potential ameloblastomas. Since Cahn's paper many such cases have been recorded, amongst others by Carpenter and Thoma (1933), Jacobs (1935), Thoma and Proctor (1937), Hankey (1938), Kaletsky (1938), Thoma (1940), Bailey (1951), Cameron (1951), Forsberg (1954), Hodson (1957), Castner, McCully and Hiatt (1967), Quinn and Fournett (1969), Taylor and colleagues (1971) and Byrd, Aden and Dunsworth (1973). Some quite large series have also been published, including Sonesson's (1950) report on 39 cases of ameloblastoma, at least 10 of which were considered to have arisen from odontogenic cysts. Bernier and Tiecke (1951), in another review, found that approximately 33 per cent of ameloblastomas originated in dentigerous or follicular cysts. There is thus a considerable body of opinion supporting the view that ameloblastoma arises not infrequently from odontogenic cysts. Nevertheless, the evidence is somewhat equivocal, despite the relatively large number of published cases, and it is also apparent that not all authors have the same ideas as to what should be described as an odontogenic cyst. The matter is further discussed below.

Histological Diagnosis

While typical tumours present no problems in microscopic diagnosis, difficulties may arise in connection with some conditions in which there is non-neoplastic epithelial proliferation (Fig. 22). The question of the relationship to dentigerous cysts has also to be considered, as well as differential diagnosis from certain other neoplasms.

Non-neoplastic Epithelial Proliferation. Epithelial overgrowth occurs very frequently in the walls of cysts of dental origin, probably as a result of the chronic inflammation that is so often present in these lesions, but sometimes proliferation is seen in the absence of any very marked inflammatory activity. Churchill (1934) demonstrated that the walls of dentigerous cysts may show proliferation somewhat comparable in appearance to the ameloblastic layer of the normal enamel organ and suggestive of ameloblastoma, but he emphasised that the

Fig. 22   **a,** radicular cyst. This common non-neoplastic lesion often shows quite extensive proliferation of its epithelial lining. This should not be mistaken for plexiform ameloblastoma. × 30. **b,** a cystic area in an ameloblastoma that shows proliferation superficially similar to that in the wall of the cyst in **a.** × 30. **c,** the cyst wall of a monocystic ameloblastoma. Note that the flattened tumour epithelium could be mistaken for non-neoplastic squamous epithelium. The gross specimen is shown in Fig. 16e, and the radiograph in Fig. 15b. × 80. **d,** a primordial cyst of the mandible. Degenerative changes in the squamous epithelial lining, due to inflammation, produce a superficial resemblance to the stellate cells of ameloblastoma. × 200.

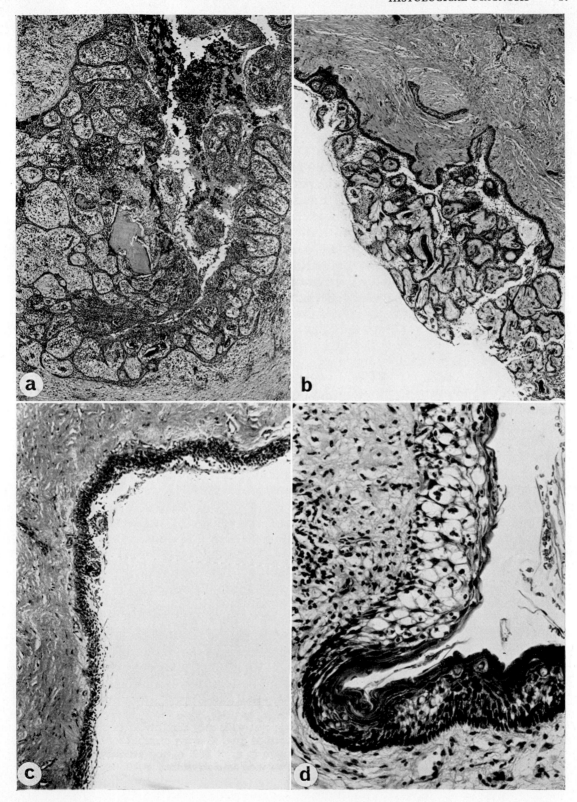

two lesions were separate entities and histologically distinct. More recently Vickers and Gorlin (1970) have drawn attention to the changes in epithelium that indicate neoplasia. As well as simulation of ameloblastoma by the non-neoplastic proliferation of the lining of odontogenic cysts, it is possible for the tumour epithelium lining a cystic ameloblastoma to undergo squamous metaplasia or to become so flattened by pressure of the cyst contents that there may be considerable difficulty in distinguishing it from non-neoplastic squamous epithelium (Lucas, 1952; 1954).

Epithelial proliferation may be noted in the form of islets of epithelium in the walls of radicular and dentigerous cysts, at some distance from the epithelial lining of the cavity itself. This type of appearance is illustrated in Fig. 23. The islets show a superficial resemblance to ameloblastoma follicles, with apparent differentiation into stellate cells and peripheral ameloblast layer, and with cyst formation. Close examination, however, shows that though the cells of the peripheral layers may appear to be distinct from the remainder they do not show the ameloblast-like appearance of the peripheral cells of the true ameloblastoma follicle. In fact, the distinct appearance of the peripheral cells of the non-neoplastic islet, when this is present, is due to these cells being smaller than the remainder since they are basal cells, and also, possibly, due to compression during the growth of the islet or to cyst formation in it, so that the nuclei come to lie very close together, resembling a distinct outer layer. Moreover, the small pyknotic nuclei of the degenerating cells that give rise to the stellate reticulum-like appearance in the non-neoplastic islet are readily distinguished from the larger vesicular nuclei of the stellate cells of the true tumour follicle.

In some cysts and non-cystic chronic inflammatory lesions anastomosing strands of epithelium, rather than islets, penetrate into the underlying connective tissue. The general appearance may be not dissimilar to the plexiform type of ameloblastoma but careful examination shows that the epithelium lacks the characteristics associated with that of the neoplasm, retaining in all essentials the appearances of a non-neoplastic, though hyperplastic, epithelial tissue.

Relationship to Dentigerous Cysts. As mentioned earlier, it is generally believed that a proportion of ameloblastomas originate in dentigerous cysts. The accuracy of this belief depends on one's concept of the meaning of the term "dentigerous cyst." If by this term no more is meant than a cystic lesion that arises in enamel organ epithelium in connection with an unerupted or partially erupted tooth, then it is certainly true that some ameloblastomas can be described in this way. In fact, Stanley, Krogh and Pannuk (1965) have shown that the lining of third molar follicles is mainly of enamel organ type below the age of 22 years, while later squamous epithelium predominates, and it has also been found (Stanley and Diehl, 1965) that when ameloblastoma occurs in association with an impacted or unerupted tooth, it does so in most cases in patients under 30 years of age. But in ordinary usage the term "dentigerous cyst" connotes a non-neoplastic lesion, and thus the statement that ameloblastoma may arise in dentigerous cysts implies neoplastic change in an initially non-neoplastic lesion.

In some of the published cases no definite evidence is offered to show that a neoplasm has developed from what was previously a simple cyst. For example, a lesion diagnosed clinically and radiologically as a dentigerous cyst is removed, but no histological examination is made, or if this has been done no photomicrographs are shown. Later, there is a recurrence, and the histological appearance is now that of ameloblastoma. Obviously, such a lesion could have been neo-

Fig. 23   Discrete islets of epithelium in non-neoplastic cyst walls may simulate ameloblastoma follicles. **a,** islets of squamous epithelium in the wall of a dentigerous cyst, showing central cyst formation. × 30. **b,** higher magnification of an islet similar to those shown in **a.** × 200. **c,** non-neoplastic islets showing cyst formation and degenerative changes in the cells, simulating ameloblastoma. × 80. **d,** higher magnification of a field from **c.** × 200.

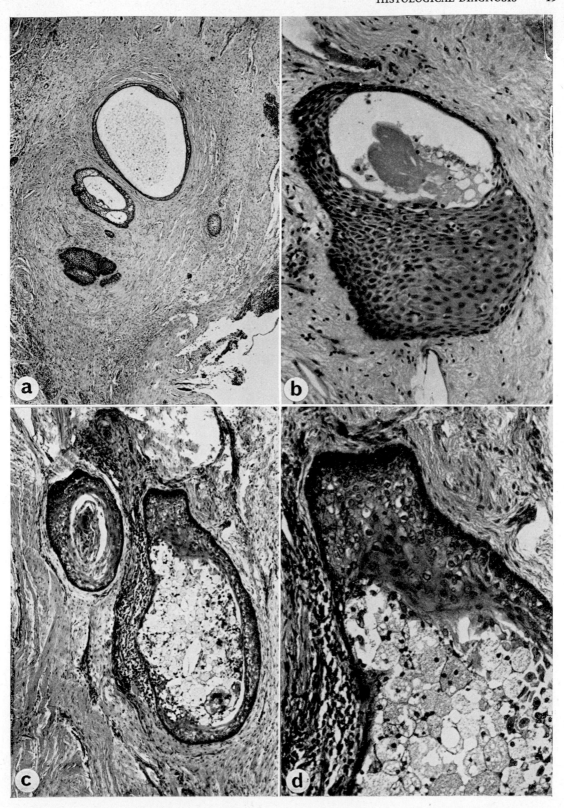

plastic from the outset, as Blum, Kaletsky and Gettinger (1940) recognised in reporting a case of this type, though many other authors ignore this possibility. In other cases photomicrographs purport to show ameloblastomatous tissue arising from the squamous epithelial lining of a simple cyst, but in many cases the appearances are not convincing. Often, what is thought to be non-neoplastic squamous epithelium could well be tumour epithelium, compressed and flattened by intracystic pressure. It is also possible that squamous metaplasia in a monocystic ameloblastoma may occur to such an extent that most of the lesion resembles a simple cyst, in which case the lesion could easily be interpreted as primarily of simple cystic nature with subsequent neoplastic change. Hewer (1952) has suggested that certain cystic lesions represent complete squamous metaplasia in a cystic ameloblastoma, but admits that there is no proof that a cyst of such type has ever had an ameloblastomatous pattern. It is probable that lesions of this type are in most cases primordial or keratocysts which, when large, often give clinical and radiological findings very similar to those of ameloblastoma.

From the point of view of microscopic diagnosis the position may be summarised by saying that a monocystic lesion with the clinical and radiological characteristics of a dentigerous cyst may prove histologically to be either a simple cyst or an ameloblastoma. It is particularly necessary to make a thorough examination of the cyst wall, with special attention to all mural nodules or thickenings, in order to avoid being misled by the resemblance of flattened tumour epithelium to non-neoplastic squamous epithelium, and to avoid missing the small tumour outgrowths that may be present in mural nodules. If, after such examination, nothing other than non-neoplastic squamous epithelium can be found, it is most unlikely that a recurrence at some future time will be in the form of ameloblastoma.

Other Neoplasms. The tumours most likely to be confused with ameloblastoma are squamous cell carcinoma, basal cell carcinoma and salivary gland tumours of the adenoid cystic carcinoma type. Squamous cell carcinoma may be diagnosed as ameloblastoma with well marked squamous metaplasia, and probably this accounts for some reports of metastasising ameloblastoma. On the other hand, squamous cell carcinoma may undergo changes which lead to some resemblance to stellate reticulum. This is what probably occurs in the case of certain extraoral tumours that have been diagnosed as ameloblastomas (see below). Basal cell carcinoma may sometimes be closely simulated by ameloblastoma. This resemblance has led some authors to classify the ameloblastoma as a type of basal cell carcinoma. Adenoid cystic carcinoma has been misdiagnosed as adenomatoid odontogenic tumour or as ameloblastoma with metastases. This occurs generally in the maxilla, where a tumour growing from sinus or nasal mucous glands may not be readily distinguishable clinically or radiologically from a tumour originating in the alveolar process. Salivary tumours may also occur in the mandible.

Finally, the possibility of metastatic carcinoma in the jaws should be kept in mind, for such deposits may be discovered before the primary growth and may simulate ameloblastoma.

EXTRAOSSEOUS AMELOBLASTOMA

Rarely, there occur tumours that are extraosseous but otherwise resemble ameloblastoma. Although there are some earlier reports (Gullifer, 1936; Ch'in, 1938; Braunstein, 1949), Stanley and Krogh (1959) were the first to provide acceptable illustrative evidence supporting their case of a tumour occurring in the soft tissues on the lingual surface of the molar-premolar area of the mandible. Subsequently, a few more cases have been recorded. Klinar and McManis (1969) report a tumour in the buccal mucosa and Russell (1966) and Wallen (1972) tumours in the maxillary tuberosity area. Lee and colleagues (1970) and Simpson (1974) report tumours in the gingivae. In Wertheimer and Stroud's (1972) case, the patient had a squamous cell papilloma of the lingual gingiva in the mandibular incisor area, and in this tumour the ameloblastoma appeared to arise. The entire lesion was excised, but the ameloblastomatous element recurred. Two apparently unrelated gingival growths in the same patient have been reported by Balfour, Loscalzo and Sulka (1973).

The possible sources of origin for these extraosseous tumours are the oral mucosa or cell rests. Other extraosseous lesions also considered to arise, wholly or in part, from similar sources include those described as peripheral odontogenic fibroma and odontogenic gingival epithelial hamartoma, and as Gardner (1973) points out, it is by no means certain that some of the reported extraosseous ameloblastomas are not related to them. In fact, epithelial tumours of local origin and growing in the jaws may present appearances very similar to ameloblastoma, although their biological behaviour is different. Thus, areas of the calcifying odontogenic cyst (p. 73, Fig. 28) can be practically identical to ameloblastoma, and primary intra-alveolar epidermoid carcinoma (p. 150) can resemble ameloblastoma.

Although these tumours are so uncommon, from the reports already published it would seem reasonable to assume that they do not require excessively drastic treatment. Complete excision should be done, but the extensive operations sometimes appropriate for intraosseous tumours are not likely to be necessary.

EXTRAORAL TUMOURS RESEMBLING AMELOBLASTOMA

Tumours somewhat similar in structure to ameloblastoma occur in the pituitary gland, the tibia and ulna, the ovary and elsewhere.

Craniopharyngioma. The pituitary craniopharyngiomas occur in the anterior lobe, which is of ectodermal origin. The lobe is derived from Rathke's pouch, an outgrowth of the oral ectoderm. The pouch gives rise to the craniopharyngeal duct, which itself degenerates in due course, but has been considered to leave as residues the collections of squamous epithelial cells that are to be found on the anterior and lateral surfaces of the infundibulum and the upper surface of the gland in the pars tuberalis. Erdheim (1904, 1925) put forward this view of the origin of the squamous epithelial cells, and from them derived the ameloblastoma-like tumours of this region. However, although he demonstrated the presence of the cell rests in most of the adult pituitary glands that he examined, he could not find them in newborn infants. Similarly, other workers have failed to find the rests in patients under 20 years of age (Kiyono, 1924; Carmichael, 1931; Susman, 1932). Because of this, and the particular incidence of tumours in younger patients, other theories have been put forward. Biggart (1961) considered that the cell rests are not derived from squamous epithelium but represent areas of metaplastic development of the cells of the pars tuberalis. Kernohan and Sayre (1956) also held this view and observed apparent transitions between chromophobe cells and the cells resembling squamous epithelium. It is not known why so many of the tumours occur before the age at which the so-called squamous epithelial cells are normally to be found in the gland. Grinker and Bucy (1949) suggested that the cells represent very slowly growing or arrested tumours, developing from pituitary cells.

The craniopharyngiomas have been described in detail by Critchley and Ironside (1926) and Peet (1927), and later cases have been reported by Frazier and Alpers (1931), McCallum (1941), Love and Marshall (1950), Campbell and Hudson (1960) and others. Gorlin and Chaudhry (1959) compare craniopharyngioma with ameloblastoma. Although craniopharyngioma can occur at any age, its greatest incidence is in children and young adults below the age of 25 years, whereas ameloblastoma occurs particularly in the third and fourth decades. Craniopharyngiomas frequently show macroscopic cystic change; although this occurs in ameloblastoma, it does so only to a minor extent in the great majority of cases. Microscopically, the resemblance between craniopharyngioma and ameloblastoma can be very close (Fig. 24). On the other hand, Russell and Rubenstein (1959) agree with Willis (1967) that craniopharyngiomas are not distinguishable from epitheliomas in which squamous and basal cells are both present. The columnar cells, these authors point out, have central nuclei, whereas the nuclei of the columnar cells in ameloblastoma are basal. Furthermore, these cells in craniopharyngioma have the longitudinal cytoplasmic fibrils that characterise basal epithelial cells in general. The central areas of the trabeculae of cells that compose the tumour consist of squamous cells showing intercellular bridges, but degeneration and oedema are common, and produce an appearance superficially similar to stellate reticulum. However, not all craniopharyngiomas show these features, and polarization of the nuclei in the columnar cells in the same manner as in ameloblastoma can often be noted.

A further difference between craniopharyngioma and ameloblastoma is the frequent presence of calcified material in the former tumour. Squamous metaplasia occurs in the central stellate area in both tumours, though much more extensively in craniopharyngioma, and keratinisation is again much more frequent and extensive in the cranial tumour. The cornified masses in the craniopharyngioma often excite a foreign body reaction and not infrequently undergo calcification, and sometimes bony metaplasia is seen. The calcification is rarely in the form of prismatic enamel, but it may have enameloid features (Kalnins and Rossi, 1965; Kalnins, 1971). Calcification and the presence of bone are seen only exceptionally in ameloblastoma, but when they do occur the resemblance to craniopharyngioma is very close indeed. It is not possible, therefore, to accept the view that the appearances in craniopharyngioma merely mimic those of ameloblastoma, any resemblances being due merely to degenerative changes. On the grounds of histology alone, the two tumours can often be seen to present an identical picture. Moreover, the occurrence of teeth in craniopharyngioma, although rare, must be regarded as strong evidence of the close link between the two tumours. Seemayer, Blundell and Wigglesworth (1972) report a case and review those previously reported. Another similarity has been demonstrated by Timperley and colleagues (1968, 1971), who have shown that both tumours, like the normal developing tooth, contain a high activity of alkaline phosphatase. However, this was not confirmed by Mori and colleagues (1969).

"Adamantinoma" of the Tibia. The first so-called adamantinoma occurring extraorally in bone was a tumour of the tibia reported by Fischer (1913). Hebbel collected some twenty or so cases in the literature up to 1940 and tumours of comparable type have been reported in the ulna (Anderson and Saunders, 1942) and the femur (Bell, 1942; Baker, Dockerty and Coventry, 1954; Moon, 1965).

Various theories have been put forward to explain the occurrence of an ameloblastoma-like tumour far away from the oral cavity. Epithelial rests misplaced during the course of development and later giving rise to tumours have been postulated, or trauma causing implantation of epithelium, with subsequent tumour formation (Ryrie, 1932; Dockerty and Meyerding, 1942). It has also been suggested that the tumour is not epithelial at all, but is a synovial sarcoma (Hicks,

---

Fig. 24   **a, b,** craniopharyngioma. **a,** the general pattern is very similar to that of the plexiform type of ameloblastoma. × 80. **b,** higher magnification, showing how closely the histology resembles that of ameloblastoma, except for the presence of keratin, which is common in craniopharyngioma but rare in ameloblastoma. × 200. "Adamantinoma" of the tibia. Two fields from the same tumour, showing in one field, **c,** appearances very similar to ameloblastoma while in the other, **d,** the picture may well be described as angioblastomatous. × 200 and × 80.

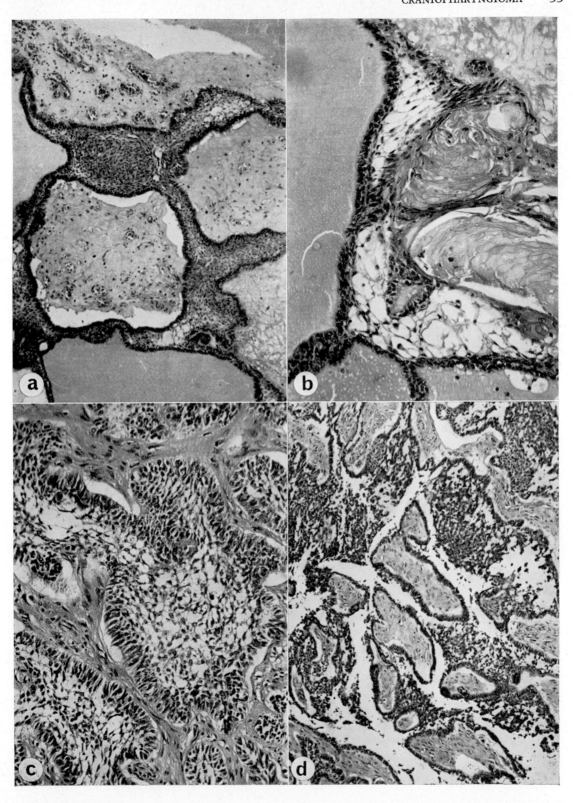

1954; Lederer and Sinclair, 1954) or other type of sarcoma (Naji and colleagues, 1964) or a malignant angioblastoma (Changus, Speed and Stewart, 1957; Elliot, 1962). Jaffe (1958) considers the arguments for and against these theories and also points out that the alveoli and tubules—which give the lesion a resemblance to ameloblastoma of the jaws—are probably formed because of liquefaction of the more centrally placed cells. Willis (1967) also believes that these tumours are epithelial and, indeed, examples have been reported in which squamous differentiation with intercellular bridges and pearl formation have been prominent (Donner and Dikland, 1966). Electron microscopic evidence also points towards the epithelial nature of the tumours (Rosai, 1969). Certainly, none of the illustrations of the published cases can strongly detract from Willis's and Jaffe's views (Fig. 24).

In a few cases lesions showing all the histological criteria of fibrous dysplasia of bone have been noted in either one or both of the long bones of a leg affected by the ameloblastoma-like tumour. The nature of this relationship is still unknown (Baker, Dockerty and Coventry, 1954; Cohen, Dahlin and Pugh, 1962).

The ameloblastoma of the ovary reported by Zajewloschin (1931) may have arisen from the dental formative elements in an ovarian dermoid.

REFERENCES

Akinosi, J. O., and Williams, A. O. (1969) Ameloblastoma in Ibadan, Nigeria. *Oral Surg.*, **27**, 257.

Aisenberg, M. S. (1950) Adamantinohemangioma. *Oral Surg.*, **3**, 798.

Aisenberg, M. S. (1953) Histopathology of ameloblastoma. *Oral Surg.*, **6**, 1111.

Anderson, C. E., and Saunders, J. B. de C. M. (1942) Primary adamantinoma of the ulna. *Surg. Gynec. Obstet.*, **75**, 351.

Ardoin, G. (1936) Histogénèse de l'adamantinome spongiocytaire (épulis congénitale). *Bull Ass. franç. Cancer*, **25**, 513.

Bailey, J. W. (1951) Dentigerous cyst with ameloblastoma. Report of a case. *Oral Surg.*, **4**, 1122.

Baden, E. (1965) Terminology of the ameloblastoma: history and current usage. *J. oral Surg.*, **23**, 40.

Baker, P. L., Dockerty, M. B., and Coventry, M. B. (1954) Adamantinoma (so-called) of the long bones. Review of the literature and a report of three new cases. *J. Bone Jt. Surg.*, **36A**, 704.

Balfour, R. S., Loscalzo, L. J. and Sulka, M. (1973) Multicentric peripheral ameloblastoma. *J. oral Surg.*, **31**, 535.

Bell, A. L. (1942) A case of adamantinoma of the femur. *Brit. J. Surg.*, **11**, 330.

Bernier, J. L., and Tiecke, R. W. (1951) A compilation of the material received by the registry of oral pathology. *J. oral Surg.*, **9**, 341.

Biggart, J. H. (1961) *Pathology of the Nervous System. A Student's Introduction.* 3rd Edition. Edinburgh and London. E. & S. Livingstone Ltd.

Bland-Sutton, J. (1922) *Tumours Innocent and Malignant.* 7th Edition. London. Cassell & Co. Ltd.

Blum, T., Kaletsky, T., and Gettinger, R. (1940). An ameloblastoma. *Arch. clin. oral Path.*, **4**, 374.

Boyle, P. D., and Kalinins, V. (1960) Enamel formation in ameloblastomas. *Arch. oral Biol.*, **2**, 285.

Braunstein, E. (1949) Case report of an extraosseous adamantinoblastoma. *Oral Surg.*, **2**, 726.

Broca, P. (1868) Recherches sur un nouveau groupe de tumeurs designées sous le nom d'odontomes. *Gaz. hebd. Sci méd.*, **5**, 70.

Bump, W. (1927) Adamantine epithelioma. *Surg. Gynec. Obstet.*, **44**, 173.

Byars, L. T., and Sarnat, B. G. (1945) Surgery of the mandible: the ameloblastoma. *Surg. Gynec. Obstet.*, **81**, 575.

Byrd, D. L., Allen, J. W., and Dunsworth, A. R. (1973) Ameloblastoma originating in the wall of a primordial cyst; report of case. *J. oral Surg.*, **31**, 301.

Cahn, L. R. (1933) The dentigerous cyst is a potential adamantinoma. *Dent. Cosmos*, **74**, 889.

Cameron, D. A. (1951) Adamantinomata: a brief discussion of their pathology with a report of three cases. *Dent. J. Aust.*, **23**, 183.

Campbell, J. A. H. (1956) Adamantinoma containing tissue resembling granular-cell myoblastoma. *J. Path. Bact.*, **71**, 45.

Campbell, J. B., and Hudson, F. M. (1960) Craniobuccal origin, signs and treatment of craniopharyngiomas. *Surg. Gynec. Obstet.*, **111**, 183.

Carmichael, H. T. (1931) Squamous epithelial rests in the hypophysis cerebri. *Arch. Neurol. Psychiat.*, **26**, 966.

Carpenter, L. S., and Thoma, K. H. (1933) Adamantinoma formed from a radicular cyst. *Dent. Items*, **55**, 716.

Carr, R. F., and Halperin, V. (1968) Malignant ameloblastomas from 1953 to 1966. Review of the literature and report of a case. *Oral Surg.*, **26**, 514.

Castner, D. V., McCully, A. C., and Hiatt, W. R. (1967) Intracystic ameloblastoma in the young patient. Report of a case. *Oral Surg.*, **23**, 127.

Champion, A. H. R., Moule, A. W., and Wilkinson, F. C. (1951) An ameloblastoma of the mandible. *Brit. dent. J.*, **90**, 143.

Changus, G. W., Speed, J. S., and Stewart, F. W. (1957) Malignant angioblastoma of bone. A reappraisal of adamantinoma of long bone. *Cancer*, **10**, 540.

Ch'in, K. Y. (1938) Adamantinoma in Chinese. A pathological study of 41 cases. *Chinese med. J.*, Suppl. II, 91.

Chung, D. H., Kinnman, J. E. G., Lee, B. C., and Lee, Y. T. (1969) Tumours of the jaws in Korea. Report of 147 cases. *Oral Surg.*, **27**, 716.

Churchill, H. R. (1929) Cited by Baden.

Churchill, H. R. (1934) Histological differentiation between certain dentigerous cysts and ameloblastomata. *Dent. Cosmos*, **76**, 1173.

Clausen, F., Philipsen, H. P., and Pindborg, J. J. (1961) Comparative histochemical investigations of ameloblastoma and enamel organs. *Acta. path. microbiol. scand.*, Suppl. 114, **51**, 109.

Clemmessen, J. (1965) Statistical studies in the aetiology of malignant neoplasms—II. Basic tables. *Acta path. microbiol. scand.*, Suppl. 174, 2.

Cohen, D. C., Dahlin, D. C., and Pugh, D. G. (1962) Fibrous dysplasia associated with adamantinoma of the long bones. *Cancer*, **15**, 575.

Critchley, M., and Ironside, R. N. (1926). The pituitary adamantinomata. *Brain*, **49**, 437.

Csiba, A., Ökros, I., Dzsinich, Cs., and Szabo, D. (1970) Virus-like particles in a human ameloblastoma. *Arch. oral Biol.*, **15**, 817.

Dahlgren, S. E., Ekström, C., and Mossberg, B. (1971) Mandibular ameloblastoma with pulmonary and mediastinal lymph node metastases. *Acta Otolaryngol.*, **72**, 220.

Davies, A. G. M., and Davies, J. N. P. (1960) Tumours of the jaw in Uganda Africans. *Acta Unio internat. contra Cancrum*, **16**, 1320.

Dockerty, M. B., and Meyerding, H. W. (1942) Adamantinoma of tibia; report of two new cases. *J. amer. med. Ass.*, **119**, 932

Dodge, O. G. (1965) Tumours of the jaw, odontogenic tissues and maxillary antrum (excluding Burkitt lymphoma) in Uganda Africans. *Cancer*, **18**, 205.

Donner, R., and Dikland, R. (1966) Adamantinoma of the tibia. A long-standing case with unusual histological features. *J. Bone Jt. Surg.*, **48B**, 138.

Elliott, G. B. (1962) Malignant angioblastoma of long bone. So-called "tibial adamantinoma." *J. Bone Jt. Surg.*, **44B**, 25.

England, L. C. (1960) Ameloblastoma of the mandible. Report of a case. *Oral Surg.*, **13**, 648.

Erdheim, J. (1904) Über Hypophysenganggeschwülste und Hirncholesteatome. *S. B. Akad. Wiss. Wien.*, **113 (Sect. III)**, 537.

Erdheim. J. (1925) Pathologie der Hypophysengeschwülste. 1. Normale Anatomie, Histologie und Entwicklung der Hypophyse. *Ergebn. allg. Path.*, **21**, 482.

Falkson, R. (1879) Zur Kenntniss der Kiefercysten. *Virchows Arch.*, **76**, 504.

Fischer, B. (1913) Über ein primares Adamantinom der Tibia. *Z. Pathopsych.*, **12**, 422.

Fish, E. W. (1948) *Surgical Pathology of the Mouth.* London. Sir Isaac Pitman & Sons Ltd.

Forsberg, A. (1954) A contribution to the knowledge of the histology, histogenesis and etiology of adamantinomas. *Acta odont. scand.*, **12**, 39.

Frantz, V. K., and Stix, L. (1932) Adamantinoma: a case of fifty-one years' duration. *Arch. Surg.*, **25**, 890.

Frazier, C. H., and Alpers, B. J. (1931) Adamantinoma of the craniopharyngeal duct. *Arch. Neurol. Psychiat.*, **26**, 905.

Gardner, D. G. (1973) An ameloblastoma and a hamartoma of the dental lamina in two siblings. *J. oral Surg.*, **31**, 697.

E

Gardner, D. G., and Spouge, J. D. (1966) Simple ameloblastoma with an interesting vascular component. *J. canad. dent. Ass.*, **32**, 589.

Geschickter, C. F. (1935) Tumors of the jaws. *Amer. J. Cancer*, **26**, 90.

Gorlin, R. J., and Chaudhry, A. P. (1959) The ameloblastoma and the craniopharyngioma—their similarities and differences. *Oral Surg.*, **12**, 199.

Grinker, R. R., and Bucy, P. C. (1949) *Neurology*. 4th Edition. Oxford. Blackwell Scientific Publishers.

Grover, C. J., Kruger, G. D., Reynolds, D. C., and Bernier, J. L. (1971) Hemangioblastoma: a vascular odontogenic tumor. *J. oral Surg.*, **29**, 23.

Gullifer, W. (1936) Adamantinoma *Dent. Cosmos*, **78**, 1256.

Gurney, C. E. (1958) The use of a tube graft to repair a palatal defect. *Amer. J. Surg.* **95**, 301.

Hair, J. A. G. (1963) Radiosensitive adamantinoma. *Brit. med. J.*, **i**, 105.

Hankey, G. T. (1938) Three unusual affections of the jaws. *Proc. roy. Soc. Med.*, **31**, 1137.

Harrer, W. V., and Patchefsky, A. S. (1970) Mandibular ameloblastoma with intracerebral and pulmonary metastasis. *Oral Surg.*, **29**, 893.

Hartman, K. S. (1974) Granular-cell ameloblastoma. A survey of twenty cases from the Armed Forces Institute of Pathology. *Oral Surg.*, **38**, 241.

Hebbel, R. (1940) Adamantinoma of the tibia. *Surgery*, **7**, 860.

Hertz, J. (1951) Adamantinoma. Histo-pathologic and prognostic studies. *Acta chir. scand.*, **102**, 405.

Hewer, T. F. (1952) Primary epithelial tumours of the jaw. *J. clin. Path.*, **5**, 225.

Hicks, J. D. (1954) Synovial sarcoma of the tibia. *J. Path. Bact.*, **67**, 151.

Hodson, J. J. (1957) Observations on the origin and nature of the adamantinoma with special reference to certain muco-epidermoid variations. *Brit. J. plast. Surg.*, **10**, 38.

Hodson, J. J. (1961) An intraosseous tumour combination of biological importance—invasion of a melanotic schwannoma by an adamantinoma. *J. Path. Bact.*, **82**, 257.

Hodson, J. J. (1961) A morphological study of dermal melanocytes and cytocrine activity in relation to certain Schwann cells and epithelial cells. *J. Path. Bact.*, **82**, 267.

Hodson, J. J. (1962) Epithelial residues of the jaw with special reference to the edentulous jaw. *J. Anat.*, **96**, 16.

Hoke, H. F., and Harrelson, A. B. (1967) Granular cell ameloblastoma with metastasis to the cervical vertebrae. Observations on the origin of the granular cells. *Cancer*, **20**, 991.

Ikemura, K., Tashiro, H., Fujino, H., Ohbu, D., and Nakajima, K. (1972) Ameloblastoma of the mandible with metastasis to the lungs and lymph nodes. *Cancer*, **29**, 930.

Ivy, R. H., and Churchill, H. R. (1930) The need of a standardized surgical and pathological classification of the tumors and anomalies of dental origin. *Trans amer. Ass. dent. Schools*, 240.

Jacobs, M. H. (1935). Adamantinomata. *Dent. Cosmos*, **77**, 239.

Jaffe, H. L. (1958) *Tumors and Tumorous Conditions of the Bones and Joints*. London. Henry Kimpton.

Jones, J. H. (1966) Soft tissue oral tumours in children: their structure, histogenesis and behaviour. *Proc. roy. Soc. Med.*, **59**, 673.

Kaletsky, T. (1938) Cystic adamantinoma with recurrence. *Arch. clin. oral Path.*, **2**, 150.

Kalnins, V. (1971) Calcification and amelogenesis in craniopharyngiomas. *Oral Surg.*, **31**, 366.

Kalnins, V., and Rossi, E. (1965) Odontogenic craniopharyngioma. *Cancer*, **18**, 899.

Kegel, R. F. C. (1932) Adamantine epithelioma. *Arch Surg.*, **25**, 498.

Kernohan, J. W., and Sayre, G. P. (1956) *Tumors of the pituitary gland and infundibulum*. Atlas of Tumor Pathology. Section 10. Fascicle 36. Washington, D. C. Armed Forces Institute of Pathology.

Kiyono, H. (1934) Über das Vorkommen von Plattenepithelherden in der Hypophyse (Zugleich ein Beitrag zur Kenntnis der Hypophysenganggewächse). *Virchows Arch.*, **252**, 118.

Klinar, K. L., and McManis, J. C. (1969) Soft-tissue ameloblastoma. Report of a case. *Oral Surg.*, **28**, 266.

Kotanyi, E. (1936) Case of adamantinoma. *J. dent. Res.*, **15**, 352.

Kovi, J., and Laing, W. N. (1966) Tumours of the mandible and maxilla in Accra, Ghana. *Cancer*, **19**, 1301.

Kramer, I. R. H. (1961) Personal communication.

Krompecher, E. (1918) Zur Histogenese und Morphologie der Adamantinome und sonstiger Kiefergeschwülste. *Beitr. path. Anat.*, **64**, 165.

Kronfeld, R. (1930) Adamantinoma. *J. amer. dent. Ass.*, **17**, 681.

Kühn, A. (1932) Über eine Kombination von Adamantinom mit Hämangiom als zentrale Kiefergeschwulst. *Dtsch. Mschr. Zahnheilk.*, **50**, 49.

Lederer, H., and Sinclair, A. J. (1954) Malignant synovioma simulating "adamantinoma of the tibia." *J. Path. Bact.*, **67**, 163.

Lee, K. W., Ch'in, T. C., and Paul, G. (1970) Peripheral ameloblastoma. *Brit. J. oral Surg.*, **8,** 150.

Lee, K. W., El-Labban, N. G., and Kramer, I. R. H. (1972) Ultrastructure of a simple ameloblastoma. *J. Path.*, **108,** 173.

Lee, R. E., White, W. L., and Totten, R. S. (1959) Ameloblastoma with distant metastases. *Arch. Path.*, **68,** 23.

Lewin, M. L. (1966) Nonmalignant maxillofacial tumors in children. *Plast. reconstr. Surg.*, **38,** 186.

Love, J. G., and Marshall, T. H. (1950) Craniopharyngiomas (pituitary adamantinomas). *Surg. Gynec. Obstet.*, **90,** 591.

Lucas, R. B. (1952) The pathology of epithelial cysts and tumours in the jaws. *Brit. J. Cancer*, **6,** 356.

Lucas, R. B. (1954) Neoplasia in odontogenic cysts. *Oral Surg.*, **7,** 1227.

Lucas, R. B. (1957) A vascular ameloblastoma. *Oral Surg.*, **10,** 863.

Lucas, R. B. (1969) Odontongenic tumours in polyoma virus-infected mice. *Fourth Proc. internat. Acad. oral Path.*, New York.

Lucas, R. B., and Thackray, A. C. (1951) The histology of adamantinoma. *Brit. J. Cancer*, **5,** 289.

Lucas, R. B., and Thackray, A. C. (1952) Cyst formation in adamantinomata. *Brit. dent. J.*, **93,** 62.

McCallum, H. M., and Cappell, D. F. (1957) Adamantinoma with granular cells. *J. Path. Bact.*, **74,** 365.

MacCallum, W. G. (1941) Adamantinoma of the hypophyseal duct. *J. Mt. Sinai Hosp.*, **8,** 798.

McFarland, J., and Patterson, H. M. (1931). Adamantinomata. A review of one hundred and ninety-six cases reported in the medical and dental literature. *Dent. Cosmos*, **73,** 656.

McGregor, K. (1935) A report of eleven instances of adamantinoma with a review of the malignant cases in the literature. *Acta radiol.*, **16,** 254.

McWhirter, R. (1952) Symposium on the treatment of adamantinoma. *Proc. roy. Soc. Med.*, **45,** 701.

Main, J. H. P., and Dawe, C. J. (1966) Tumor induction in transplanted tooth buds infected with polyoma virus. *J. nat. Cancer Inst.*, **36,** 1121.

Malassez, L. (1885) Sur le rôle des débris épithéliaux paradentaires. *Arch. Physiol.*, **6,** 379.

Mallik, K. C. B. (1957) An atypical adamantinoma. An adamantinoma with cells resembling granular-cell myoblastoma. *Arch. Path.*, **64,** 158.

Manley, E. B. (1954) Adamantinoma in relationship to tooth development. *Aust. J. Dent.*, **58,** 137.

Mehlisch, D. R., Dahlin, D. C., and Masson, J. K. (1972) Ameloblastoma: a clinicopathologic report. *J. oral Surg.*, **30,** 9.

Mincer, H. H., and McGinnis, J. P. (1972) Ultrastructure of three histologic variants of ameloblastoma. *Cancer*, **30,** 1036.

Moe, H., Clausen, F., and Philipsen, H. P. (1961) The ultrastructure of the simple ameloblastoma. *Acta path. microbiol. scand.*, **52,** 140.

Moon, N. F. (1965). Adamantinoma of the appendicular skeleton. A statistical review of reported cases and inclusion of 10 new cases. *Clin. Orthop.*, **43,** 189.

Mori, M., Okamoto, Y., Oka, R., and Mizushima, T. (1964) Enzymatic histochemical demonstration of ameloblastoma. *Oral Surg.*, **17,** 235.

Mori, M., Sugimura, M., and Matsuura, H. (1969) Histochemical comparisons of enzymes in craniopharyngioma and ameloblastoma. *Ann. Histochim.*, **14,** 349.

Mori, M., Tamari, Y., Sugimura, M., Fukui, A., and Kawakatsu, K. (1965) Histochemical detection of three dehydrogenase systems in ameloblastoma. *Oral Surg.*, **20,** 776.

Naji, A. F., Murphy, J. A., Stasney, R. J., Neville, W. E., and Chrenka, P. (1964) So-called adamantinoma of long bones. Report of a case with massive pulmonary metastasis. *J. Bone Jt. Surg.*, **46A,** 151.

Navarette, A. R., and Smith, M. (1971) Ultrastructure of granular cell ameloblastoma. *Cancer*, **27,** 948.

New, G. B. (1915) Cystic odontomas. *J. amer. med. Ass.*, **64,** 34.

Oesterreich, H. (1936) Cited by Thoma and Goldman (1960).

Oliver, R. T., McKenna, W. F., and Shafer, W. G. (1961) Hemangio-ameloblastoma: report of case. *J. oral Surg.*, **19,** 245.

Peet, M. M. (1927) Pituitary adamantinomas. *Arch. Surg.*, **15,** 829.

Pindborg, J. J., and Kramer, I. R. H. (1971). *International Histological Classification of Tumours No. 5. Histological Typing of Odontogenic Tumours, Jaw Cysts, and Allied Lesions.* Geneva. World Health Organization.

Pindborg, J. J., and Weinmann, J. P. (1958) Squamous cell metaplasia with calcification in ameloblastomas. *Acta path. microbiol. scand.*, **44,** 247.

Quinn, J. H., and Fournet, I. F. (1969) Dentigerous cyst with mural ameloblastoma: report of case. *J. oral Surg.*, **27,** 662.

Quinn, J. H., and Fullmer, H. M. (1953) A small ameloblastoma of the mandible. *Oral Surg.*, **6,** 949.

Robinson, H. B. G. (1937) Histologic study of the ameloblastoma. *Arch. Path.*, **23**, 664.

Robinson, H. B. G. (1937) Ameloblastoma. A survey of the three hundred and seventy-nine cases from the literature. *Arch. Path.*, **23**, 831

Robinson, H. B. G., and Lefkowitz, W. (1958) The ameloblastomatous potentiality of odontogenic epithelium demonstrated in tissue culture. *Oral Surg.*, **11**, 630.

Rosai, J. (1969) Adamantinoma of the tibia. Electron miscroscopic evidence of its epithelial origin. *Amer. J. clin. Path.*, **51**, 786.

Russell, A., (1966). Ameloblastoma of mucosal origin. *New Zealand dent. J.*, **62**, 116.

Russell, D. S., and Rubenstein, L. J. (1959) *The Pathology of Tumours of the Nervous System*. London. Edward Arnold (Publishers) Ltd.

Ryrie, B. J. (1932) Adamantinoma of the tibia: aetiology and pathogenesis. *Brit. med J.*, **2**, 1000.

Schroff, J. (1931) Preliminary report of an interesting case of adamantinoma. *J. dent. Res.*, **11**, 635.

Schweitzer, F. C., and Barnfield, W. F. (1943) Ameloblastoma of the mandible with metastasis to the lungs: report of a case. *J. oral Surg.*, **1**, 287.

Seemayer, T. A., Blundell, J. S., and Wigglesworth, F. W. (1972) Pituitary craniopharyngioma with tooth formation. *Cancer*, **29**, 423.

Sehdev, M. K., Huvos, A. G., Strong, E. W., Gerold, F. P., and Willis, G. W. (1974) Ameloblastoma of maxilla and mandible. *Cancer*, **33**, 324.

Shafer, W. G., and Spivey, A. W. (1954) Ameloblastoma. Report of a case. *Oral Surg.*, **7**, 32.

Sharp, G. S., Bullock, W. K., and Binkley, F. C. (1955) Ameloblastoma of the jaws. *Oral Surg.*, **8**, 1013.

Shatkin, S., and Hoffmeister, F. S. (1965) Ameloblastoma: a rational approach to therapy. *Oral Surg.*, **20**, 421.

Shear, M. (1969) Primary intra-alveolar epidermoid carcinoma of the jaw. *J. Path.*, **97**, 645.

Siegmund, H. (1929) Pathologische histologie. *Fortschr. Zahnheilk.*, **5**, 243.

Siegmund, H., and Weber, R. (1926) *Pathologische Histologie der Mundhohle*. Leipzig. Hirzel.

Simmons, C. C. (1928) Adamantinoma. *Ann. Surg.*, **88**, 693.

Simpson, H. E. (1974) Basal-cell carcinoma and peripheral ameloblastoma. *Oral Surg.*, **38**, 239.

Small, I. A., and Waldron, C. A. (1955) Ameloblastomas of the jaws. *Oral Surg.*, **8**, 281.

Sonesson, A. (1950) Odontogenic cysts and cystic tumours of the jaws. *Acta radiol.*, Suppl. 81.

Spouge, J. D. (1967) The adenoameloblastoma. *Oral Surg.*, **23**, 470.

Spouge, J. D. (1967) Embryonal significance of epithelial odontogenic tumours. *J. canad. dent. Ass.*, **33**, 200.

Sprawson, E. (1937) Odontomes. *Brit. dent. J.* **62**, 177.

Sprawson, E., and Keizer, W. R. (1933) On the similarity of rodent ulcers (basal-celled carcinomata), multilocular cysts of the jaws ("adamantinomata"), and epithelial tumours of the anterior (suprasellar) portion of the pituitary body. *Dent. Rec.*, **53**, 369.

Stanley, H. R., and Krogh, H. W. (1959) Peripheral ameloblastoma. Report of a case. *Oral Surg.*, **12**, 760.

Stanley, H. R., Baer, P. N., and Kilham, L. (1965) Oral tissue alterations in mice inoculated with the Rose substrain of polyoma virus. *Periodontics*, **3**, 178.

Stanley, H. R., Daw, C. J., and Law, L. W. (1964) Oral tumors induced by polyoma virus in mice. *Oral Surg.*, **17**, 547.

Stanley, H. R., and Diehl, D. L. (1965) Ameloblastoma potential of follicular cysts. *Oral Surg.*, **20**, 260.

Stanley, H. R., Krogh, H., and Pannkuk, E. (1965) Age changes in the epithelial components of follicles (dental sacs) associated with impacted third molars. *Oral Surg.*, **19**, 128.

Stoll, H. C., Marchetta, F. C., and Shobinger, R. (1957) Malignant epithelial tumors of the mandible and maxilla. *Arch. Path.*, **64**, 239.

Sugimura, M., Yamauchi, T., Yashikawa, K., Takeda, N., Sakita, M., and Miyazaki, T. (1969) Malignant ameloblastoma with metastasis to the lumbar vertebra: report of case. *J. oral Surg.*, **27**, 350.

Susman, W. (1932) Embryonic epithelial rests in the pituitary. *Brit. J. Surg.*, **19**, 571.

Taylor, R. N., Callins, J. F., Menell, H. B., and Williams, A. C. (1971) Dentigerous cyst with ameloblastomatous proliferation: report of case. *J. oral Surg.*, **29**, 2.

Thoma, K. H. (1940) Follicular cysts and tumors associated with impacted third molars. *Arch. clin. oral. Path.*, **4**, 292.

Thoma, K. H. (1944) Adamantoblastoma of mandible. *Amer. J. Orthodont.* (Oral Surg. Sect.), **20**, 248.

Thoma, K. H., and Goldman, H. M. (1960) *Oral Pathology*. 5th Edition. London. Henry Kimpton.

Thoma, K. H., and Proctor, C. H. (1937) Adamantinoma developing from odontogenic cyst. *Int. J. Orthod.*, **23**, 307.

Timperley, W. R. (1968) Histochemistry of Rathke pouch tumours. *J. Neurol. Neurosurg. Psychiat.*, **31**, 589.

Timperley, W. R., Turner, P., and Davies, S. (1971) Alkaline phosphatase in craniopharyngiomas. *J. Path.*, **103**, 257.

Topazian, R. G. (1964) Ameloblastoma in a 4 year old child. *Oral Surg.*, **17**, 581.

Tsukada, Y., de la Pava, S., and Pickren, J. W. (1965) Granular-cell ameloblastoma with metastasis to the lungs. Report of a case and review of the literature. *Cancer*, **18**, 916.

Vickers, R. A., and Gorlin, R. J. (1970) Ameloblastoma: delineation of early histopathologic features of neoplasia. *Cancer*, **26**, 1970.

Vorzimer, J., and Perla, D. (1932) An instance of adamantinoma of the jaw with metastases to the right lung. *Amer. J. Path.*, **8**, 445.

Wallen, N. G. (1972) Extraosseous ameloblastoma. *Oral Surg.*, **34**, 95.

Wertheimer, F. W., and Stroud, D. E. (1972) Peripheral ameloblastoma in a papilloma with recurrence: report of case. *J. oral Surg.*, **30**, 47.

Wilkinson, F. C. (1952) Adamantinoma: a review of twelve cases. *Med. Pr.*, **228**, 90.

Willis, R. A. (1967) *Pathology of Tumours.* 4th Edition. London. Butterworth & Co. (Publishers) Ltd.

Wunderer, S. (1953) Zur Frage maligner Odontome. *Öst. Z. Stomatol.*, **50**, 567.

Young, D. R., and Robinson, M. (1962) Ameloblastomas in children. *Oral Surg.*, **15**, 1155.

Zajewloschin, M. N. (1931) Adamantinoma primarium malignum Ovarii. *Frankfurt. Z. Path.*, **41**, 100.

Zegarelli, E. V. (1944) Adamantoblastomas in the Slye stock of mice. *Amer. J. Path.*, **20**, 23.

4. Adenomatoid Odontogenic Tumour

This tumour, like some others of odontogenic origin, has had a chequered terminological career. The earliest cases appear to have been reported by Dreibladt (1907) as pseudo-adenoma adamantinum and by L'Esperance (1910) as glandular adamantinoma. Stafne (1948) reported three cases as epithelial tumours associated with developmental cysts and Miles (1951) published a case as a cystic complex composite odontome. Further examples were reported as adenoameloblastoma by Bernier and Tiecke (1950, 1956), Aisenberg (1953) and Thoma (1955). Oehlers (1956) described the lesion as a pleomorphic adenoma-like tumour and a case was reported as a tumour of enamel organ epithelium (Lucas, 1957). The literature is reviewed by Gorlin and Chaudhry (1958) and further reviews taking in the more recent cases have been published by Philipsen and Birn (1969), Tehertkoff, Daino and Ehrenreich (1969), Giansanti and colleagues (1970) and Courtney and Kerr (1975).

Clinical Features

The tumour occurs typically in young persons in the second or third decade, but older patients are occasionally seen. A tumour in a woman of 82 years has been reported by Meyer and Giunta (1974). Females are more commonly affected than males.

There are few symptoms apart from a gradually increasing swelling, more often in the upper than in the lower jaw. Occasionally there may be pain. The tumour is generally situated in the lateral incisor, canine or premolar region though it has also been seen near the angle of the mandible. It is frequently associated with an unerupted tooth but may occur in a normally erupted dentition. The tumour expands the bone and fluctuation may be elicited. Very uncommonly, however, as reported by Gorlin and Chaudhry and by Abrams, Melrose and Howell (1968), the tumour may develop extraosseously, in the gingiva. Radiographs generally show a clearly demarcated radiolucent lesion; although there is frequently some calcification in the tumour this is often insufficient to produce detectable radiopacity (Fig. 25). Accordingly, the lesion is usually diagnosed clinically as a dentigerous or lateral periodontal cyst.

Pathology

Most tumours are quite small, measuring in the region of 1 to 3 cm in diameter, though much larger examples have been reported. There is a well defined fibrous capsule. The cut

---

Fig. 25 Adenomatoid odontogenic tumour in a girl of 19 years. There was a painless swelling in the maxillary canine-premolar region of recent duration. This was thought to be a small dentigerous cyst and was excised. The patient was well with no recurrence 7 years later, **a,** the radiograph shows a rounded soft tissue lesion in the canine-premolar area. The canine and first premolar were missing. The lesion is well demarcated but there is no surrounding bony condensation. The substance of the lesion shows numerous small convoluted areas and a number of very small areas of calcification, **b,** low power view of the lesion. It is well encapsulated, and its partly solid, partly cystic, nature can be seen. × 6·5. **c,** tubule-like structures are a prominent feature, with intervening solid areas and areas with a looser cribriform pattern. × 80. **d,** an area of solid growth. × 80. **e,** higher magnification of the tubule-like structures, showing the radially arranged columnar cells that resemble ameloblasts and the homogeneous material in the central cystic space, forming a thin layer in contact with the columnar cells. × 200.

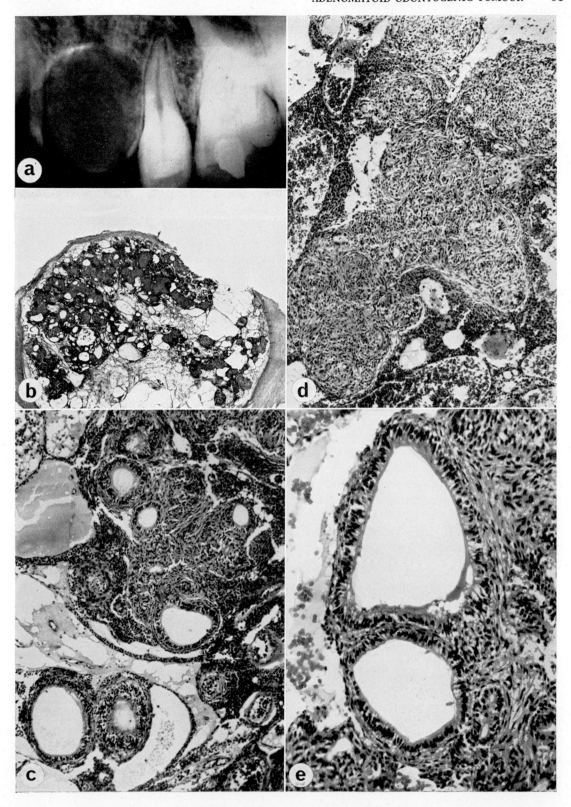

surface shows a variegated appearance with small areas of haemorrhage in a greyish-white tissue. Small or large cystic spaces may be present and these may contain yellowish gelatinous material or blood-stained fluid. In some cases the tumour may be almost entirely cystic. A tooth or teeth may be embedded in the tumour or attached to it.

Microscopically, the tumour consists of sheets and strands of epithelial cells that differentiate in places into columnar cells very similar to ameloblasts. These cells form structures of tubular appearance, distributed throughout the tumour. The tubule-like structures consist of a central space enclosed by the columnar cells, which are disposed radially, in a single layer. The nuclei of the columnar cells are situated towards the ends of the cell bodies farthest from the central space and the space itself usually contains some homogeneous eosinophilic material that forms a thin layer in contact with the free ends of the cells (Figs. 25 and 26).

In addition to forming tubule-like structures the columnar cells also form convoluted bands arranged in complicated patterns. These bands consist of a double row of cells and appear to represent tubule-like structures which have not yet expanded to include a central space. However, the homogeneous eosinophilic material can again be seen as a thin layer between the ends of the opposed columnar cells. The areas intervening between the tubular and band formations are occupied by small cells with oval nuclei and clear cytoplasm that form continuous sheets of tissue, except in some areas where they form slender strands that intercommunicate to enclose cystic spaces. In these areas the appearance is not unlike the cribriform pattern seen in some salivary tumours. The cystic spaces tend to coalesce, due to degeneration of the intervening cellular strands, to form larger cystic areas.

Very little stroma is present in the tumour. The solid areas appear to be almost entirely epithelial and are avascular. Such stroma as may be present is situated mainly in the cribriform areas, where it undergoes cystic degeneration, and small haemorrhages may be seen.

Small foci of calcification are scattered throughout the tumour. Oehlers (1961) has demonstrated that these are not merely dystrophic deposits but represent attempted enamel formation, since they often occur in close relationship to groups of tall columnar cells that particularly resemble ameloblasts. They also show the morphological appearance and staining reactions of the "enameloid" tissue that Mezl (1959) has described as occurring in the development of enamelomas. Spouge and Spruyt (1968) have demonstrated that the calcified deposits commence intracellularly as minute multifocal diastase-PAS-positive globules that subsequently fuse to form the calcific masses. Lee's (1974) ultrastructure studies indicated that there may well be different components in the calcified material. He found evidence of amyloid-like fibrils and also of dentine-like material. True tubular dentine has been found in some tumours (Dunlap and Fritzlen, 1972).

Histogenesis

The close resemblance of the columnar cells to ameloblasts and the frequent association of the tumour with unerupted teeth indicate its origin from dental epithelium. The actual point of origin of the lesion in the dental tissues is unknown. Like the ameloblastoma, it could theoretically derive from the enamel organ or its remnants, or from a dentigerous cyst. As to the last-named possibility, the position is again comparable to the relationship between ameloblastoma

Fig. 26   **a,** a tubular formation showing an ingrowth or invagination. × 200. **b,** the solid areas consist of convoluted and infolded tubular structures with intervening sheets of small cells. × 200. **c,** columnar cells forming a folded band-like structure. × 200. **d,** higher magnification from **c.** The homogeneous material is seen between the columnar cells and in close relation to them. × 500.

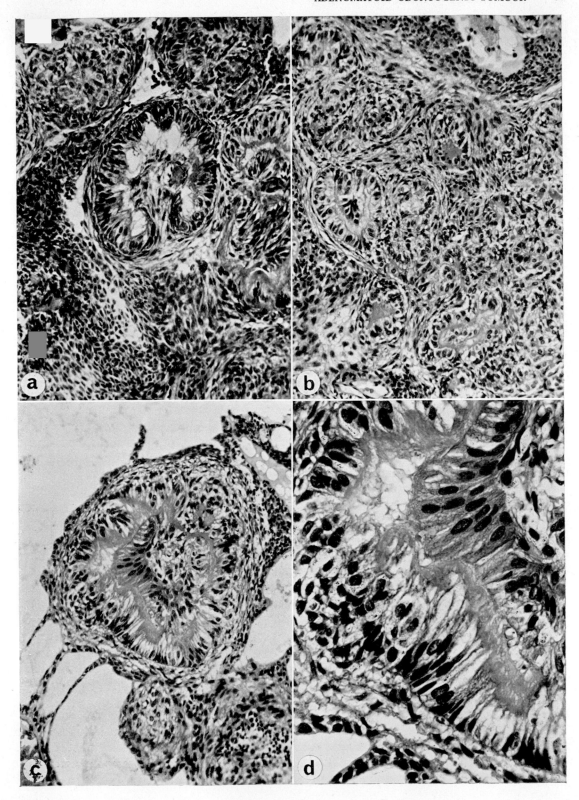

and dentigerous cyst. That is to say, the lesion quite frequently presents in the anatomical form of a dentigerous cyst, but there is no evidence that it represents the subsequent development of neoplasia in the wall of a cyst that was originally of simple nature. Bhaskar (1964) has examined 50 primordial and follicular cysts, and has found areas similar to the tumour in 4 per cent. He concludes that the lesion arises from odontogenic epithelium at the stage of follicle formation, specifically from the outer enamel epithelium.

It seems not unreasonable to suppose that in some cases at least cyst formation might be a secondary phenomenon, resulting from extension of the stromal degeneration seen in the cribriform areas.

Until relatively recently most authors followed the earlier reports in regarding the tumour as a type of ameloblastoma with differentiation towards glandular structures. It is now generally recognised, however, that there are significant differences between the two lesions. Not only are the pathological appearances quite distinctive, but the clinical features also, with the young age incidence and benign behaviour, serve clearly to establish the tumour as a separate entity. So far as the so-called adenomatous element is concerned, since it was pointed out (Lucas, 1957) that the similarity to glandular structure is superficial only, there has been general agreement that this is indeed the case and that the tumour is neither an ameloblastoma nor an adenoma. The tubule-like structures, which bear some resemblance to ducts, are in fact abortive attempts at the formation of enamel organs and, as Oehlers (1961) has shown in serial sections, are "blind" and do not interconnect to form a ductular system.

The nature of the eosinophilic material apparently secreted by the columnar cells, which as Miles (1951) has stressed, are in fact more like ameloblasts than the columnar cells of the ameloblastoma, is still in doubt. It may be a pre-enamel since it occurs in the correct morphological relationship to the ameloblast-like cells and it is an acid mucopolysaccharide (Gorlin and Chaudhry). Moreover, the small cells situated between the tubule-like structures are alkaline phosphatase-positive, as is the stratum intermedium of the normal tooth germ. On the other hand, Shear (1962) considered the homogeneous material to represent pre-dentine matrix, since it is reticulin-positive and may be traced in occasional fields to an apparent continuity with what little stroma is present. Ishikawa and Mori (1962) also found this material to give the staining reactions of mesenchymal connective tissue, and consider that the duct-like spaces represent stromal cysts. However, Spouge and Spruyt (1967, 1968), while agreeing that the homogeneous material in the tumour does not appear to be pre-enamel, consider that any analogy with pre-dentine matrix is doubtful. They point out that the silver-staining material in the tumour is homogeneous, whereas reticulin not only fixes silver salts but is also fibrillar. Furthermore, there are a number of histochemical similarities between the epithelium of normal developing teeth and the cells of the tumour to indicate that these represent the preameloblastic stage of development. Another suggestion ascribes the homogenous material to basement membrane. As Courtney and Kerr (1975) point out, the synthesis of basement membrane precedes the induction of the mesenchyme to differentiate into odontoblasts .The apparent absence, or extreme scantiness, of mesenchyme in the tumour would inhibit further amelogenesis, and this might result in continued production of basement membrane and subsequent pooling of this material as eosinophilic droplets.

Behaviour

Although long duration follow-up data are not as yet available for many cases, the tumour appears to be benign, not recurring after such conservative procedures as simple enucleation. Halperin, Carr and Peltier (1967) have checked the follow-up times of 35 cases reported in the literature and found that only one had been followed for more than 5 years. Moreover, in most cases the condition has been noticed at quite an early stage and has been treated promptly. Thus there have been few opportunities of studying the natural history of the condition, uninfluenced by treatment. However, there are some cases in which the lesion has been observed over quite a long period, when it has been noted to show continued growth and has attained a fairly large size by the time of removal. Thus it would appear that the lesion exhibits persistence of growth, and is neoplastic. On the other hand, Miles (1951) and Cahn (1955) have suggested that the lesion is hamartomatous, while in two of Oehler's cases tumour tissue was known to have been left *in situ* after operation, but in each case the lesion subsequently regressed. In any event, it is important to note that this lesion lacks entirely the propensities for recurrence of the ordinary ameloblastoma, and does not demand radical surgery.

REFERENCES

Abrams, A. M., Melrose, R. J., and Howell, F. V. (1968) Adenoameloblastoma. A clinical pathologic study of ten new cases. *Cancer*, **22**, 175.

Aisenberg, M. S. (1953) Histopathology of ameloblastomas. *Oral Surg.*, **6**, 1111.

Bernier, J. L., and Tiecke, R. W. (1950) Adeno-ameloblastoma. *J. oral Surg.*, **8**, 259.

Bernier, J. L., and Tiecke, R. W. (1956) Adenoameloblastoma. *Oral Surg.*, **9**, 1304.

Bhaskar, S. N. (1964) Adenoameloblastoma; its histogenesis and report of 15 new cases. *J. oral Surg.*, **22**, 218.

Cahn, L. R. (1955) Discussion of Thoma, K. H., in *Oral Surg.*, **8**, 441.

Courtney, R. M., and Kerr, D. A. (1975) The odontogenic adenomatoid tumor. A comprehensive study of twenty new cases. *Oral Surg.*, **39**, 424.

Dreibladt, H. (1907) Cited by Langer.

Dunlap, C. L., and Fritzlen, T. J. (1972) Cystic odontoma with concomitant adenoameloblastoma (adenoameloblastic odontoma). *Oral Surg.*, **34**, 450.

Giansanti, J. S., Someren, A., and Waldron, C. A. (1970) Odontogenic adenomatoid tumor (adenoameloblastoma). Survey of 111 cases. *Oral Surg.*, **30**, 69.

Gorlin, R. J., and Chaudhry, A. P. (1958) Adenoameloblastoma. *Oral Surg.*, **11**, 762.

Halperin, V., Carr, R. F., and Peltier, J. R. (1967) Follow-up of adenoameloblastomas. Review of thirty-five cases from the literature and report of two additional cases. *Oral Surg.*, **24**, 642.

Ishikawa, G., and Mori, K. (1962) A histopathological study on the adenomatoid ameloblastoma. Report of four cases. *Acta odont. scand.*, **20**, 419.

Lee, K. W. (1974) A light and electron microscopic study of the adenomatoid odontogenic tumor. *Int. J. oral Surg.*, **3**, 183.

L'Esperance, E. (1910) A preliminary report of eight cases of adamantinoma. *Proc. N. Y. path. Soc.*, **10**, 136.

Lucas, R. B. (1957) A tumor of enamel organ epithelium. *Oral Surg.*, **10**, 652.

Meyer, I., and Giunta, J. L. (1974) Adenomatoid odontogenic tumor (adenoameloblastoma): report of case. *J. oral Surg.*, **32**, 448.

Mezl, Z. (1959) Pathologic amelogenesis. *Canad. dent. Ass. J.*, **25**, 364.

Miles, A. E. W. (1951) A cystic complex composite odontome. *Proc. roy. Soc. Med.*, **44**, 51.

Oehlers, F. A. C. (1956) An unusual pleomorphic adenoma-like tumor in the wall of a dentigerous cyst. *Oral Surg.*, **9**, 411.

Oehlers, F. A. C. (1961) The so-called adenoameloblastoma. *Oral Surg.*, **14**, 712.

Oehlers, F. A. C. (1961) So-called adenoameloblastoma. *Oral Surg.*, **14**, 1961.

Philipsen, H. P., and Birn, H. (1969) The adenomatoid odontogenic tumor. Ameloblastic adenomatoid tumor or adenoameloblastoma. *Acta path. microbiol. scand.*, **75**, 375.

Shear, M. (1962) The histogenesis of the "tumour of enamel organ epithelium." *Brit. dent. J.*, **112**, 494.

Spouge, J. D. (1967) The adenoameloblastoma. *Oral Surg.*, **23**, 470.

Spouge, J. D., and Spruyt, C. L. (1968) Odontogenic tumors. Histochemical comparison of the adenoameloblastoma and developing tooth. *Oral Surg.*, **25**, 447.

Stafne, E. C. (1948) Epithelial tumors associated with developmental cysts of the maxilla. *Oral Surg.*, **1**, 887.

Tehertkoff, V., Daino, J. A., and Ehrenreich, T. (1969) Ameloblastic adenomatoid tumor (adenoameloblastoma). Case reports and review of the literature. *Oral Surg.*, **27**, 72.

Thoma, K. H. (1955) Adenoameloblastoma. *Oral Surg.*, **8**, 441.

5. Calcifying Epithelial Odontogenic Tumour

Pindborg (1958) described under the designation of "calcifying epithelial odontogenic tumour" an uncommon lesion of distinctive pathology that seemed previously to have been considered as a type of ameloblastoma or odontome. Some 70 cases have now been reported (Krolls and Pindborg, 1974).

Clinical Features

Reviews of the literature (Pindborg, 1966; Vap, Dahlin and Turlington, 1970) show that the tumour is rather commoner in males than in females. The average age of patients is about 42 years, with a range from 8 to 92 years. The mandible is affected much more often than the maxilla, the site of election being the premolar-molar region. The growth is symptomless, apart from the progressive swelling of the jaw, and examination shows a hard tumour that may be diffuse or well defined. Radiographic examination shows a translucent zone with areas of radio-pacity, which may or may not be well demarcated from surrounding normal tissues. In about half the cases an unerupted tooth is associated with the tumour. The preoperative diagnosis may be dentigerous cyst or ameloblastoma, because of the radiographic appearances. However, at operation an invasive tumour that destroys the bone may be found, the apparent cystic spaces being filled with soft tumour tissue. In other cases, the tumour appears to be well circumscribed.

Recently there have been reports of tumours occurring extraosseously in the gingiva. These lesions correspond very closely in structure to the intraosseous growths (Pindborg, 1966; Abrams and Howell, 1967; Decker and Laffitte, 1967; Patterson and colleagues, 1969). They occur most often in the anterior region of the jaw.

Pathology

The tumour consists of sheets of polyhedral epithelial cells in a connective tissue stroma The epithelial cells tend to be closely packed in most areas, though sometimes they show a cribriform arrangement enclosing areas of hyaline stroma. The cell outlines are distinct and the cytoplasm is slightly eosinophilic and homogeneous in appearance. Intercellular bridges are often present. The nucleus is vesicular, with distinct nucleoli. There is much variation in nuclear size and giant nuclei, measuring up to 100 μ in diameter, can be seen. Many cells have two or more nuclei. Mitoses are rare. The homogeneous hyaline areas have been demonstrated by Vickers, Dahlin and Gorlin (1965), Ranløv and Pindborg (1966) and Gardner, Michaels and Liepa (1968) to have many of the attributes of amyloid. Thus, they show green birefringence with congo red, fluorescence with thioflavin T and, electron microscopically, a finely fibrillar structure. However, the fibrillar appearance differs from that characteristic of the amyloid that is associated with reticuloendothelial cells. Chaudhry and colleagues (1972) suggest that the amyloid-like material might be an altered structural protein such as keratin, or an enamel matrix. The ultra-structure of the lesion has been investigated by Anderson, Kim and Minkowitz (1969), Main-wairing and colleagues (1970) and Chaudhry and colleagues (1972). The tumour cells show intercellular bridges with desmosomes, intracytoplasmic tonofilaments and well-developed hemidesmosomes. These commonly observed features of epidermal cells are in keeping with a possible origin of the tumour from enamel organ or oral epithelium.

The homogeneous material appears to be the matrix in which occurs the calcification that is such a striking feature of the tumour. The calcium is deposited in concentric masses in and around the epithelial cells, which appear to be undergoing degeneration, with a surrounding collagenous tissue that is partially mineralised. In the older parts of the tumour the calcified areas are confluent, forming large masses (Fig. 27).

Not infrequently, there are variations from the typical pattern just described. Thus the tumour may be almost entirely cellular, with little or no calcification, and the cells may form large sheets or they may be arranged in smaller sheets and strands. In other cases there may be a moderate amount of calcification with a similar type of cellular pattern. Occasionally calcification may be partly in the form of the calcified dental tissues. Chaudhry, Holte and Vickers (1962) noted a tubular appearance suggestive of dentine in the calcified areas in their case and, in fact, cases occur in which quite large masses of dentine may be present, even forming recognisable tooth-like structures. Areas of clear cells have been noted by Krolls and Pindborg (1974).

Histogenesis

Before the tumour was recognised as an entity, earlier authors had supposed it to be a type of ameloblastoma (Thoma and Goldman, 1946; Ivy, 1948), or because of the calcification, an odontome (Wunderer, 1953; Stoopack, 1957). However, Pindborg has shown that there are no ameloblast-like cells in the tumour. Its frequent occurrence in connection with an embedded tooth indicates its dental nature, and Pindborg suggests that it develops from the reduced enamel epithelium of the embedded tooth or from stratum intermedium. This view is supported by Gon's (1965) morphological and histochemical investigations.

Behaviour

There is as yet insufficient evidence to indicate the long-term behaviour of this tumour. However, from what is known, it does appear that while incomplete removal is likely to be followed by recurrence, effective cure can be obtained by complete resection of the lesion. One case, reported by Stimson, Luna and Butler (1968), has been followed for 15 years following partial maxillary resection. The patient is alive and well, with no recurrence.

REFERENCES

Abrams, A. M., and Howell, F. V. (1967) Calcifying epithelial odontogenic tumors: report of four cases. *J. amer. dent. Ass.*, **74**, 1231.

Anderson, H. C., Kim, B., and Minkowitz, S. (1969) Calcifying epithelial odontogenic tumor of Pindborg. An electron microscopic study. *Cancer*, **24**, 585.

Chaudhry, A. P., Hanks, C. T., Leifer, C. and Gargiulo, E. A. (1972) Calcifying epithelial odontogenic tumor. A histochemical and ultrastructural study. *Cancer*, **30**, 519.

Fig. 27   Calcifying odontogenic epithelial tumour in a man of 28 years. The tumour, which had been present for 18 months, painless but increasing in size, was situated in the maxilla. A tooth had been extracted at the site of the tumour 7 years previously. The maxilla was resected and 10 years later the patient was well with no recurrence. **a,** the radiograph shows replacement of the normal bony structure in the incisor-premolar area by ill-defined spherical opacities, varying in size and density. The lesion involved the whole alveolus in the angle between the nasal fossa and the antrum. **b,** the tumour consists of sheets of epithelial cells in which are extensive deposits of calcified material. × 80. **c,** degeneration of the epithelial cells frequently produces a cribriform pattern. × 200. **d,** in other areas the epithelium is arranged in broad bands or sheets. × 200. **e,** higher magnification of an area with calcification. × 200.

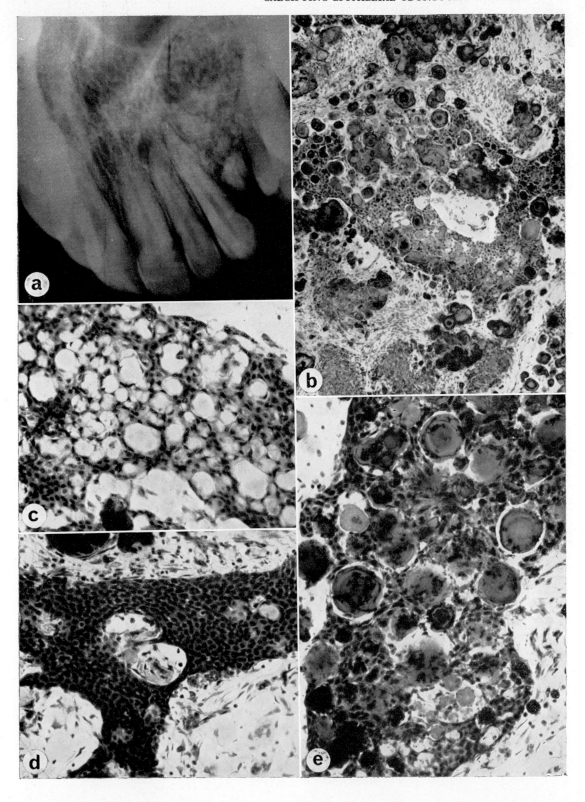

Chaudhry, A. P., Holte, N. O., and Vickers, R. A. (1962) Calcifying epithelial odontogenic tumor. Report of a case. *Oral Surg.*, **15**, 843.

Decker, R. M., and Laffitte, H. B. (1967) Peripheral calcifying epithelial odontogenic tumor. *Oral Surg.*, **23**, 398.

Gardner, D. G., Michaels, L., and Liepa, E. (1968) Calcifying epithelial odontogenic tumor: an amyloid-producing neoplasm. *Oral Surg.*, **26**, 812.

Gon, F. (1965) The calcifying epithelial odontogenic tumor. Report of a case and a study of its histo-genesis. *Brit. J. Cancer*, **19**, 39.

Ivy, R. H. (1948) Unusual case of ameloblastoma of mandible. Resection followed by restoration of continuity by iliac bone graft. *Oral Surg.*, **1**, 1074.

Krolls, S. O., and Pindborg, J. J. (1974) Calcifying epithelial odontogenic tumor. A survey of 23 cases and discussion of histomorphologic variations. *Arch. Path.*, **98**, 206.

Mainwairing, A. R., Ahmed, A., Hopkinson, J. M., and Anderson, P. (1971) A clinical and electron microscopic study of a calcifying epithelial odontogenic tumour. *J. clin. Path.*, **24**, 152.

Patterson, J. T., Martin, T. H., DeJean, E. K., and Burzynski, N. J. (1969) Extraosseous calcifying epithelial odontogenic tumor. Report of a case. *Oral Surg.*, **27**, 363.

Pindborg, J. J. (1958) A calcifying epithelial odontogenic tumor. *Cancer*, **11**, 838.

Pindborg, J. J. (1966) The calcifying epithelial odontogenic tumor. Review of literature and report of an extraosseous case. *Acta odont. scand.*, **24**, 419.

Ranløv, P., and Pindborg, J. J. (1966) The amyloid nature of the homogeneous substance in the calcifying epithelial odontogenic tumor. *Acta path. microbiol. scand.*, **68**, 169.

Stimson, P. G., Luna, M. A., and Butler, J. J. (1968) Seventeen-year history of a calcifying epithelial odontogenic (Pindborg) tumor. *Oral Surg.*, **25**, 204.

Stoopack, J. C. (1957). Cystic odontoma of the mandible. *Oral Surg.*, **10**, 807.

Thoma, K. H., and Goldman, H. M. (1946) Odontogenic tumors. A classification based on observations of the epithelial, mesenchymal, and mixed varieties. *Amer. J. Path.*, **22**, 433.

Vap, D. R., Dahlin, D. C., and Turlington, E. G. (1970) Pindborg tumor: the so-called calcifying epithelial odontogenic tumor. *Cancer*, **25**, 629.

Vickers, R. A., Dahlin, D. C., and Gorlin, R. J. (1965) Amyloid-containing odontogenic tumors. *Oral Surg.*, **20**, 476.

Wunderer, S. (1953) Zur Frage maligner Odontome. *Öst. Z. Stomatol.*, **50**, 567.

6. Calcifying Odontogenic Cyst

This lesion, which has histological similarities to ameloblastoma, was characterised by Gorlin and colleagues (1962, 1964) as a distinctive entity. Further reports have appeared from Gold (1963), Sycamore (1964), Smith and Blankenship (1965), Chaves and Pessoa (1968), Johnson and Topazian (1968), Komiya and colleagues (1969), Herd (1972), Sauk (1972) and others. Ulmansky, Azaz and Sela (1969) and Freedman, Lumerman and Gee (1975) review the more recent reports. The few cases that can be traced in the earlier literature appear to have been described as atypical ameloblastomas or as types of odontome.

The terminology proposed by Gorlin is not altogether appropriate, although it is difficult at present to find a suitable alternative. The lesion is not invariably cystic and the similarity of nomenclature leads to confusion with the calcifying epithelial odontogenic tumour, which is a separate entity. Some authors use the designation keratinising ameloblastoma (Bhaskar, 1965), but this is also inappropriate. Although the lesion has histological similarities to ameloblastoma, its behaviour is different.

Clinical Features

The lesion usually occurs as a slowly enlarging, frequently painless and non-tender swelling of the jaw. However, in an appreciable number of cases it is not intraosseous, but arises in the gingiva. In the 70 cases reviewed by Freedman, Lumerman and Gee, males and females were, overall, equally affected, but before the age of 41 the lesion was much more common in females, while after that age it was much more common in males. The youngest patient so far reported was 7 years of age and the oldest 82 (Jones, McGowan and Gorman, 1968), but most patients are under the age of 40. Freedman and colleagues also noted that before the age of 41 most of the lesions occurred in the maxilla (70 per cent), while in patients over 41 most lesions (80 per cent) were in the mandible. Seventy five per cent of the lesions were situated anterior to the first molar.

Radiologically, the intrabony lesion appears as a radiolucent area, perhaps with spotty calcification. An embedded tooth may be noted, or denticle-like structures may be present. The radiolucency may appear unilocular or multilocular and is usually well defined. Some lesions, however, may be poorly demarcated. The clinical diagnosis may therefore be dentigerous cyst, adenomatoid odontogenic tumour, compound or complex odontome or calcifying epithelial odontogenic tumour. Lesions occurring in the soft tissues only may cause saucerisation of the adjacent bone.

Pathology

The lesion is frequently cystic but occasionally it presents as a solid mass. Microscopically, the cyst cavity, which in some cases may be potential only, is lined by epithelium with a deeply staining basal layer of cubical or columnar cells somewhat resembling ameloblasts (Fig. 28). When the cells are columnar it can be seen that the nucleus is situated at the end of the cell distant from the basement membrane. Above this basal layer is a zone of varying width composed of basophilic cells rather more loosely arranged and having some resemblance to stellate reticulum. The epithelium thus appears not dissimilar to that of the ameloblastoma, but there are also present the characteristic features of this lesion, the ghost cells. These are epithelial cells which enlarge, become eosinophilic and undergo an aberrant type of keratinisation, and since many

F

cells are affected in this way, large masses of keratin accumulate. The cells often show a central pale area formerly occupied by the nucleus, and they do not become markedly flattened, as in normal keratinisation. The keratin stains poorly and the outlines of the keratinised cells can often still be discerned, but with some difficulty. Hence the term, ghost cells. As increasing numbers of cells become changed in this way, masses of keratin form which fill the cyst lumen on one side and push through the basement membrane on the other, into the underlying connective tissue. When this occurs, there is a foreign body reaction and numerous giant cells are seen in relation to the keratin masses. In addition, calcification of the ghost cells may occur (Fig. 29). Although the ghost cells are a characteristic feature of calcifying odontogenic cyst, they are not pathognomonic since they also occur, although much less obviously, in other odontogenic lesions. They have been observed in odontomes (Levy, 1973; Sedano and Pindborg, 1975), in ameloblastoma and in ameloblastic fibroma (Regezi, Courtney and Kerr, 1975).

In some lesions there may be additional features. The basal layer of the epithelium may proliferate, with the formation of strands of cells growing into the surrounding connective tissue. Sometimes discrete islets of cells are seen in the connective tissue at some little distance from the cyst lining proper. Dentine-like material may be present, and even true tubular dentine and enamel. In some cases these hard dental tissues may form tooth-like structures, and cases of this type have been reported as composite odontomes (Forest and Mercier, 1967). The presence of melanin pigment has been reported in a few cases (Gorlin and colleagues, 1964; Duckworth and Seward, 1965; Abrams and Howell, 1968; Chandi and Simon, 1970). Lurie's (1961) case of melanotic progonoma in an adult would also appear to fall into this group.

Histogenesis. There can be little doubt as to the odontogenic origin of this lesion in view of its characteristic histological appearance. Moreover, in three cases Gorlin and colleagues have demonstrated its origin in the dental epithelium of a developing or unerupted tooth. In those lesions arising in an extraosseous situation, it seems reasonable to postulate an origin from the remnants of odontogenic epithelium that may be present in the gingiva or alveolar mucosa. The ultrastructure of the tumour has been investigated by Fejerskov and Krogh (1972), who found that the ghost cells were similar in fine structure to the keratinised masses in craniopharyngioma. Ultrastructure studies have also been reported by Chen and Miller (1975).

The remarkable resemblance of some aspects of the lesion to the calcifying epithelioma of Malherbe has been noted by a number of authors (Spirgi, 1960; Gorlin and colleagues, 1962; Peterson and Gorlin, 1964). This tumour occurs usually on the face and arms of young women, and may arise from hair matrix cells. The basophilic cells that appear to constitute the principal element of the tumour undergo changes similar to those seen in the calcifying odontogenic cyst, becoming eosinophilic and losing their nuclear staining. These "shadow" cells undergo cornification and calcification and a foreign body giant cell reaction occurs in relation to them. However, these similarities, although of considerable interest, do not at present contribute to our understanding of the histogenesis of the calcifying odontogenic cyst.

Behaviour. Recurrence of the lesion, even after procedures so conservative as enucleation, seems to be exceptional. So far as can be judged, therefore, it appears to be benign.

Fig. 28   Calcifying odontogenic cyst. **a,** the cyst wall is lined by epithelium resembling that seen in ameloblastoma. × 50. **b,** higher magnification shows the basal layer of columnar cells and the adjacent stellate cells, with areas of keratinisation. × 200. **c,** the epithelium may penetrate the connective tissue, in anastomosing strands. × 50. **d,** details of the epithelium. × 80.

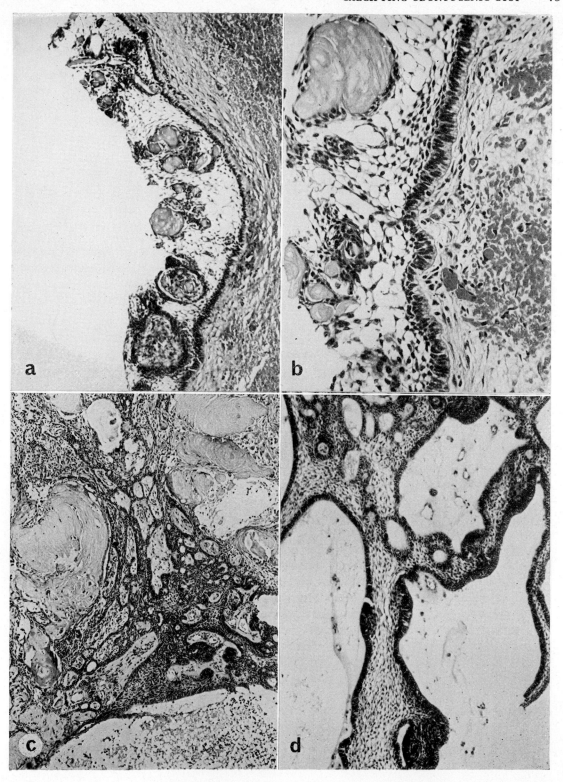

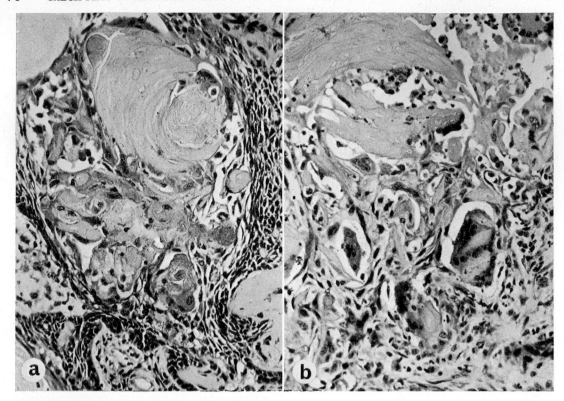

Fig. 29 **a, b,** showing the ghost cells and keratinisation with accompanying foreign body reaction. Both × 200.

REFERENCES

Abrams, A. M., and Howell, F. V. (1968) The calcifying odontogenic cyst. Report of four cases. *Oral Surg.*, **25,** 594.

Bhaskar, S. N. (1965) Gingival cyst and the keratinizing ameloblastoma. *Oral Surg.*, **19,** 796.

Chandi, S. M., and Simon, G. T. (1970) Calcifying odontogenic cyst. Report of two cases. *Oral Surg.*, **30,** 99.

Chaves, E. and Pessoa, J. (1968) The calcifying odontogenic cyst. Report of two cases. *Oral Surg.*, **25,** 849.

Chen, S-Y., and Miller, A. S. (1975) Ultrastructure of the keratinizing and calcifying odontogenic cyst. *Oral Surg.*, **39,** 769.

Duckworth, R., and Seward, G. R. (1965) A melanotic ameloblastic odontoma. *Oral Surg.*, **19,** 73.

Fejerskov, O., and Krogh, J. (1972) The calcifying ghost cell odontogenic tumor—or the calcifying odontogenic cyst. *J. oral Path.*, **1,** 273.

Forest, D., and Mercier, P. (1967) Compound composite odontome associated with keratinizing masses. *J. canad. dent. Ass.*, **33,** 487.

Freedman, P. D., Lumerman, H., and Gee, J. K. (1975) Calcifying odontogenic cyst. A review and analysis of seventy cases. *Oral Surg.*, **40,** 93.

Gold, L. (1963) The keratinizing and calcifying odontogenic cyst. *Oral Surg.*, **16,** 1414.

Gorlin, R. J., Pindborg, J. J., Clausen, F. P., and Vickers, R. A. (1962) The calcifying odontogenic cyst— a possible analogue of the cutaneous calcifying epithelioma of Malherbe. An analysis of fifteen cases. *Oral Surg.*, **15,** 1235.

Gorlin, R. J., Pindborg, J. J., Redman, R. S., Williamson, J. J., and Hansen, L. S. (1964) The calcifying odontogenic cyst. A new entity and possible analogue of the cutaneous calcifying epithelioma of Malherbe. *Cancer*, **17,** 723.

Herd, J. R. (1972) The calcifying odontogenic cyst. *Austr. dent. J.*, **17,** 6.

Johnson, R. H., and Topazian, R. G. (1968) Calcifying odontogenic cyst: report of case. *J. oral Surg.*, **26,** 394.

Jones, J. H., McGowan, D. A., and Gorman, J. M. (1968) Calcifying epithelial odontogenic and keratinizing odontogenic tumors. *Oral Surg.*, **25,** 465.

Komiya, Y., Susa, A., Kawachi, H., Yamamura, T., Eda, S., and Kawachi, Y. (1969) Calcifying odontogenic cyst. Report of a case. *Oral Surg.*, **27,** 90.

Levy, B. A. (1973) Ghost cells and odontomas. *Oral Surg.*, **36,** 851.

Lurie, H. I. (1961) Congenital melanocarcinoma, melanotic adamantinoma, retinal anlage tumor, progonoma, and pigmented epulis of infancy. Summary and review of the literature and report of the first case in an adult. *Cancer*, **14,** 1090.

Peterson, W. C., and Gorlin, R. J. (1964) Possible analogous cutaneous and odontogenic tumors. *Arch. Dermatol.*, **90,** 255.

Regezi, J. A., Courtney, R. M., and Kerr, D. A. (1975) Keratinization in odontogenic tumors. *Oral Surg.*, **39,** 447.

Sedano, H. O., and Pindborg, J. J. (1975) Ghost cell epithelium in odontomas. *J. oral Path.*, **4,** 27.

Smith, J. F., and Blankenship, J. (1965) The calcifying odontogenic cyst. Report of a case. *Oral Surg.*, **20,** 624.

Spirgi, M. (1960) Un cas d'épithélioma adamantin calcifié au niveau de la mugueuse buccale. *Schweiz. Monatschr. Zahnheilk.*, **70,** 1077.

Sauk, J. J. (1972) Calcifying and keratinizing odontogenic cyst. *J. oral Surg.*, **30,** 893.

Sycamore, E. M. (1964). Calcifying odontogenic cyst. Report of a case. *Brit. dent. J.*, **116,** 164.

Thoma, K. H., and Goldman, H. M. (1946) Odontogenic tumors. A classification based on observations of the epithelial, mesenchymal, and mixed varieties. *Amer. J. Path.*, **22,** 433.

Ulmansky, M., Azaz, B., and Sela, J. (1969) Calcifying odontogenic cyst: report of cases. *J. oral Surg.*, **27,** 415.

7. Ameloblastic Fibroma

This tumour contains both epithelial and mesenchymal neoplastic elements, the former deriving from the enamel organ or its epithelial remnants and the latter from the dental papilla or the dental follicle. Because of the presence of the two tissues the lesion was formerly referred to as a mixed tumour or as a soft (i.e., noncalcifying) odontome.

Clinical Features

The ameloblastic fibroma is much less common than ameloblastoma. The reported cases are reviewed by Shafer (1955) and Gorlin, Chaudhry and Pindborg (1961), and Trodahl (1972) has analysed twenty-four cases from the files of the American Armed Forces Institute of Pathology.

The tumour occurs in patients of the younger age groups, generally between the ages of 15 and 25 years. Huebsch and Stephenson (1956) report a case in which the tumour appeared at the age of $1\frac{1}{2}$ years. There is no sex predilection.

The tumour grows slowly and painlessly, expanding the jaw. The mandible is more often affected than the maxilla, the usual site being the canine-molar region. Radiologically, the tumour appears as a unilocular area of translucency with smooth outline that is not distinguishable from a unilocular ameloblastoma or dentigerous cyst. Sometimes the radiolucency is multilocular. Unerupted teeth may be present.

Pathology

The tumour forms a mass expanding the bone, but not invading it. On section, it has the appearance and consistency of a soft fibroma. There may or may not be a definite capsule but the growth is circumscribed and has a smooth surface. Microscopically, the tumour consists of strands and groups of epithelial cells in an abundant connective tissue background (Fig. 30). The epithelial cells are generally cubical or low columnar in type and are similar to the cells that form the peripheral layer of the follicles in ameloblastoma. They are arranged in irregularly branching strands that have some resemblance to the dental lamina. These strands frequently consist only of a double row of cells, but in some of the larger strands a central area of stellate cells is present. Thus there is some similarity to ameloblastoma, with the epithelial elements consisting of a peripheral layer of cubical or columnar cells enclosing a stellate reticulum. However, the stellate cells, when present, are never so abundant as in ameloblastoma and cyst formation is unusual.

The connective tissue element generally takes the form of a very cellular fibroblastic tissue that resembles the dental papilla in the developing tooth, though in some cases thick collagen bands may be present. There may be acellular hyaline zones around some of the epithelial strands, possibly indicating an inductive effect of the epithelium upon the connective tissue. Chaudhry and colleagues (1962) have described an ameloblastic fibroma in which large areas were myxomatous and foci of predentine were present. Myxomatous areas have also been reported by Hammarström and colleagues (1971).

In some tumours fully formed tubular dentine may occur. Where this is a notable feature the designation *ameloblastic fibro-odontoma* has been used by some workers, who have held that such lesions represent an independent category. However, this is arguable. Structural variations occurring in more or less familiar lesions do not constitute grounds for the creation of a new class of lesion, unless accompanied by distinctive clinical or behavioural characteristics. It has

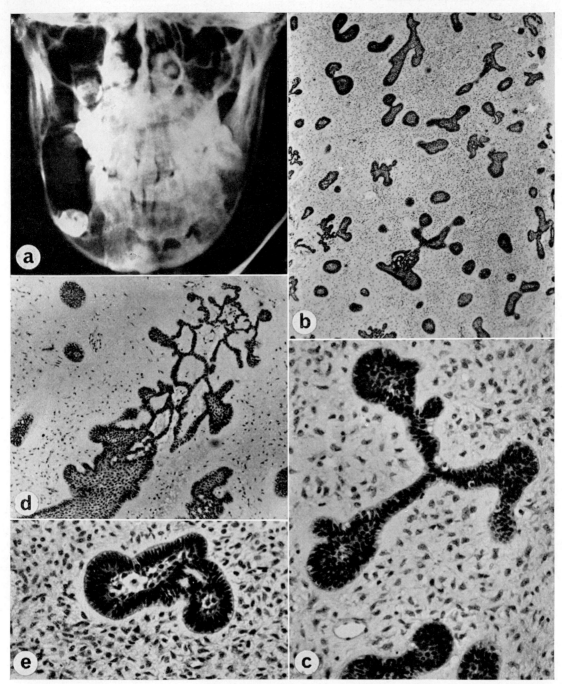

Fig. 30   Ameloblastic fibroma in a girl of 17 years. The tumour formed a painless swelling of the mandible of 6 weeks' duration. The affected segment of mandible was excised and the patient was well with no recurrence 5 years later. **a,** the radiograph shows a large unilocular translucency associated with an unerupted tooth, resembling a dentigerous cyst. **b,** the tumour consists of groups of epithelial cells in a cellular matrix. × 30. **c,** the epithelial cells are low columnar in type and form irregularly branched strands. The fibroblastic element of the tumour is well seen here. × 200. **d,** occasionally, the cellular strands form small networks. × 80. **e,** some cell groups show central areas resembling the central stellate cells of the ameloblastoma follicle. × 200.

not been demonstrated that the so-called ameloblastic fibro-odontoma is essentially different in behaviour to the ameloblastic fibroma.

Couch, Morris and Vellios (1962) reported the occurrence of granular cells, similar to the granular cells of congenital epulis, in two cases that they diagnosed as ameloblastic fibroma. They consider that the granular cells arise from the fibroblastic element of the tumour. A similar case has been reported by Waldron, Thompson and Conner (1963).

Behaviour

It has been suggested by Cahn and Blum (1952) that the lesion represents the immature stage of a complex odontome and that in the course of time calcified tissues would appear. That is to say, with the appearance of dentine the tumour would evolve to what is sometimes called ameloblastic fibro-odontoma and finally, with the formation of enamel, to a complex or compound odontome. However, no such evolution has been noted, even in older patients. Eversole, Tomich and Cherrick (1971) have analysed the cases in the literature reported as ameloblastic fibroma, ameloblastic fibroma with dentinoid, and ameloblastic fibro-odontoma, and find that in all these conditions males are more often affected than females, whereas for the complex and compound odontomes the sexes are equally affected or females predominate. Clearly, if some of these lesions are to evolve into others, the sex ratios must agree. Moreover, if ameloblastic fibroma evolves into the odontomes, it should occur in younger patients, and the odontomes should occur in older patients. It was found, however, that all these lesions occur in patients of the same general age group. Thus, the available evidence indicates that ameloblastic fibroma and the odontomes are separate entities to the extent that they represent differing end points of a disturbance of growth, although this itself may indeed be of the same fundamental nature for the various lesions.

Ameloblastic fibroma is a benign lesion. It has generally been considered that the recurrence rate is low; in Gorlin, Chaudhry and Pindborg's (1961) report on twenty-three cases there were only two recurrences, but in Trodahl's (1972) recent series, which probably had a more extensive follow-up, the recurrence rate was 43·5 per cent. Individual reports of recurrent tumours include those of Carr and colleagues (1970) and Tanaka and colleagues (1972). It thus appears that the ameloblastic fibroma might be rather more difficult to extirpate completely than had been originally thought. But the available evidence does not appear to call for heroic measures such as extensive resections; simple excision should be adequate in most cases.

Ameloblastic Sarcoma

This rare lesion may be regarded as the malignant counterpart of the ameloblastic fibroma. Leider and colleagues (1972) have collected the reports from the literature; together with their own series they give an analysis of 17 cases. Subsequent case reports have been published by Forman and Garrett (1972) and Hatzifotiadis and Economou (1973).

The tumour usually occurs in young adults, of either sex, and in the mandible more often than the maxilla. Pain and swelling are nearly always prominent features and the rate of growth is usually rapid. Radiographically, there is irregular bone destruction.

Microscopically, the general picture resembles ameloblastic fibroma, with epithelial follicles set in cellular fibroblastic tissue. Other than the occasional occurrence of dystrophic calcification, the epithelial component shows no marked difference to that of ameloblastic fibroma. The fibroblastic element, however, is highly cellular and pleomorphism and numerous mitoses, some atypical, are prominent features. Tumour giant cells may be present.

In some cases there is evidence that the tumour has developed in an originally benign ameloblastic fibroma. Cina, Dahlin and Gores (1962) report two cases of this type, and in one of

Leider's cases the tumour, originally an ameloblastic fibroma, showed transition in consecutive recurrences to ameloblastic sarcoma and eventually fibrosarcoma without epithelium. Evidently the epithelial element had been submerged by the increasingly anaplastic mesenchymal element. The authors suggest that some tumours reported as fibrosarcomas of the jaws may have commenced as ameloblastic fibromas and may thus indeed be of odontogenic origin. Mori and colleagues (1972) have reported a similar case.

The tumour appears to be of low grade malignancy: no metastases have occurred in any of the cases so far reported. There is probably a reasonable chance of effecting a cure if the tumour can be wholly removed, but recurrences may appear even after a considerable length of time. One patient was alive and well after 12 years, having had one recurrence (Hertz, 1952); another died after 18 years with two recurrences (Cina and colleagues). The invasive capacity of the tumour is illustrated by Pindborg's (1960) case of a 17-year-old male with a maxillary tumour. This grew rapidly, recurred several times and finally proved fatal some two years after diagnosis, with destruction of the base of the skull and invasion of the hypophysis.

Ameloblastic odontosarcoma. These very rare tumours resemble ameloblastic sarcoma but in addition dentine and enamel are present. Examples of tumours probably coming into this group have been reported by Thoma (1951) and Villa (1955).

REFERENCES

Cahn, L. R., and Blum, T. (1952) Ameloblastic odontoma; case report critically analyzed. *J. oral Surg.*, **10**, 169.

Carr, R. F., Halperin, V., Wood, C., Krust, L., and Schoen, J. (1970) Recurrent ameloblastic fibroma. *Oral Surg.*, **29**, 85.

Chaudhry, A. P., Stickel, F. R., Gorlin, R. J., and Vickers, R. A. (1962) An unusual odontogenic tumor. Report of a case. *Oral Surg.*, **15**, 86.

Cina, M. T., Dahlin, D. C., and Gores, R. J. (1962) Ameloblastic sarcoma. Report of two cases. *Oral Surg.*, **15**, 969.

Couch, R. D., Morris, E. E., and Vellios, F. (1962) Granular cell ameloblastic fibroma. Report of two cases in adults, with observations on its similarity to congenital epulis. *Amer. J. clin. Path.*, **37**, 398.

Eversole, L. R., Tomich, C. E., and Cherrick, H. M. (1971) Histogenesis of odontogenic tumors. *Oral Surg.*, **32**, 569.

Forman, G., and Garrett, J. (1972) Ameloblastic sarcoma: report of case. *J. oral Surg.*, **30**, 50.

Gorlin, R. J., Chaudhry, A. P., and Pindborg, J. J. (1961) Odontogenic tumors. Classification, histopathology, and clinical behavior in man and domesticated animals. *Cancer*, **14**, 73.

Hammarström, L., Molin, C., and Pretorius-Clausen, F. (1971) Ameloblastic fibroma with hyalinisation and myxomatous changes. *Swed. dent. J.*, **64**, 633.

Hatzifotiadis, D., and Economou, A. (1973) Ameloblastic sarcoma in the maxilla. A case report. *J. max. fac. Surg.*, **1**, 62.

Hertz, J. (1952) Adamantinoma. Studies in histo-pathology and prognosis. *Acta Med. scand.*, **142**, (Suppl. 266), 529.

Huebsch, R. F., and Stephenson, T. D. (1956) Recurrent ameloblastic fibroma in a 3-year old boy. *Oral Surg.*, **9**, 707.

Leider, A. S., Nelson, J. F., and Trodahl, J. N. (1972) Ameloblastic fibrosarcoma of the jaws. *Oral Surg.*, **33**, 559.

Mori, M., Shimozato, T., Kawano, S., and Kawakatsu, K. (1972) Ameloblastic fibroma and ameloblastic sarcoma—a report of the cases, histopathology and histochemistry. *J. Osaka Univ. dent. Schl.*, **12**, 91.

Pindborg, J. J. (1960) Ameloblastic sarcoma in the maxilla. Report of a case. *Cancer*, **13**, 917.

Shafer, W. G. (1955) Ameloblastic fibroma. *J. oral Surg.*, **13**, 317.

Tanaka, S., Mitsui, Y., Mizuno, Y., and Emori, S. (1972) Recurrent ameloblastic fibroma. Report of a case. *Oral Surg.*, **30**, 944.

Thoma, K. H. (1951) The pathogenesis of the odontogenic tumors. *Oral Surg.*, **4,** 1262.

Trodahl, J. N. (1972) Ameloblastic fibroma. A survey of cases from the Armed Forces Institute of Pathology. *Oral Surg.*, **33,** 547.

Villa, V. G. (1955) Ameloblastic sarcoma in the mandible. Report of a case. *Oral Surg.*, **8,** 123.

Waldron, C. A., Thompson, C. W., and Conner, W. A. (1963) Granular-cell ameloblastic fibroma. Report of two cases. *Oral Surg.*, **16,** 1202.

8. Odontoma

It has already been noted (p. 24) that the term "odontome" or "odontoma," which was originally used as a general description for any tumour of the dental tissues has, in the course of time, come to be employed in a much more restricted sense. It is now taken to denote tumours that contain both enamel and dentine, and when used in general parlance without further qualification, it is usually with reference to the complex and the compound odontomes. These lesions, when completely developed, consist principally of fully formed enamel and dentine, but during the period of active growth ameloblastic epithelium and odontoblastic tissue is present. Enamel and dentine and their precursor tissues are also present in a number of other lesions, and this is indicated by the inclusion of "odonto" or "odontoma" in the names of these lesions. They include ameloblastic fibro-odontoma (p. 76), odontoameloblastoma (p. 38), ameloblastic odontosarcoma (p. 79) and other lesions which are difficult to classify at present.

COMPLEX AND COMPOUND ODONTOMES

The complex odontome consists of a mass of irregularly arranged dentine, enamel, cementum and connective tissue. The compound odontome is an agglomeration of often large numbers of small though morphologically recognisable teeth. Many lesions, however, occupy an intermediate position, and all gradations between an unorganised mass of dental tissues and the formation of complete teeth may be encountered. Thus, most of a lesion may consist of irregularly arranged enamel, dentine and cementum, but here and there a more recognisably tooth-like structure may be embedded in the general mixture of tissues, while at almost the other end of the scale the lesion may consist of a number of small teeth, but with some areas of irregular dental tissues also present. Frequently, the lesions take the place of a missing tooth, that is to say, an odontome is formed in the place of a normal tooth, or alternatively if all the teeth are present an odontome may represent a supernumerary tooth.

Clinical Features

The majority of odontomes are discovered in children and adolescents, more often in females than in males, and more often in the mandible than in the maxilla. Gorlin, Chaudhry and Pindborg (1961) have found that complex odontomes occur particularly in the molar area while compound odontomes occur for the most part in the incisor-canine region. Generally, the lesions are quite small and symptomless, being discovered only on routine radiographic examination, though occasionally quite large dimensions may be attained. In most cases the lesion is associated with permanent teeth, but Hitchin and Dekonor (1963), Noonan (1971) and Malik and Khalid (1974) report odontomes associated with the primary dentition. Multiple odontomes are rare. In Bader's (1967) patient they were associated with multiple malformations in other parts of the body. Thompson, Hale and McLeran (1968), Malik and Khalid (1974) and Mani (1974) have also reported cases. Browne (1970) reports the occurrence of six odontomes in three members of the same family. Familial lesions, associated with other abnormalities, have also been reported by Schmidseder and Hausamen (1975).

Radiologically, the complex odontome appears as an area of opacity that may be similar to that caused by osteosclerosis. That is to say, the mass of calcified dental tissues of which it is composed shows merely as an irregular dense area. The compound odontome shows numerous small tooth-like structures, but of course a great variety of appearances can be met with, according to the degree of organisation of the hard tissues.

Pathology

The complex odontome occurs as a roughly spherical or ovoid mass that may expand the jaw but is often not much larger than a normal tooth, causing no deformity. The outer surface is smooth and slightly, or sometimes markedly, lobulated. On section, the entire lesion is seen to be solid, resembling an osteoma, but instead of the homogeneous, ivory-like appearance of the compact osteoma, or the trabeculae of the cancellous tumour, the cut surface shows a striated appearance, with radially arranged markings. Most lesions are quite small, measuring a centimetre or less in diameter, but some specimens measuring many centimetres across have been reported.

Microscopically, the lesion is surrounded by a fibrous capsule. Not infrequently the capsule is partially separated from the lesion by fluid; the resultant cyst is usually lined by squamous epithelium. The lesion itself consists of enamel, dentine and cementum, forming an extensive mass and arranged quite irregularly. Much of the enamel is fully calcified, and thus in routine sections of decalcified material its participation in the lesion is indicated by the empty spaces that remain after its removal by decalcification. In some of these spaces, where the enamel had not fully matured, enamel matrix may be seen. This is recognised by its faintly haematoxyphil staining and its fibrillar or whorled appearance, due to the enamel prisms. If the section cuts transversely across the prisms, the matrix appears to consist of numerous overlapping fish scale-like structures, or of tiny incomplete hexagons. In specimens that come under examination during the period of active growth ameloblastic epithelium can be seen, but in mature specimens, as in normal completed amelogenesis, this is absent (Fig. 31). Epithelial "ghost" cells, similar to those seen in the calcifying odontogenic cyst, may be present (Levy, 1973; Sedano and Pindborg, 1975; Regezi, Courtney and Kerr, 1975).

Dentine is present in relatively large quantities and generally forms the bulk of the odontome. It is usually well formed with regular tubules. In contact with the masses of dentine is connective tissue similar to normal pulp, and displaying odontoblasts. Cementum of cellular or acellular type is also present, generally in moderate quantity (Figs. 32, 33 and 34).

The qualitative normality of the ameloblastic epithelium and dentine that are present in a developing complex odontome is an important feature. Although these tissues are irregularly disposed and are likely to be quantitatively excessive in comparison with a developing normal tooth, they do not greatly differ in other respects from the normal odontogenic tissues. This

---

Fig. 31   Developing odontome in a girl of 16 years. The tumour appeared as a painless swelling, of about a year's duration, in the region of the tuberosity of the maxilla. The second and third molar teeth were absent. The tumour was excised locally and the patient was well with no recurrence 8 years later. **a,** much of the tumour consists of areas of fibroblastic connective tissue, with numerous small strands and groups of cubical or low columnar epithelial cells. × 80. **b,** in some areas the epithelial cells form structures resembling enamel organ, with an outer layer of low columnar or cubical cells enclosing a central zone of stellate cells. × 80. **c,** the epithelial cells also form small solid masses. Dentine is present in this field. × 80. **d,** a field showing a mixture of the hard dental tissues. The clear areas indicate the site of enamel prior to decalcification. Enamel matrix can be seen to the left of the largest of these areas. × 80.

ES Enamel space remaining after decalcification.   EM Enamel matrix.   D Dentine.

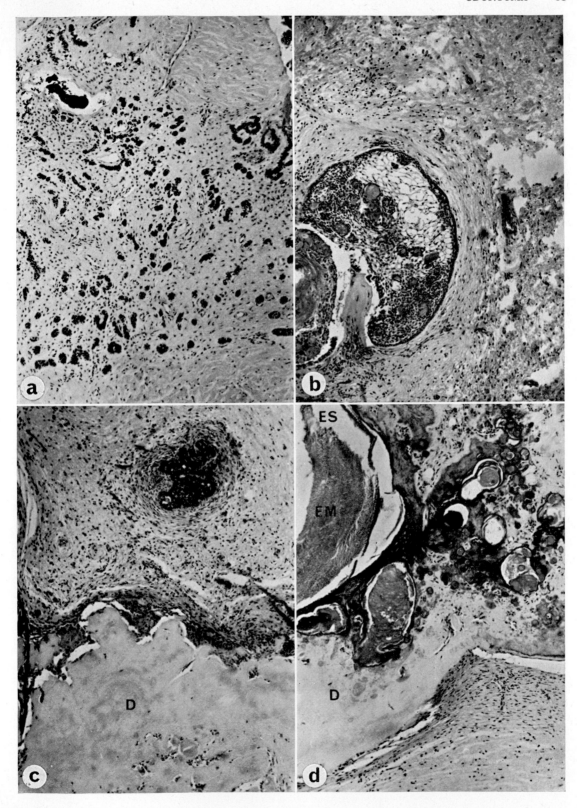

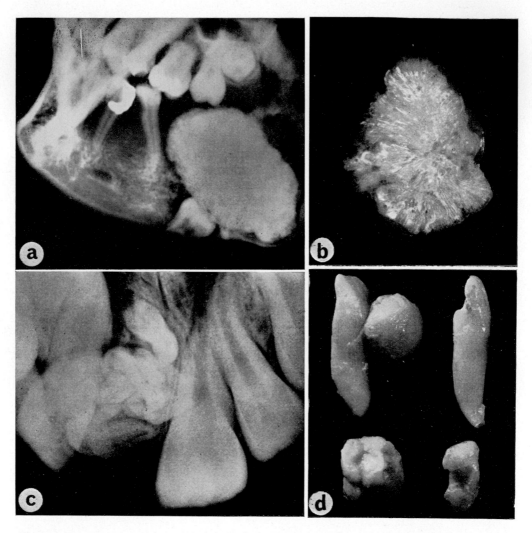

Fig. 32 **a** and **b,** complex odontome. **a,** the radiograph shows a well circumscribed ovoid area of radiopacity in the left mandibular region, composed of many irregular areas of density. **b,** the gross specimen. It was bony hard, with a smooth, slightly lobulated outer surface. The cut surface, shown here, displays a striated pattern. Some of the striae are greyish-white rather than the grey-yellow of the remainder of the lesion, and suggest enamel. Natural size. **c** and **d,** compound odontome. **c,** the radiograph shows a lesion composed of a number of small denticles. **d,** denticles from a compound odontome. × 1·5.

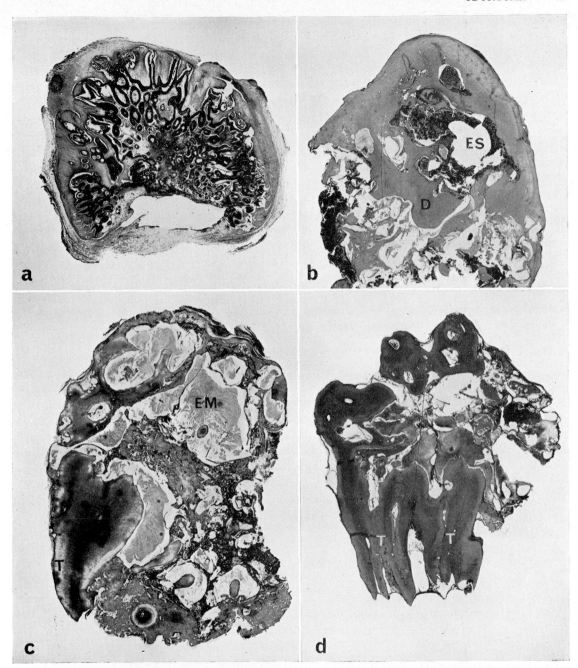

Fig. 33   A series of complex odontomes illustrating the variations in degree of organisation of the hard tissues that occur in these growths. **a,** this lesion consists of an irregular mixture of the hard and soft dental tissues. It is still growing and much developing enamel is present, seen as dark zones around the more lightly staining dentine. × 3·5. **b,** a mature lesion, in which active mineralisation has ceased. The hard tissues still form an irregular, unorganised mass. × 5·5. **c,** though most of the hard tissues in this odontome are irregularly disposed, a definite tooth-like structure has also developed. × 7. **d.** a number of tooth-like structures have been formed in this lesion. × 6·5.

ES Space remaining after mature enamel has been removed by decalcification

D Dentine   T Tooth-like structure   EM Enamel matrix

differentiates the immature complex odontome from ameloblastic fibro-odontoma, in which the enamel and dentine are accompanied by tissue resembling ameloblastic fibroma, and from odonto-ameloblastoma, in which as well as enamel and dentine there is epithelium resembling that of ameloblastoma.

The compound odontome is generally enclosed in a fibrous capsule and consists of a number of separate small teeth or denticles embedded in fibrous tissue in which there may be trabeculae of bone. The denticles vary in number from a few up to some hundreds in exceptional cases. Very often they are recognisable macroscopically as teeth, though much smaller than normal and irregular in shape, and are not identifiable as teeth of the normal series (Hitchin and Mason, 1958).

Microscopically the denticles consist of enamel, dentine, cementum and pulp arranged regularly on the whole, but showing many small divergences from the normal pattern (Fig. 34).

Ameloblastic odontoma. It seems probable that many of the lesions reported in the literature under the heading of ameloblastic odontoma have been immature complex odontomes and thus do not represent a different category of lesion. Others were probably examples of ameloblastic fibroma with dentine formation, or of odontoameloblastoma. For this reason, the category of ameloblastic odontoma has been omitted from the World Health Organization classification (Pindborg and Kramer, 1971). The cases reported under this designation have been reviewed by Olech and Alvares (1967) and subsequent reports include those of Hamner and Pizer (1968), Jacobsohn and Quinn (1968) and Worley and McKee (1972).

Behaviour

The complex and compound odontomes have a limited growth potential, even though during the active growth period quite large dimensions may be attained, as noted. Occasionally, the rate of growth during this period may be quite rapid, as in Bramley and Marsland's (1963) case.

The maturation of the odontomes from an early, chiefly cellular, stage to a final calcified state has not been objectively demonstrated by serial biopsies, since occasion for such procedures hardly ever occurs. However, Rushton (in Riddett, 1944) was able to study a lesion that occurred in a child of 22 months, in which microscopic examination of a biopsy specimen showed proliferating odontogenic epithelium as well as enamel and dentine. The lesion was not removed at the time, but some months later, when excision was carried out, no odontogenic epithelium remained and the lesion had undergone complete calcification.

OTHER LESIONS CONTAINING ENAMEL AND DENTINE

Since normal odontogenesis with its interaction of epithelial and connective tissues is a rather complicated process, it is not surprising that when abnormalities and anomalies occur,

---

Fig. 34   **a,** from the lesion shown in Fig. 33a. Most of the growth consists of dentine, but ameloblastic epithelium and developing enamel are also present. × 80. **b,** in this odontome the tissues show some evidence of organisation, with the formation of structures having some resemblance to teeth. In some of these, cut in cross-section and obliquely, can be seen a central core of pulp tissue × 30. **c,** little evidence of organised dental structures can be discerned in this specimen. Enamel dentine and cementum form a heterogeneous mixture. × 80. **d,** section of denticles from a compound odontome. These small teeth consist of the normal dental tissues, but they are irregular in shape and form. × 4.

ES Space remaining after mature enamel has been removed by decalcification
C Cementum   EM Enamel matrix   P Pulp   D Dentine

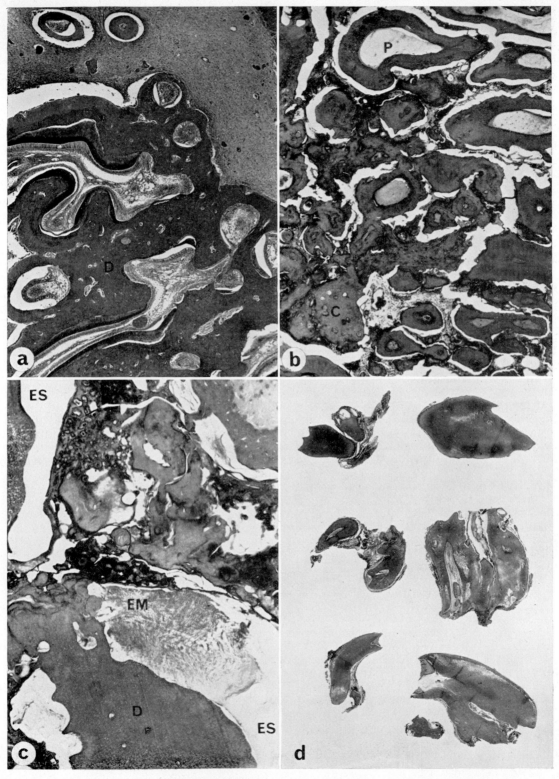

some of these should present unusual appearances. In addition to the recognised entities that have been described in this chapter, other tumours or tumour-like lesions containing enamel and dentine have been observed from time to time. Lesions in which the features of calcifying odontogenic cyst were combined with those of odontoameloblastoma, ameloblastic fibroma and complex odontoma have been observed. A tumour combining the features of adenomatoid odontogenic tumour with a cystic odontoma has been reported by Dunlap and Fritzlen (1972). Mohamed and Waterhouse (1973) have reported an atypical ameloblastic fibroma containing amyloid-like material. Eversole and colleagues (1971) give an informative discussion of the way in which the "mixed" odontogenic tumours can be related to normal odontogenesis.

REFERENCES

Bader, G. (1967) Odontomatosis (multiple odontomas). *Oral Surg.*, **23,** 770.

Bramley, P., and Marsland, E. A. (1963) An aggressive odontome of infancy. *Brit. J. oral Surg.*, **1,** 33.

Browne, W. G. (1970) Familial compound composite odontomes. *Oral Surg.*, **29,** 428.

Dunlap, C. L., and Fritzlen, T. J. (1972) Cystic odontoma with concomitant adenoameloblastoma (adeno-ameloblastic odontoma). *Oral Surg.*, **34,** 450.

Eversole, L. R., Tomich, C. E., and Cherrick, H. M. (1971) Histogenesis of odontogenic tumors. *Oral Surg.*, **32,** 569.

Gorlin, R. J., Chaudhry, A. P., and Pindborg, J. J. (1961) Odontogenic tumors. Classification, histopathology, and clinical behavior in man and domesticated animals. *Cancer*, **14,** 73.

Hamner, J. E., and Pizer, M. E. (1968) Ameloblastic odontome. Report of two cases. *Amer. J. Dis. Child.*, **115,** 332.

Hitchin, A. D., and Dekonor, E. (1963) Two cases of compound composite odontomes associated with deciduous teeth. *Brit. dent. J.*, **114,** 26.

Hitchin, A. D., and Mason, D. K. (1958) Four cases of compound composite odontomes. *Brit. dent. J.*, **104,** 269.

Jacobsohn, P. H., and Quinn, J. H. (1968) Ameloblastic odontomas. Report of three cases. *Oral Surg.*, **26,** 829.

Levy, B. A. (1973) Ghost cells and odontomes. *Oral Surg.*, **36,** 851.

Malik, S. A., and Khalid, M. (1974) Odontomatosis (multiple odontomas)—a case report. *Brit. J. oral Surg.*, **11,** 262.

Mani, N. J. (1974) Odontoma syndrome: report of an unusual case with multiple multiform odontomas of both jaws. *J. Dentistry*, **2,** 149.

Mohamed, A. H., and Waterhouse, J. P. (1973) A light and electron microscopic study of an atypical calcifying odontogenic tumor containing "amyloid." *J. oral Path.*, **2,** 150.

Noonan, R. G. (1971) A compound odontoma associated with a deciduous tooth. *Oral Surg.*, **32,** 740.

Olech, E., and Alvares, O. (1967). Ameloblastic odontoma. *Oral Surg.*, **23,** 487.

Pindborg, J. J., and Kramer, I. R. H. (1971) *International Histological Classification of Tumours, No. 5. Histological Typing of Odontogenic Tumours, Jaw Cysts, and Allied Lesions.* Geneva. World Health Organization.

Regezi, J. A., Courtney, R. M., and Kerr, D. A. (1975) Keratinization in odontogenic tumors. *Oral Surg.*, **39,** 447.

Riddett, S. A. (1944) A composite odontome at a very early age. *Brit. dent. J.*, **77,** 129.

Schmidseder, R., and Hausamen, J. E. (1975) Multiple odontogenic tumors and other anomalies. An autosomal dominantly inherited syndrome. *Oral Surg.*, **39,** 249.

Sedano, H. O., and Pindborg, J. J. (1975). Ghost cell epithelium in odontomas. *J. oral Path.*, **4,** 27.

Thompson, R. D., Hale, M. L., and McLeran, J. H. (1968) Multiple compound composite odontomas of maxilla and mandible: report of case. *J. oral Surg.*, **26,** 478.

Worley, R. D., and McKee, P. E. (1972). Ameloblastic odontoma: report of case. *J. oral Surg.*, **30,** 764.

9. Dens Invaginatus

During the course of odontogenesis a portion of the enamel organ may protrude, or invaginate, into the dental papilla. Thus, when development has been completed, the affected tooth contains a cavity that is lined by enamel. The cavity itself opens to the exterior on the surface of the tooth and the enamel that lines it is continuous with the normal enamel covering of the tooth. The presence of the enamel-lined cavity within the tooth produces a complicated appearance on section, which led the earlier investigators to believe that they were dealing with a tooth forming within a tooth, hence the synonym *dens in dente*. In some cases the invagination cavity may be of considerable size, as a result of which the whole tooth is enlarged and appears to be distended (Fig. 35). This type of appearance occasioned the synonyms *dilated odontome* and *gestant odontome*. Severe degrees of invagination of this type are, however, rare, but mild forms in which there is only a very small cavity are not uncommon. Recent investigations, such as that of Amos (1955), indicate that if all grades of invagination, mild and severe, be considered, evidence of the condition will be found in about 5 per cent of all patients examined.

Clinical Features

Since invagination is a developmental defect it is often diagnosed in children or adolescents, either on routine examination or because pulpitis and subsequent apical infection have given rise to symptoms. Pulpitis and its sequelae are in fact very common complications of invagination and from the practical standpoint are among its most significant features.

There appears to be no difference in sex incidence. In most cases there is no definite evidence of a familial incidence, though Grahnén and colleagues (1958, 1959) have shown that there may be a genetic factor concerned in cases of invagination affecting the maxillary lateral incisors.

Invagination occurs only in the teeth of the permanent dentition and in most cases the tooth affected is a maxillary lateral incisor. The central incisors or the canines may also be involved, though much less frequently, and less often still the condition occurs in the premolar or molar teeth. Invagination in mandibular teeth is much less frequent than in maxillary teeth.

The condition can occur bilaterally. Swanson and McCarthy (1947) described the first instance of such an occurrence, but it is obvious from Hallett's (1953) investigations that minor degrees of invagination occurring bilaterally are not uncommon.

Pathology

In many cases, and particularly where the invagination is of minor degree, very little alteration in the normal appearance of the tooth can be detected on naked-eye examination. The entrance to the invagination cavity will be seen on the surface, but it is often very small indeed. It may be filled with debris and in some cases caries is present. Sometimes, however, the entrance to the cavity may be very wide, being practically of the same diameter as the cavity itself.

In the more extensive forms of invagination the crown may be bulbous or conical, and where the invaginating epithelium has "ballooned" out the tooth may be considerably enlarged in diameter, particularly in its more rootward part. The roots in invaginated teeth may be normal or may be incompletely developed, with a wide apical foramen.

The general configuration to be seen on the cut surface varies considerably (Fig. 36). The invagination cavity itself may be relatively shallow or it may be so deep and extensive as to reach far into the root, and as noted previously, its formation may have caused expansion of much of the tooth. The cavity extends into the tooth as a single process in the great majority of cases, though instances of two invaginations in the same tooth have been described by Colyer (1926), Rushton (1936) and Pappo (1950). Hitchin and McHugh (1954) describe a case with three coronal invaginations and Miller's (1901) well-known specimen showed fifteen coronal invaginations.

In most cases the cavity is empty, apart from food debris which has been forced into it during mastication. Sometimes, however, a mass of bone may be found, the result of ossification in the connective tissue which once occupied the cavity. At an early stage in the development of the affected tooth, when the infolding of the enamel organ occurred, a core or pedicle of connective tissue was drawn in with the invaginating epithelium. On eruption, this connective tissue lost its connection with that of the submucosa and hence underwent necrosis. Specimens are very rarely obtained in which the core still remains, owing to its early isolation and necrosis. Rushton (1958) has described specimens of this type.

The lining of the cavity consists of enamel, and at the opening of the cavity this is continuous with the enamel that covers the exterior of the tooth. The enamel lining the cavity may form a continuous layer or it may be partially, or even largely, absent.

The pulp chamber is seen in the cut surface as a second cavity. Where the invagination is of relatively small dimensions the pulp chamber is of little less than normal size, though its coronal aspect is to some degree indented by the invagination cavity. In invagination of severe degree, however, the pulp cavity is grossly encroached upon and may be represented by a mere slit in the dentine on each side of the invagination cavity.

Though the enamel covering the exterior of the tooth is normal, that lining the invagination cavity is invariably defective owing to poor mineralisation and it may be totally absent in areas, particularly at the bottom of the cavity. Here, enamel matrix can often be seen. It is generally quite normal in appearance, as the defect in the enamel of the invagination is one of mineralisation rather than of the organic matrix. In young specimens the remains of enamel organ epithelium may also be seen.

Numerous fine channels, around which the calcification of the dentine is defective, have been observed in some cases running between the invagination and the pulp, or there may be actual cracks in the dentine, but complete communication between the invagination cavity and the pulp is very seldom seen. Nevertheless, infection of the pulp is almost invariable and the majority of specimens show the acute pulpitis, often with abscess formation, which may have drawn attention to the condition, or else by the time the tooth is removed the pulp has already been necrotic for some time. Stephens (1953) has found that despite infection there may be remarkably few symptoms. Kramer (1953) has shown in a series of teeth with minor degrees of invagination that the enamel lining the invagination cavity is almost constantly absent over a small area at the deepest part. The unprotected dentine here may well permit the access of bacteria to the underlying pulp.

Well-illustrated accounts of the gross and microscopic anatomy of invagination, in addition to those already mentioned, have been given by Shafer and Hine (1952) and Oehlers (1957). Gustafson and Sundberg (1950) also give a very full bibliography and review of the literature.

Pathogenesis

In many cases invagination represents an exaggeration of the same process that gives rise to the lingual pit. This normal anatomical feature occurs on the lingual or palatal aspect of incisor teeth and varies considerably in extent, from a barely perceptible depression to a definite cavity. Sections of developing normal incisor teeth show the infolding of the enamel organ that produces the pit, and it may be inferred that an infolding of comparable but more pronounced nature is

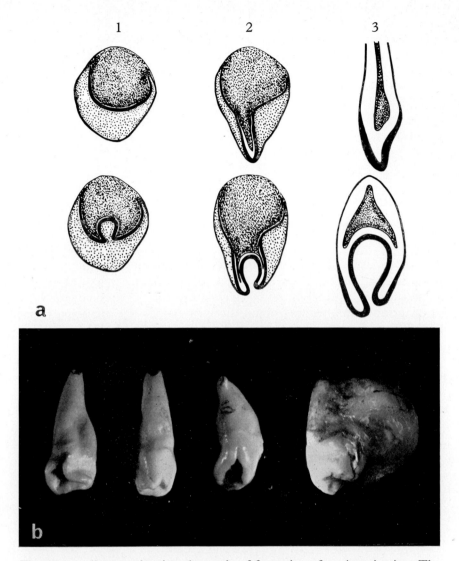

Fig. 35 **a,** diagram showing the mode of formation of an invagination. The upper row of figures represent the normal development of a tooth, from the tooth germ, 1 to the fully formed tooth, 3. The lower figures show protrusion of the enamel organ into the dental papilla at 1, which leads to the formation of a cavity lined by enamel, 2 and 3. **b,** examples of dens invaginatus. The enamel-lined cavities in the crown are shown, and the general enlargement of the tooth caused by the presence of the cavity.

responsible for invaginated teeth. As well as occurring as an exaggeration of the lingual pit invagination may occur from the region of the incisal edge of the tooth. Much less commonly, the condition may occur in the root. When this is the case it is often posterior teeth that are affected.

The mechanism of the invagination process is not clear. Kronfeld (1934), Kitchen (1935, 1949) and others have considered that a relative retardation in growth of a portion of the enamel organ occurs, with the result that this part of the enamel organ remains stationary, the remainder growing around, and more or less burying it. Gustafson and Sundberg (1950) also support this theory, believing that localised absence of ameloblasts is the cause of the retardation of growth. There are good arguments against the retardation theory, however. Thus it cannot explain the pathogenesis of the severe forms of invagination in which the entire tooth, or the greater part of it, may be expanded or dilated. Further, as Swanson and McCarthy pointed out, the enamel which lines the invagination cavity does not terminate at the level of the external enamel-cementum junction, which it would do if the invagination were due to retardation of growth.

Rushton (1936, 1937) put forward the view that the invagination was due to active proliferation of an area of enamel organ, which then grew into the dental papilla, as a sort of adenoma. Bøhn (1948), however, suggested the possibility of increased internal pressure resulting from stasis and Rushton (1958) later accepted this view in the light of his studies on unerupted specimens. These specimens showed the presence of extravascular fluid in the soft tissue that fills the potential invagination cavity of the tooth before it erupts, suggesting that there is increased venous pressure within the invagination. This could be due to pressure on the blood vessels as they pass through the entrance channel of the invagination cavity where enamel is forming concentrically and centripetally, thus tending progressively to narrow the entrance. Expansion of the invagination could then result from the increased venous pressure and transudation, though the initiation of the invagination is not explained by this theory. Rushton suggested that invagination may occur in tooth germs in which there happens to be a deep, narrow entry of the enamel organ into the dental papilla, either as the result of some disturbance of growth or slight variation of the normal pattern.

Local causes of invagination have also been suggested, for example infection of the deciduous predecessor (Fischer, 1936) or trauma (Hoepfel, 1936; Gustafson and Sundberg, 1950); but there is insufficient evidence for such views to be accepted, at any rate with regard to most cases. Pressure on the growing teeth by disproportionately small jaws has also been suggested (Atkinson, 1943). On the whole, it seems justifiable to regard invagination as one expression of a growth disturbance which may not infrequently affect a wider field, generally in the region of the premaxilla. Other expressions of the disturbance are the occurrence of supernumerary teeth and of invagination in the laterally opposite tooth.

Little is known of the pathogenesis of invagination in the root. Oehlers (1958) believes that

---

Fig. 36   **a,** ground section of a maxillary incisor tooth with a small invagination. This palatal invagination is an exaggeration of the normal lingual pit. × 4. **b,** a deep invagination from the incisal edge. Decalcified section. Some enamel matrix remains at the deepest part of the invagination cavity. × 6. **c,** transverse section of a tooth, showing the invagination cavity and the pulp chamber. × 10. **d** and **e,** ground section of a tooth with a large invagination cavity at the incisal edge, CAV 1, and a prolongation of the cavity, CAV 2, running rootwards from it. × 4·5.

E	Enamel	CAV	Invagination cavity
EM	Enamel matrix	P	Pulp

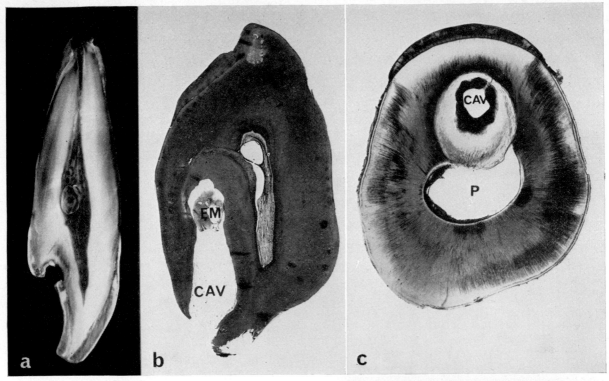

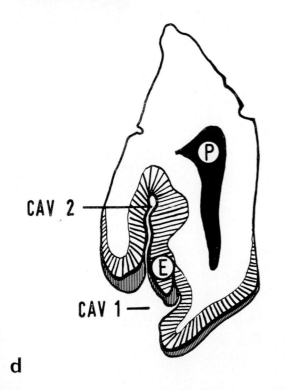

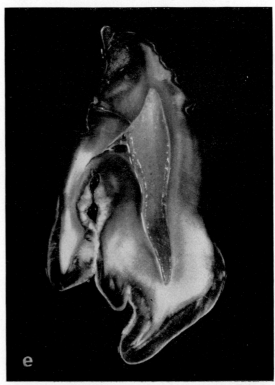

the published cases include two distinct conditions. In the first place, there are the cases of the type described by Cohen (1919) in which the invagination is merely the exaggeration of a groove that is normally present on the roots of the mandibular first premolars. An increase of depth of this groove leads to its floor being buried quite deeply. This type of invagination, if it may be so called, is of course lined by cementum. Tratman (1950) and Oehlers (1958) have found the condition to be very frequent in Chinese and Malays, and regard it as an attempt at root bifurcation.

In the other type of root invagination—and the only one that should be properly so called, according to Oehlers—the invagination cavity is lined by enamel and not by cementum. It is thought that the condition is due to the ingrowth of Hertwig's root sheath to the dental papilla, and subsequent amelogenesis by its cells. This type of invagination is rare. It is demonstrated in some of Rushton's (1937) cases and other examples have been reported by Beust and Freericks (1935), Oehlers (1948), and Bhatt and Dholakia (1975).

REFERENCES

Amos, E. R. (1955) Incidence of the small dens in dente. *J. amer. dent. Ass.*, **51**, 31.

Atkinson, S. R. (1943) The permanent maxillary lateral incisor. *Amer. J. Orthodont.*, **29**, 685.

Beust, T. B., and Freericks, F. H. (1935) Dens in dente. *J. dent. Res.*, **15**, 158.

Bhatt, A. P., and Dholakia, H. M. (1975) Radicular variety of double dens invaginatus. *Oral Surg.*, **39**, 284.

Bøhn, A. (1948) Dens in dente. *Acta odont. scand.*, **8**, 53.

Cohen, T. E. De J. (1919) A contribution to the morphogeny of the "dens in dente." *Dent. Cosmos*, **61**, 224.

Colyer, F. (1926) Abnormally-shaped teeth from the region of the premaxilla. *Proc. roy. Soc. Med. (Sect. Odont.)*, **19**, 39.

Fischer, C. H. (1936). Zur Frage des Dens in dente. *Dtsch. Zahn- Mund- u. Kieferheilk*, **3**, 621.

Grahnén, H., Lindahl, B., and Omnell, K. Å. (1958) Palatinal invaginations ("dens in dente") of the second maxillary permanent incisors. *Odont. Rev.*, **9**, 163.

Grahnén, H., Lindahl, B., and Omnell, K. Å. (1959) Dens invaginatus. I. A clinical, roentgenological and genetical study of permanent upper lateral incisors. *Odont. Rev.*, **10**, 115.

Gustafson, G., and Sundberg, S. (1950) Dens in dente. *Brit. dent. J.*, **88**, 83.

Hallett, G. E. M. (1953) The incidence, nature and clinical significance of palatal invaginations in the maxillary incisor teeth. *Proc. roy. Soc. Med.*, **46**, 491.

Hitchin, A. D., and McHugh, W. D. (1954) Three coronal invaginations in a dilated composite odontome. *Brit. dent. J.*, **97**, 90.

Hoepfel, W. (1936) Der Dens in dente. *Dtsch. Zahn- Mund- u. Kieferheilk*, **3**, 67.

Kitchen, P. C. (1935) Dens in dente. *J. dent. Res.*, **15**, 117.

Kitchen, P. C. (1949) Dens in dente. *Oral Surg.*, **2**, 1181.

Kramer, I. R. H. (1953) The pathology of pulp death in non-carious maxillary incisors with minor palatal invaginations. *Proc. roy. Soc. Med.*, **46**, 503.

Kronfeld, R. (1934) Dens in dente. *J. dent. Res.*, **14**, 49.

Miller, W. D. (1901) A study of some dental anomalies with reference to eburnitis. *Dent. Cosmos*, **43**, 845.

Oehlers, F. A. C. (1957) Dens invaginatus (dilated composite odontome). I. Variations of the invagination process and associated anterior crown forms. *Oral Surg.*, **10**, 1204. II. Associated posterior crown forms and pathogenesis. *Oral Surg.*, **10**, 1302.

Oehlers, F. A. C. (1958) The radicular variety of dens invaginatus. *Oral Surg.*, **11**, 1251.

Pappo, H. (1950) *Dens in Dente*. Paris. Julien Prélat.

Rushton, M. A. (1936) Some dilated composite odontomes. *Dent. Rec.*, **56**, 766.

Rushton, M. A. (1937) A collection of dilated composite odontomes. *Brit. dent. J.*, **63**, 65.

Rushton, M. A. (1958) Invaginated teeth (dens in dente): contents of the invagination. *Oral Surg.*, **11**, 1378.

Shafer, W. G., and Hine, M. K. (1952) Dens in dente. Reports of nine cases. *Oral Surg.*, **5,** 306.

Stephens, R. R. (1953) The diagnosis, clinical significance and treatment of minor palatal invaginations in maxillary incisors. *Proc. roy. Soc. Med.*, **46,** 499.

Swanson, W. F., and McCarthy, F. M. (1947) Bilateral dens in dente. *J. dent. Res.*, **26,** 167.

Tratman, E. K. (1950) A comparison of the teeth of people. Indo-European racial stock with the mongoloid racial stock. *Dent. Rec.*, **70,** 31, 63.

10. Enameloma and Dentinoma

ENAMELOMA

Small deposits of enamel are not infrequently found on the roots of teeth, either in continuity with the normal enamel of the crown or as quite separate masses, at some distance from the normal enamel. These deposits are termed enamelomas or enamel drops or pearls. They are thought to be the result of a disturbance during odontogenesis, which has caused a localised area of Hertwig's sheath to form enamel.

Enamelomas occur most often in maxillary permanent molar teeth, between the roots. Occasionally, they are situated near the apex. Macroscopically, they are seen as small circumscribed masses, of the same general appearance as normal enamel. Microscopically, the structure varies. In some cases the enameloma consists entirely of enamel, but there may be a small core of dentine and even a small amount of pulp tissue (Fig. 37). The lesion is described in some detail by Cavanha (1965).

DENTINOMA

The dentinoma is an odontogenic tumour consisting essentially of connective tissue and dentine, although epithelium may also be present in some cases. The first example was recorded by Straith (1936).

Clinical Features

Straith's patient was a woman of 30 with a swelling of the jaw, due to the presence of a calcified mass situated immediately above the crown of an unerupted mandibular third molar. On removal, this mass was found to consist of dentine and bone, but no enamel was present.

Subsequent cases have been of similar type. The lesion has occurred most often in the mandible and usually in association with unerupted molar teeth. The patients have generally been young adults, up to the age of 36, but examples in children have been reported (Thoma and Goldman, 1946; Hitchin and White, 1955; Azaz, Ulmansky and Lewin-Epstein, 1967). Azaz notes that in the four cases in which anterior teeth were implicated, these were deciduous teeth. In the remaining cases posterior permanent teeth were involved.

Pain is a variable feature, but when present is not severe. Swelling of the jaw is also variable. In some cases there is redness of the overlying mucosa, with discharge. In two cases in which the maxilla and maxillary sinus were involved there was nasal obstruction and discharge. On the other hand, the condition may be symptomless.

Radiologically, the usual finding is the presence of a radiopaque mass, or several small masses, over the crown of an unerupted molar tooth. This may be surrounded by a radiolucent area. In one case (Ingham, 1952), the lesion was associated with the root of a molar tooth.

Pathology

The tumour consists of a single mass, or several portions, of hard tissue surrounded by or embedded in connective tissue. In the published cases the hard tissue has been described as dentine or osteodentine, and though dentinal tubules may be seen, in most cases these have been

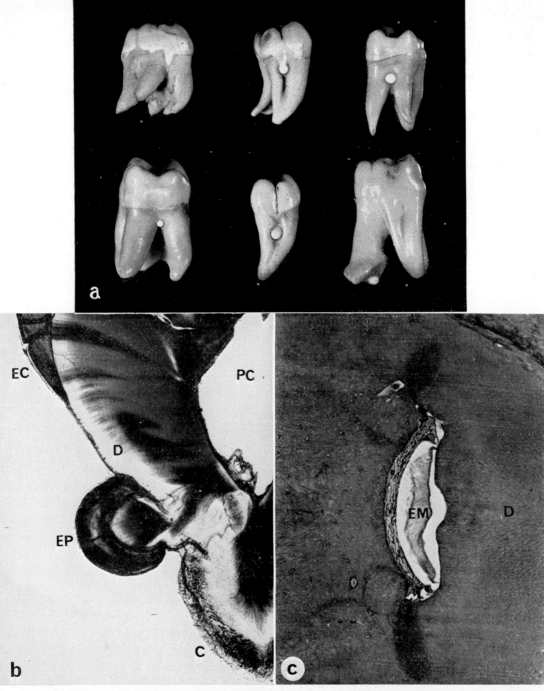

Fig. 37 Enameloma. **a,** examples of teeth with enamelomas in various situations. × 1·5. **b,** ground section showing an enameloma on the root of a tooth, just below the junction of the normal enamel of the crown and the cementum. The enameloma has a core of dentine. × 12. **c,** decalcified section of tooth with an enameloma between the roots. The mature enamel has been removed by decalcification but some enamel matrix remains. × 80.

EC	Normal enamel of the crown	C	Cementum	D	Dentine
EP	Enamel of the enameloma	PC	Pulp cavity	EM	Enamel matrix

only rudimentary or even totally absent. The characterisation of the tissue as dentine or osteo-dentine has then rested on its similarity to the osteodentine that forms in the pulp in certain circumstances. However, in Manning and Browne's (1970) case, an area of orthodentine was present. No morphologically recognisable odontoblasts are seen, though some flattened cells may be noted around the periphery and lacunae may be present in the calcified matrix. These represent cells that are entrapped as the hard tissue increases, in the same way as occurs in bone and cementum (Stafne, 1943; Sirsat, 1952). The connective tissue in which the hard tissue develops has in some cases resembled dental pulp. A thin layer of cementum on the osteodentine has sometimes been noted. Odontogenic epithelium may be present (Ingham, 1952; Pindborg, 1955) or even enamel (Stafne, 1946). The epithelium may be present as small islands of cells, or in a more extensive arrangement similar to that found in ameloblastoma.

Histogenesis

The existence of the dentinoma as an independent entity is not fully accepted. This is partly due to the fact that the identification of the hard tissue as dentine has not always been unequiv-ocal, and also because of histogenetic objections. In normal dental development odontoblasts differentiate from the cells of the dental papilla only on the inductive stimulus of the enamel epithelium and subsequently enamel itself is not laid down until dentine has been deposited. Hence it can be argued that dentine cannot occur alone; that odontogenic epithelium must be present, or have been present, to induce its formation. In some of the reported cases, as noted, odontogenic epithelium and even enamel have been seen and Pindborg suggests that epithelium must in fact have been present in all lesions that subsequently appear to be composed only of den-tine. In these cases, he postulates, the epithelium originally present has subsequently degener-ated. Thus the lesion may be considered as really a type of odontome rather than a pure growth of one dental tissue. Gorlin, Chaudhry and Pindborg (1961) refer to lesions in which epithelium is present as immature dentinomas. They consider that these lesions are essentially ameloblastic fibromas in which further inductive action on the mesenchyme by the epithelium has resulted in the production of dentine or osteodentine. The lesions in which no epithelium is present are referred to as mature dentinomas.

Behaviour

Dentinomas have recurred in some cases where removal was incomplete, but adequate local excision is curative.

REFERENCES

Azaz, B., Ulmansky, M., and Lewin-Epstein, J. (1967) Dentinoma. Report of a case. *Oral Surg.*, **24,** 659.
Cavanha, A. O. (1965) Enamel pearls. *Oral Surg.*, **19,** 373.
Gorlin, R. J., Chaudhry, A. P., and Pindborg, J. J. (1961) Odontogenic tumors. Classification, histo-pathology, and clinical behavior in man and domesticated animals. *Cancer*, **14,** 73.
Hitchin, A. D., and White, J. W. (1955) A dentinoma related to the deciduous dentition. *Brit. dent. J.*, **98,** 163.
Ingham, G. G. (1952) Detinoma. *Oral Surg.*, **5,** 353.
Manning, G. L., and Browne, R. M. (1970) Dentinoma. *Brit. dent. J.*, **128,** 178.
Pindborg, J. J. (1955) On dentinomas. With report of a case. *Acta path. microbiol. scand.*, Suppl. 105, 135.
Sirsat, M. V. (1952) Odontogenic tumors. *Ind. J. med. Res.*, **40,** 555.
Stafne, E. C. (1943) Dentinoma. Report of two cases. *Amer. J. Orthodont. (Oral Surg. Sect.)*, **29,** 156.
Stafne, E. C. (1946) Dentinoma: report of a case. *J. oral Surg.*, **4,** 145.
Straith, F. E. (1936) Odontoma: a rare type: report of a case. *Dent. Digest*, **42,** 196.
Thoma, K. H., and Goldman, H. M. (1946) Odontogenic tumors. A classification based on observations of the epithelial, mesenchymal, and mixed varieties. *Amer. J. Path.*, **22,** 433.

11. Hypercementosis and Cementoma

Overgrowth of cementum occurs in response to a variety of stimuli, some of known nature, like infection, others unknown. The morphological appearances of the proliferated cementum also vary, and terms such as cementosis or hypercementosis, cementoma, cementifying fibroma, periapical fibrous dysplasia and others have been used.

HYPERCEMENTOSIS

Cementum is normally deposited on the roots of the teeth continuously throughout life, and thus in later years the layer of cementum around the tooth roots is thicker than in younger persons. This is a necessary physiological process, for the elongation of the tooth that results from the additional cementum at the apex helps to compensate for the loss of dental substance at the occlusal end of the tooth, due to normal wear. Deposition of cementum in excess of this physiological amount constitutes hypercementosis.

In some cases, hypercementosis is a reaction to chronic periapical inflammation and here the excessive cementum often forms a more or less uniformly thick layer ensheathing the root (Fig. 38). Hypercementosis may also affect teeth that are not in function and here again the excessive tissue may be deposited uniformly around the root, or it may be irregularly deposited in separate areas. Localised spikes or spurs of cementum may form as a reaction to increased stress, their function being to provide an increased area for the attachment of periodontal fibres. Hypercementosis may also occur for unknown reasons. An important, though uncommon, cause of hypercementosis is Paget's disease.

Hypercementosis is symptomless, apart from the difficulty in extraction which may result when a great excess of tissue has been deposited, as in some cases of Paget's disease. Localised hypercementoses of the spur or spike type and mild degrees of hypercementosis affecting the root diffusely produce little detectable change on naked-eye examination. Moderate degrees of hypercementosis lead to increased thickness of the root, sometimes affecting its whole length or perhaps localised to the region of the apex. In marked hypercementosis the root is buried in a mass of cementum and this may have ankylosed with the alveolar bone.

Spurs or prongs of cementum may occur singly or in a series, growing out from the side of the tooth. This is the type of hypercementosis that results from increased functional stress, the outgrowths giving additional attachment to the periodontal fibres and thus being analogous to the exotoses that may form at muscle insertions under conditions of increased stress.

The more diffuse types of hypercementosis appear as in Fig. 38. Here, the thick layers of the additional tissue are seen to line the root quite uniformly. Prominent resting lines are seen between successive layers.

CEMENTICLES

Cementicles are small calcified bodies that form in the periodontal ligament, sometimes singly, sometimes in numbers. Probably the foci around which calcification occurs are in many cases degenerating epithelial cells; such cells are normally present in the periodontal ligament

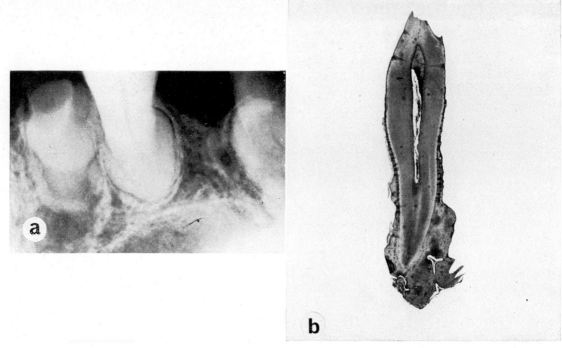

Fig. 38   Hypercementosis. **a,** the radiograph shows thickening of the roots of the teeth, with blunting and rounding of the apices. **b,** longitudinal section of a tooth, showing excessive cementum around the root. ×3.

as epithelial rests. In other cases small splinters of cementum or alveolar bone, detached as a result of trauma from the root of the tooth or the alveolar wall, may become cementicle-like bodies, and there is also evidence to show that cementicles may develop from calcified thrombosed capillaries in the periodontal ligament (Mikola and Bauer, 1949). With continued deposition of calcium salts the cementicles gradually increase in size and this, together with the increase of cementum around the root of the tooth itself, may in time bring the cementicles into contact with the root cementum, in which they gradually become incorporated. Alternatively, cementicles may reach and become included in the alveolar bone (Fig. 39).

Cementicles are symptomless. They are generally detected only when large enough to be demonstrable radiographically. The overwhelming majority of these small bodies, however, do not reach such dimensions.

CEMENTOMA

The dividing line between hypercementosis and cementoma is not always clear. Generally, however, the latter term is used when the excessive tissue forms a more or less circumscribed

Fig. 39   Hypercementosis. **a,** longitudinal section of tooth, showing excessive deposition of cementum commencing abruptly just below the enamel-cementum junction. The successive layers are clearly demarcated. × 30. **b,** longitudinal section of tooth, showing a moderate degree of hypercementosis in the region of the apex. × 30. **c,** transverse section of tooth *in situ* in the alveolus. Two cementicles are seen in the periodontal ligament. × 30. **d,** higher magnification of one of the cementicles shown in **c.** The concentric layers of successive depositions of cementum are evident. × 200. **e,** cementicles forming in epithelial rests in the periodontal ligament. × 500.

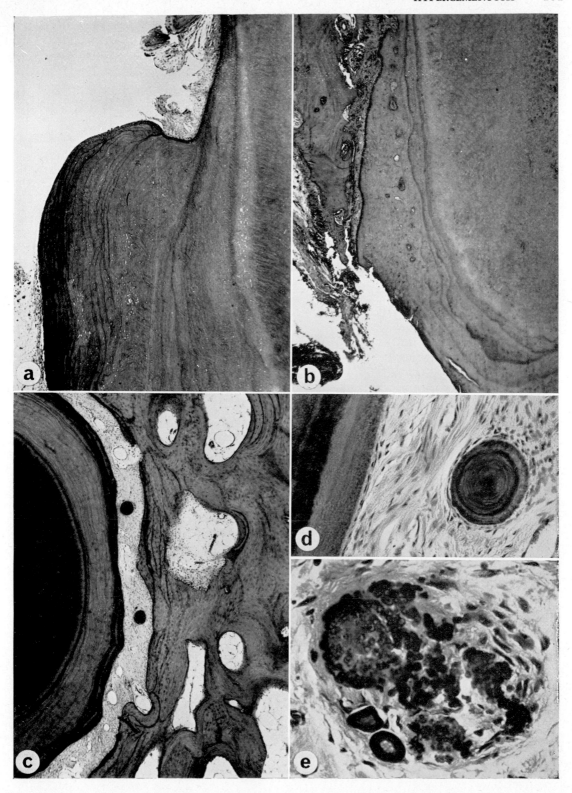

tumour-like mass at the apex of a tooth. The cemental mass may be separated from the apex by a zone of connective tissue, or it may form around the apex.

Lesions conforming in general to the above description and described as cementomas are at present placed in four categories in the World Health Organization Classification (Pindborg and Kramer, 1971). Since some of the lesions are rare, and others that would seem to come into the general category of cementoma do not readily correspond with any of the groups, it is likely that revision will be required as further experience is gained.

Cementoblastoma (benign cementoblastoma; true cementoma). The published cases of this distinctive lesion have been reviewed by Eversole and colleagues (1973) and Cherrick and colleagues (1974), and there are subsequent reports from Astacio and Méndez (1974) and Abrams and colleagues (1974). Although not common, it is probable that the tumour occurs much more frequently than the paucity of recorded cases would seem to indicate.

Males are more often affected than females and although the oldest recorded patient was aged 63, most are less than 25 years of age. The youngest patient observed so far was 12 years of age. The tumour nearly always occurs in connection with a premolar or molar tooth, more commonly in the mandible than in the maxilla. It grows slowly, forming a bulbous swelling around a root or roots of the tooth and in the course of time expands the jaw. Some patients complain of pain, but the lesion is often symptomless. Radiologically, there is a well defined radiopacity involving a root, often with a narrow surrounding radiolucent zone. The tumour can be readily enucleated, and can frequently be removed complete with the affected tooth (Fig. 40). When the specimen is bisected, the continuity of tumour tissue with the tooth root, which is nearly always partially resorbed, can often be seen with the naked eye. This is confirmed by microscopic examination, which shows the tumour to consist of a mass of calcified cementum-like tissue which has numerous deeply stained reversal lines. Small areas of vascular connective tissue are generally present here and there throughout the mass of calcified tissue, and these may contain osteoclast or osteoblast-like cells. It is these cells, entrapped in the calcifying mass as deposition proceeds, that are seen in the lacunae that are scattered throughout the tissue. Towards the periphery and elsewhere, if the tumour is still actively growing, there is a zone of uncalcified tissue. Here there are no reversal lines. When seen entire, with its related tooth, the cementoblastoma has a strikingly characteristic appearance. When small fragments only are available for microscopic examination, a purely histological diagnosis may be difficult. It should be noted that in actively growing areas the osteoblast-like cells are large and stain deeply and they may be numerous. Occasional cells may show some nuclear pleomorphism, but mitoses are absent (Fig. 41).

The general appearance of the lesion, apart from the relationship to the teeth, is very similar to that of osteoid osteoma or osteoblastoma, and some authors have raised the question as to whether the tumour tissue is indeed cementum rather than bone. There is some reason to believe that cementum is characterised by fine fibrillar birefringence (Giansanti, 1970), but neither Eversole nor Abrams and their associates were able to demonstrate this in substantial amount in their cementoblastomas. Thus the hard tissue of the cementoblastoma might appear more like osteoid. Although the distinction between bone and cementum, other than the topographical one

---

Fig. 40 Cementoblastoma. **a,** the radiograph shows a well defined radiopacity at the tooth root, with a radiolucent border distinguishable in some areas. **b,** the tumour, consisting of a mass of cementum, is attached to the tooth root. × 4. **c,** the actively growing edge of the tumour. The freshly deposited cementoid tissue stains palely, the older, mineralizing tissue is darker. Numerous cementoblasts are present. × 120. **d,** the main mass of the tumour consists of hard tissue with a few entrapped cells, and shows well marked reversal lines. × 120.

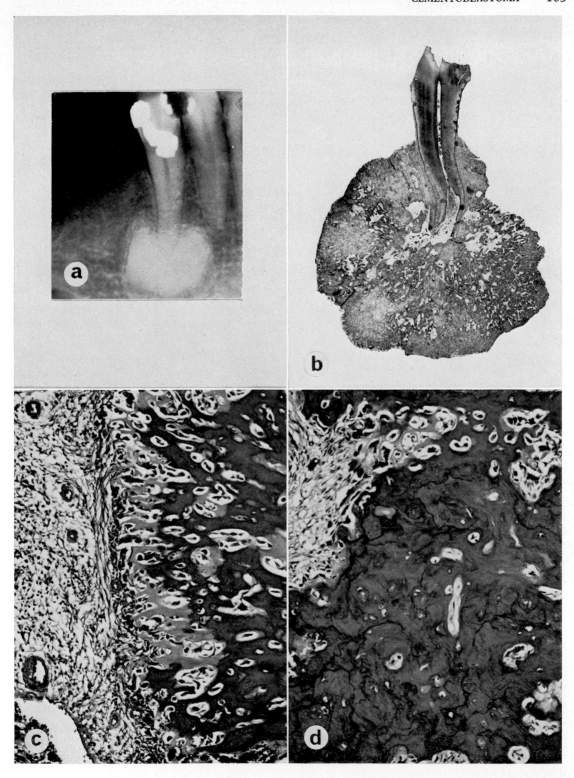

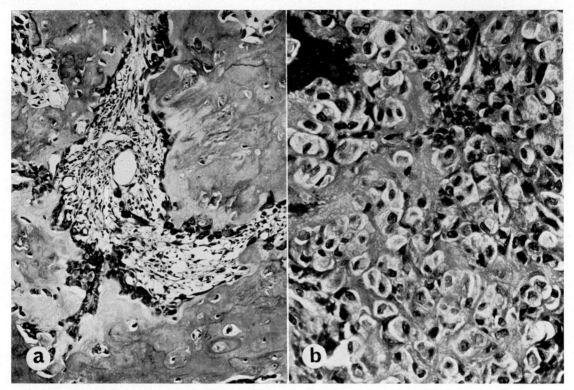

Fig. 41   **a, b,** areas from two cementoblastomas, showing the degree of cellularity that can occur where active growth is proceeding. × 120 and × 300.

of relationship to the roots of teeth, still remains ill-defined, most authors are agreed that because of its characteristic relationship to the teeth, the cementoblastoma is correctly designated.

Cementoblastoma is a benign lesion. Enucleation is sufficient treatment.

Gigantiform Cementoma. This variety of cementoma, like the cementoblastoma, is a distinctive lesion. In its most characteristic form there are multiple growths, symmetrically distributed in the jaws, but single lesions may also occur. Females are more often affected than males. Negroes appear to be more susceptible than Caucasians and there may be a familial incidence. Agazzi and Belloni (1953) have reported lesions occurring in four brothers of the same Italian family. Most patients are adults, commonly about middle age, and the usual complaint is of a painless, slowly increasing swelling or swellings in the jaws. If the lesion or lesions remain untreated, considerable deformity may ensue. Radiologically, the tumour presents as a dense lobulated radiopacity, lacking the surrounding zone of radiolucency that is seen in cemento-blastoma. Microscopically, the gigantiform cementoma consists of dense irregular or lobulated masses of highly calcified and practically acellular cementum, although many empty lacunae are present. This tissue may be continuous with the normal cementum of the root of the tooth. Some connective tissue may remain in interstices between the calcified material, but frequently such spaces contain only necrotic material (Fig. 42).

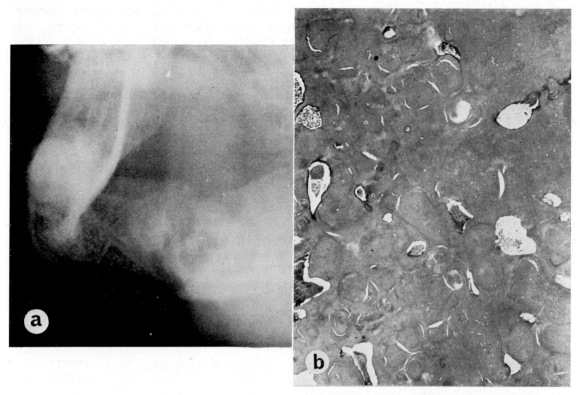

Fig. 42   Gigantiform cementoma. **a,** the radiograph shows irregular areas of radiopacity with a tendency to lobulation. There is no radiolucent border. **b,** the lesion consists of a dense mass of acellular cementum. Numerous empty lacunae are present. × 120.

Although the gigantiform cementoma can grow to large proportions, it is a benign lesion and may well be a dysplasia or hamartomatous condition rather than neoplastic, as is suggested by the multiple incidence and symmetrical distribution of the lesions in the jaws.

Periapical Cemental Dysplasia and Cementifying Fibroma. These members of the cementoma group share many features in common; the distinction between them is largely one of location, number and sex incidence. Both lesions occur in patients of middle age and over, and especially in the mandible. In periapical cemental dysplasia the lesions—they are multiple in the majority of patients—occur at the apices of the mandibular incisor teeth, in women much more commonly than in men. The condition is generally symptomless, and it has been thought that the predominance of females might indicate a causal hormonal disturbance (Zegarelli and Ziskin, 1943). However, Fontaine (1955) and others have been unable to find any evidence of this, or of the operation of any other systemic factors. Nor can local causes such as chronic inflammation or trauma be implicated, and the cause remains unknown.

The condition is usually detected on radiological examination, and Stafne (1934) and Bernier and Thompson (1946) have described the evolution of the lesion. The initial stage seems to be

REFERENCES

Abrams, A. M., Kirby, J. W., and Melrose, R. J. (1974) Cementoblastoma. A clinico-pathologic study of seven new cases. *Oral Surg.*, **38**, 394.

Agazzi, C., and Belloni, L. (1953) Gli odontomi duri dei mascellari. Contributo clinico-rôntgenologico e anatomo-microscopico con particolare riguardo alle forme ad ampia estensione e alla comparsa familiare. *Arch. ital. Otol.*, Suppl. 16, 1.

Astacio, J. N., and Méndez, J. E. (1974) Benign cementoblastoma (true cementoma). *Oral Surg.*, **38**, 95.

Bhaskar, S. N., and Cutright, D. E. (1968) Multiple enostosis: report of 16 cases. *J. oral Surg.*, **26**, 321.

Bernier, J. L., and Thompson, H. C. (1946) The histogenesis of the cementoma. Report of 15 cases. *Amer. J. Orthodont. (Oral Surg. Sect.)*, **32**, 543.

Cherrick, H. M., King, O. H., Lucatorto, F. M., and Suggs, D. M. (1974) Benign cementoblastoma. A clinicopathologic evaluation. *Oral Surg.*, **37**, 54.

Eversole, L. R., Sabes, W. R., and Dauchess, V. G. (1973) Benign cementoblastoma. *Oral Surg.*, **36**, 824.

Fontaine, J. (1955) Periapical fibro-osteoma or cementoma. *J. canad. dent. Ass.*, **21**, 10.

Giansanti, J. S. (1970) The pattern and width of the collagen bundles in bone and cementum. *Oral Surg.*, **30**, 508.

Mikola, O. J., and Bauer, W. H. (1949) "Cementicles" and fragments of cementum in the periodontal membrane. *Oral Surg.*, **2**, 1063.

Pindborg, J. J., and Kramer, I. R. H. (1971) *International Histological Classification of Tumours, No. 5. Histological Typing of Odontogenic Tumours, Jaws, Cysts, and Allied Lesions*. Geneva. World Health Organization.

Stafne, E. C. (1934). Periapical osteofibrosis with formation of cementoma. *J. amer. dent. Ass.*, **21**, 1822.

Waldron, C. A., Giansanti, J. S., and Browand, B. C. (1975) Sclerotic cemental masses of the jaws (so-called chronic sclerosing osteomyelitis, sclerosing osteitis, multiple enostosis, and gigantiform cementoma). *Oral Surg.*, **39**, 590.

Zegarelli, E. V., and Ziskin, D. E. (1943) Cementomas. A report of 50 cases. *Amer. J. Orthodont, (Oral Surg. Sect.)*, **29**, 285.

IV

TUMOURS OF DEBATABLE DENTAL ORIGIN

12. Pigmented Tumour of the Jaw of Infants

This tumour of rather obscure nature occurs exclusively in infants and, although in most cases the lesion is situated in the jaws, similar tumours have been reported in extraoral situations.

Clinical Features

The lesion occurs in infants under 12 months old, the usual age being between 1 and 3 months. The sexes are equally affected. The maxilla is affected much more often than the mandible, the tumour forming a mass that expands the bone, apparently without pain or tenderness. The rate of growth is variable, in some cases the lesion having grown to quite a large size fairly rapidly, while in others it has been described as of slow growth. Radiologically, there may be a well defined area of translucency suggesting a cyst but often the margins of the area of bone destruction are irregular, giving the impression of an invasive tumour. The developing teeth are often displaced.

Pathology

The tumour generally separates quite readily from the bone though it is unencapsulated or has only a partial fibrous capsule. The cut surface has a characteristic slate-blue to greyish-black appearance, perhaps with greyish-white streaks. Multiple tumour nodules have been reported in two cases. In one of these, three adjacent teeth were involved by apparently separate and distinct tumour nodules (Jones and Williams, 1960) and in the other, two separate maxillary tumours were associated with three teeth (Pontius, Dziabis and Foster, 1965). The possibility that seemingly separate tumour nodules are in fact offshoots from the main mass cannot, however, be excluded.

Microscopically, the tumour consists of both pigmented and non-pigmented cells in a plentiful connective tissue stroma. The pigmented cells are cubical or rather flattened and have large, pale nuclei. The cytoplasm contains melanin in the form of minute rod-shaped particles, often aggregated into large masses that obscure all internal cellular detail. These pigmented cells are arranged in solid groups, or form the lining of small cleft-like spaces. The unpigmented cells are small and round, and contain a well-stained nucleus that nearly fills the cell body. They occur in groups, often within the spaces lined by the pigmented cells. In some groups there is very little intercellular material but in others there is a fine fibrillar matrix.

Small groups of spindle-shaped cells with hyperchromatic and elongated nuclei may also be seen, scattered among the round unpigmented cells (Fig. 44).

There may be a well marked osteoblastic reaction to the tumour (Williams, 1967; Ostrander and Hayward, 1974).

Fig. 44 Tumour of the maxillary incisor region in a female infant of 6 months. **a,** general view of the tumour, showing groups of pigmented cells, sometimes enclosing small cleft-like spaces, in a fibrous stroma. × 80. **b,** the spaces may contain groups of small unpigmented cells. × 80. **c,** higher magnification of a group of unpigmented cells, showing the intercellular fibrillary matrix. × 500. **d,** higher magnification of pigmented cells. The pigment is so plentiful as to obscure cellular detail. It is composed of aggregates of minute rod-shaped particles. × 500.

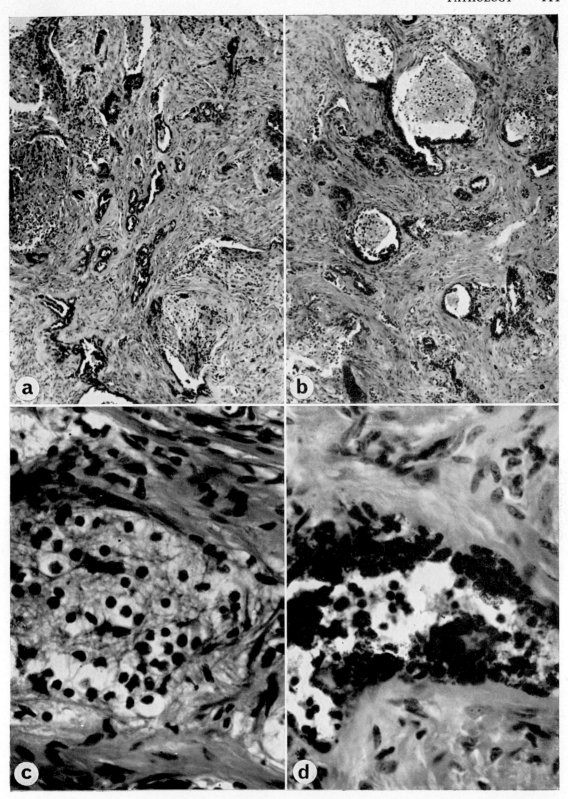

Histogenesis

Krompecher (1918) published the first report of this tumour under the designation of congenital melanocarcinoma. Dudits and Szabó (1935), Soderberg and Padgett (1941) and Notter and Söderberg (1953) also regarded their cases as melanocarcinomas or melanomas, derived from odontogenic epithelium or from epithelial rests enclaved in the process of fusion of the maxillary processes. More recently Stokke (1968) has revived this view, designating the tumour as a melanocytoma. He does not believe it to originate from odontogenic epithelium. However, it is clear that the tumour is benign.

Mummery and Pitts (1926) were the first to regard the tumour as a type of epithelial odontome and a number of subsequent authors also reported cases as variants of ameloblastoma (melanotic adamantinoma, Wass (1948); pigmented adamantinoma, Battle, Hovell and Spencer (1952); pigmented ameloblastoma, Tiecke and Bernier (1956)). This view of the origin of the tumour derives from its anatomical relationship to the tooth-bearing tissues and from the fact that in a few cases tumour tissue was found to be closely related to developing teeth, and even connected with the dental tissues, as Mummery and Pitts, Willis (1958) and Mitchell and Read (1960) have shown. Nevertheless, the histological picture bears little resemblance to odontogenic tissue, so that there are difficulties in accepting the lesion as a derivative of that tissue, and the possibility remains that the connections between tumour tissue and developing teeth are of the same fortuitous nature as, for example, may be connections between ameloblastoma and the epithelium of the overlying mucous membrane. In any event, for reasons of structure and particularly of behaviour, the tumour cannot be considered as simply a variant of the ordinary type of ameloblastoma.

The retinal anlage theory was put forward by Halpert and Patzer (1947), who suggested that the tumour was derived from retinal elements that had been misplaced in the course of development. These authors pointed out that the cleft-like spaces lined by pigmented cells sometimes contained infoldings resembling the ciliary processes of the eye and that the smaller unpigmented cells resembled those seen in the nuclear layers of the retina or the cells in neuroblastomas. MacDonald and White (1954) noted that the pigment granules in the cuboidal cells showed the characteristic bacillary morphology of retinal pigment and that there was some similarity between the tumour and the embryonic eye at an early stage when the retina is still composed of neuroblasts, and later when the optic cup has formed. They considered the small round cells to be neuroblasts, with the fibrillar intercellular material representing glial fibres. Martin and Foote (1951) thought that not all the cells of the stroma were fibroblastic. Some they considered to be transitions from the pigmented cells towards smooth muscle, possibly representing ciliary muscle. Other authors who have reported their cases as retinal anlage tumours include Shafer and Frissell (1953), Caldwell, Ernst and Thompson (1955) and Lucas (1957).

Yet another theory has been put forward by Stowens (1957), who derives the tumour from Jacobson's vomeronasal organ or from misplaced sensory neuroectoderm. He considers that the spindle cells are bipolar neurones and that the other cells may correspond to the cells in olfactory epithelium. Lurie (1961), who reported the only case so far noted in an adult, supports Stowen's neuroectodermal theory.

Willis (1958) has re-examined the theories of origin and concludes that the retinal anlage hypothesis is very improbable, both on embryological grounds and because the use of nervous tissue stains does not give a positive result with those elements of the tumour that have been described as neural in type. Henry and Bodian (1960) have also failed to demonstrate neural elements by specific staining. Willis further points to the fact that melanin-containing cells have been found in odontogenic epithelium (Mitchell and Read, 1960), and such cells have also been found in ameloblastoma (Hodson, 1961; Lurie, 1961). Willis has also demonstrated a connection between tooth germs and tumour tissue and concludes that the tumour is derived from dental epithelium.

The occurrence of tumours that appear to be similar to that of the jaw, but arising in extra-oral situations, adds to the histogenetic difficulties. In Clarke and Parsons' (1951) case the tumour arose in the soft tissues over the anterior fontanelle in an infant of 5 months of age, and grew rapidly. Structurally, it resembled the jaw tumours. Kuhn, Cabanne and Garneau's (1954) case was similar, and the illustrations in this paper in particular show a very close resemblance to the jaw tumour. In both cases, the authors postulate an origin from retinal tissue. Ashley (1964) and Best (1972) have also reported identical tumours in the skull and a possible similar example has been found in the cerebellum (Fowler and Simpson, 1962). A brain tumour has also been reported by Stowens and Lin (1974).

Eaton and Ferguson (1956) reported a pigmented tumour of the epididymis in a 5 month old infant. They considered it to be similar to the jaw tumours and thought that it might possibly represent a one-sided development of a teratoma arising from a totipotent cell rest. They note that pigmented embryonic ocular tissue has been found occasionally in testicular teratomas. Frank and Koten (1967) have also reported a tumour of the epididymis which appears identical to the jaw tumours. A pigmented tumour of the uterus has been reported by Schulz (1957). Though the author describes the tumour as resembling the "retinal anlage" tumours, his patient was a woman aged 69 years and metastases were found in the liver, adrenal and lymph nodes. Moreover, the illustrations do not suggest a close resemblance to the tumour of the jaw. A pigmented tumour associated with dental elements in an ovarian dermoid cyst in a $8\frac{1}{2}$ year old girl has been reported by Sinniah and O'Brien (1973). The authors consider the lesion to be similar to the jaw tumour, and support an odontogenic origin for the entity. However, their illustrations are not conclusive. An ovarian tumour in a woman of 64, somewhat similar to the jaw tumours, has been reported by Hameed and Burslem (1970), who think that it may represent a teratoma with particular development of melanogenic tissue. Blanc, Rosenblatt and Wolff (1958) reported a melanotic progonoma (retinal anlage tumour) in the subcutaneous tissue of the deltoid region of an infant aged 5 months, and Lurie and Isaacson (1961) report a tumour of the scapular region in a child of 4 years of age. This tumour contained ciliated columnar epithelium, which has not previously been reported in these growths, and again there must be some doubt as to whether this lesion is the same as those of the jaws.

Recently, Misugi and colleagues (1965) suggested, on the basis of ultrastructural studies of a tumour from the posterior mediastinum, that the growth is derived from the neural crest. They showed that the pigment-containing cells did not exhibit any definite characteristics of retinal pigment epithelium but had instead a structure consistent with melanocytes and melanoma cells. The small non-pigmented cells were probably neuroblasts. Hayward, Fickling and Lucas (1969) studied the ultrastructure of a typical maxillary tumour and concurred with Misugi's findings.

Biochemical and histochemical investigations also support the possibility of neural crest origin. Borello and Gorlin (1966) have demonstrated a high urinary level of vanilmandelic acid in an infant with a typical maxillary tumour, which returned to normal after removal of the growth. Vanilmandelic acid (3-methoxy, 4-hydroxymandelic acid) is a product of catecholamine metabolism and high levels in the urine have hitherto been found only in patients with tumours of neural crest derivation—phaeochromocytoma, ganglioneuroblastoma, neuroblastoma and retinoblastoma. Furthermore, Koudstaal and colleagues (1968) have demonstrated in a tumour of the temporal bone and in a maxillary tumour an enzyme pattern similar to that of tumours thought to be of neural crest origin. Thus there is a variety of evidence pointing towards a neural crest origin for the pigmented tumour of the jaws of infants, although of course much more positive proof will be required before the matter can be regarded as finally settled.

Lurie (1961) discusses the various theories of histogenesis in detail and gives the literature. Borello and Gorlin (1966) also give a very full account of the literature.

Behaviour

The tumour is benign, simple excision effecting a cure. However, untreated growths may reach large dimensions, as exemplified by Williams's (1967) case in which the tumour reached dimensions of $7 \times 3 \times 5$ cm, weighing 80 g. In Stokke's (1968) case, the tumour weighed 160 g and proved fatal because its extent precluded adequate treatment.

REFERENCES

Ashley, D. J. B. (1964) Melanotic "adamantinoma" of the skull. *J. Path. Bact.*, **87**, 179.

Battle, R. J. V., Hovell, J. H., and Spencer, H. (1952) Pigmented adamantinomata. *Brit. J. Surg.*, **39**, 368.

Best, P. V. (1972) Pigmented tumour arising in the skull of an infant. *J. Path.*, **107**, 69.

Blanc, W. A., Rosenblatt, P., and Wolff, J. A. (1958) Melanotic progonoma ("retinal anlage" tumor) of shoulder in an infant. A case report. *Cancer*, **11**, 959.

Borello, E. D., and Gorlin, R. J. (1966) Melanotic neuroectodermal tumor of infancy; a neoplasm of neural crest origin. *Cancer*, **19**, 196.

Caldwell, J. B., Ernst, K. F., and Thompson, H. C. (1955) Retinal anlage tumor of the maxilla. *Oral Surg.*, **8**, 796.

Clarke, B. E., and Parsons, H. (1951) An embryological tumor of retinal anlage involving the skull. *Cancer*, **4**, 78.

Dudits, A., and Szabó, B. (1935) Kongenitales Melanokarzinom des Oberkiefers. *Mschr. Kinderheilk.*, **63**, 294.

Eaton, W. L., and Ferguson, J. P. (1956) A retinoblastic teratoma of the epididymis. Case report. *Cancer*, **9**, 718.

Fowler, M., and Simpson, D. A. (1962) A malignant melanin-forming tumour of the cerebellum. *J. Path. Bact.*, **84**, 307.

Frank, G. L., and Koten, J. W. (1967) Melanotic hamartoma ("retinal anlage tumour") of the epididymis. *J. Path. Bact.*, **93**, 549.

Halpert, B., and Patzer, R. (1947) Maxillary tumor of retinal anlage. *Surgery*, **22**, 837.

Hameed, K., and Burslem, M. R. G. (1970) A melanotic ovarian neoplasm resembling the "retinal anlage" tumor. *Cancer*, **25**, 564.

Hayward, A. F., Fickling, B. W., and Lucas, R. B. (1969) An electron microscope study of a pigmented tumour of the jaw of infants. *Brit. J. Cancer*, **23**, 702.

Henry, T. C., and Bodian, M. (1960) A case of pigmented congenital epulis. *Brit. J. Surg.*, **47**, 547.

Hodson, J. J. (1961) An intra-osseous tumour combination of biological importance—invasion of a melanotic schwannoma by an adamantinoma. *J. Path. Bact.*, **82**, 257.

Hodson, J. J. (1961) A morphological study of dermal melanocytes and cytocrine activity in relation to certain Schwann cells and epithelial cells. *J. Path. Bact.*, **82**, 267.

Jones, P., and Williams, A. (1960) A case of multicentric melanotic adamantinoma. *Brit. J. Surg.*, **48**, 282.

Koudstaal, J., Oldhoff, J., Panders, A. K., and Hardonk, M. J. (1968) Melanotic neuroectodermal tumor of infancy. *Cancer*, **22**, 151.

Krompecher, E. (1918) Zur Histogenese und Morphologie der Adamantinome und sonstiger Kiefergeschwülste. *Beitr. path. Anat.*, **64**, 165.

Kuhn, R., Cabanne, F., and Garneau, R. (1954) Le rétinoblastome pigmentaire hétérotopique. Rapport d'un cas et étude générale. *Sem. Hôp. Paris (Arch. Anat. path.)*, **30**, A.178.

Lucas, R. B. (1957) Retinal anlage tumour of the maxilla. *Brit. J. Cancer*, **11**, 26.

Lurie, H. I. (1961) Congenital melanocarcinoma, melanotic adamantinoma, retinal anlage tumor, progonoma, and pigmented epulis of infancy. Summary and review of the literature and report of the first case in an adult. *Cancer*, **14**, 1090.

Lurie, H. I., and Isaacson, C. (1961) A melanotic progonoma in the scapula region. *Cancer*, **14**, 1088.

MacDonald, A. M., and White, M. (1954) Pigmented congenital epulides of neuro-epithelial origin. The description of a further case with successful excision and survival. *Brit. J. Surg.*, **41**, 610.

Martin, H., and Foote, F. W. (1951) A third case of so-called retinal anlage tumor. *Cancer*, **4,** 86.

Misugi, K., Okajima, H., Newton, W. A., Kmetz, D. R., and deLorimier, A. A. (1965) Mediastinal origin of a melanotic progonoma or retinal anlage tumor. Ultrastructural evidence for neural crest origin. *Cancer*, **18,** 477.

Mitchell, W. M., and Read, T. T. (1960) Congenital pigmented epulis in a three-month infant. *J. Path. Bact.*, **80,** 83.

Mummery, J. H., and Pitts, A. T. (1926) A melanotic epithelial odontome in a child. *Proc. roy. Soc. Med. (Sect. Odont.)*, **19,** 11.

Notter, G., and Söderberg, G. (1953) Ein Fall von sog. "Melanocarcinoma congenitum processus alveolaris" (Krompecher). *Acta radiol.*, **40,** 54.

Ostrander, R. B., and Hayward, J. R. (1974) Pigmented neuroectodermal tumor of infancy: report of two cases. *J. oral Surg.*, **32,** 626.

Pontius, E. E., Dziabis, M. D., and Foster, J. A. (1965) Multicentric melano-ameloblastomata of the maxilla. *Cancer*, **18,** 381.

Schulz, D. M. (1957) A malignant, melanotic neoplasm of the uterus, resembling the "retinal anlage" tumors. Report of a case. *Amer. J. clin. Path.*, **28,** 524.

Shafer, W. G., and Frissell, C. T. (1953) The melanoameloblastoma and retinal anlage tumors. *Cancer*, **6,** 360.

Sinniah, R., and O'Brien, F. V. (1973) Pigmented progonoma in a dermoid cyst of the ovary. *J. Path.*, **109,** 357.

Soderberg, N. B., and Padgett, E. C. (1941) Two unusual melanomas of the alveolus and maxilla. *Amer. J. Orthodont. (Oral Surg. Sect.)*, **27,** 270.

Stokke, T. (1968) Pigmented jaw tumor in an infant. A melanocytoma. *Acta odont. scand.*, **26,** 657.

Stowens, D. (1957) A pigmented tumour of infancy: the melanotic progonoma. *J. Path. Bact.*, **73,** 43.

Stowens, D., and Lin, T. H. (1974) Melanotic progonoma of the brain. *Human Path.*, **5,** 105.

Tiecke, R. W. and Bernier, J. L. (1956) Melanotic ameloblastoma. *Oral Surg.*, **9,** 1197.

Wass, S. H. (1948) Melanotic adamantinoma of the mandible in a child aged 5 months. *Proc. roy. Soc. Med.*, **41,** 281.

Williams, A. O. (1967) Melanotic ameloblastoma ("progonoma") of infancy showing osteogenesis. *J. Path. Bact.*, **93,** 545.

Willis, R. A. (1958) The histogenesis of the pigmented epulis of infancy. *J. Path. Bact.*, **76,** 89.

13.   Congenital Epulis

This growth of the gingiva in infants was first described by Neumann (1871). The literature has been reviewed by Custer and Fust (1952), Herschfus and Wolter (1970), and Fuhr and Krogh (1972).

The lesion occurs in newborn infants, about ten times more frequently in females than in males. It presents as a smooth swelling, generally round or oval, but sometimes showing irregular lobulation. It is usually pedunculated, but may be sessile. The maxilla is more often affected than the mandible, the incisor region being the usual location. Occasionally more than one growth may be present.

Pathology

Microscopically, the congenital epulis is very similar to the granular cell myoblastoma (p. 233). The lesion consists of large cells closely packed beneath the surface epithelium, from which they are separated by a narrow zone of connective tissue. The cells are round or polyhedral, though occasionally oval or elongated forms are seen. In some areas the cell outlines are indistinct, so that an almost syncytial appearance results, while in other parts the cells tend to be more discrete, being separated by collagen fibres. The cytoplasm of the cells contains abundant fine eosinophilic granules that give the same histochemical reactions as are obtained in myoblastoma (Campbell, 1955). The nucleus is small, vesicular and eccentrically situated, with a well defined central nucleolus. Mitoses are not seen. Numerous capillaries are usually present.

The overlying epithelium does not show the pseudoepitheliomatous hyperplasia that is often so prominent a feature in myoblastoma. On the contrary, it may be rather thinner than normal (Fig. 45).

Histogenesis

Since the appearances are similar to the myoblastoma of the tongue and other tissues in adults, it has been suggested by Bernier and Thompson (1946) and others that the two lesions are identical. Moreover, cases have been reported in which, in addition to the tumour of the gingiva, there was also a similar tumour of the tongue (Dixter and colleagues, 1975). However, a number of alternative theories have been put forward.

Massin (1894) was the first to suggest a dental origin for the lesion. He considered the possibility that it might arise from muscle, but since there was no demonstrable connection with that tissue he finally concluded that the granular cells were epithelial and derived from the enamel organ. A number of other authors have agreed, in general, with this view. Kaempfer (1911) concurred that the tumour was of dental derivation, but suggested a mesodermal origin, from the dental papilla, and Custer and Fust (1952), who review the literature in some detail, believe the lesion to represent a malformation of the developing tooth. A possible dental origin has also been suggested by the presence in some lesions of dental epithelium. Thus in Bhaskar and Akamine's

---

Fig. 45   **a,** the tumour consists of a mass of granular cells in the subepithelial connective tissue. Note that the epithelium is slightly thinner than normal. Capillaries are prominent. × 200. **b,** the large granular cells are identical to those seen in the myoblastoma of adults. × 500. **c,** most of the granular cells are round or polyhedral, but occasional elongated strap-like forms are seen. × 500.

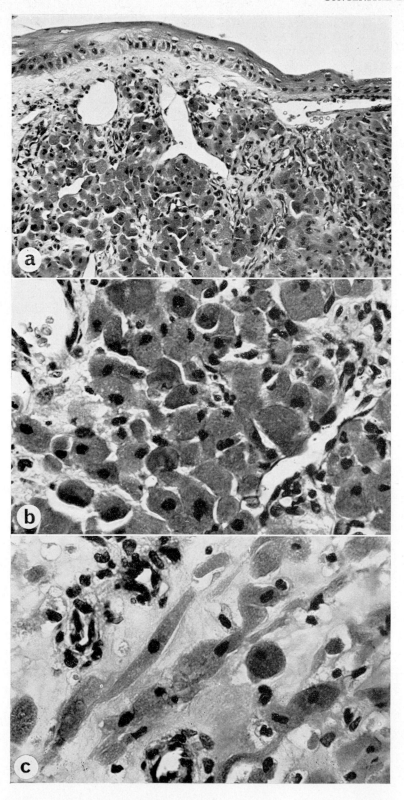

(1955) case islands of epithelium were present in the lesional tissue. These islands consisted of a peripheral layer of columnar cells arranged in a palisaded manner and a central area of squamous cells. Some islands showed calcification. Quite clearly, these epithelial formations were of dental origin, but they were present only at the periphery of the lesion and mainly under the oral epithelium. As the authors point out, epithelial islands of this type are frequently seen in normal fetal alveolar mucosa and in the alveolar crypts. Their presence does not afford sufficient evidence, therefore, to conclude that the granular cell lesion arises from dental epithelium.

Campbell (1956) suggested that there might be a relationship between ameloblastoma and congenital epulis, on the grounds that the granular cells that may be present in some ameloblastomas have identical histochemical reactions to those of the congenital epulis.

Ultrastructure studies have not yet shed much light on the nature of the lesion. Kay, Elzay and Willson (1971) found that the cells of congenital epulis are similar electron microscopically to those of myoblastoma. No Schwann cells or axon fibres were seen in their case. They suggest that the lesion may be epithelial, since junctional complexes were found between some of the cells.

Bhaskar and Akamine have noted transitions from fibroblast-like cells to large clear cells, and conclude that granules probably then form in the latter. They agree with Bauer and Bauer (1953) that the lesion is a granular cell myoblastoma. Other authors who have put forward myogenous, neural or fibroblastic theories of origin for the myoblastoma of adults generally include the congenital epulis in their arguments. The various theories are reviewed by Fuhr and Krogh (1972).

Behaviour

Though the nature and origin of the congenital epulis are still obscure its behaviour is uniformly characteristic. It is a benign lesion that is easily removed and does not recur.

REFERENCES

Bauer, W. H., and Bauer, J. D. (1953) The so-called "congenital epulis." *Oral Surg.*, **6**, 1065.

Bernier, J. L., and Thompson, H. C. (1946) Myoblastoma. *J. dent. Res.*, **25**, 253.

Bhaskar, S. N., and Akamine, R. (1955) Congenital epulis (congenital granular cell fibroblastoma). Report of a case. *Oral Surg.*, **8**, 517.

Campbell, J. A. H. (1955) Congenital epulis. *J. Path. Bact.*, **70**, 233.

Campbell, J. A. H. (1956) Adamantinoma containing tissue resembling granular-cell myoblastoma. *J. Path. Bact.*, **71**, 45.

Custer, R. P., and Fust, J. A. (1952) Congenital epulis. *Amer. J. clin. Path.*, **22**, 1044.

Dixter, C. T., Konstat, M. S., Giunta, J. L., Schreier, E., and White, G. E. (1975) Congenital granular-cell tumor of alveolar ridge and tongue. Report of two cases. *Oral Surg.*, **40**, 270.

Fuhr, A. H., and Krogh, P. H. J. (1972) Congenital epulis of the newborn: centennial review of the literature and a report of case. *J. oral Surg.*, **30**, 30.

Herschfus, L., and Wolter, J. G. (1970) Granular-cell myoblastoma of the oral cavity. *Oral Surg.*, **29**, 341.

Kaempfer, L. G. (1911) Congenital epulides (odontoblastomata). A clinical and pathological study. *Surg. Gynec. Obstet.*, **12**, 357.

Kay, S., Elzay, R. P., and Willson, M. A. (1971) Ultrastructural observations on a gingival granular cell tumor (congenital epulis). *Cancer*, **27**, 674,

Massin, W. N. (1894) Ein Fall von angeborenem Epitheliom, enstanden aus dem Schmelzorgan. *Virchows Arch.*, **136**, 328.

Neumann, E. (1871) Ein Fall von congenitaler Epulis. *Arch. Heilk.*, **12**, 189.

V

PRIMARY TUMOURS OF THE JAWS AND
SOFT TISSUES OF NON-DENTAL ORIGIN

14. Leukoplakia and White Lesions of the Oral Mucosa

LEUKOPLAKIA

The literal meaning of leukoplakia is "white plaque" and the term has been used for very many years by clinicians and pathologists for any mucosal lesion that could be described in this way. Traditionally, also, the term has carried implications of malignant potential. However, a number of conditions characterised by the formation of white or whitish patches on the oral mucous membrane are benign, or are only exceptionally associated with the subsequent appearance of malignancy, so that their designation as leukoplakia might well tend to endow them with a quite undeserved sinister prognosis. For this reason, many workers in recent years have suggested that the designation of leukoplakia should be reserved for lesions that show histological changes considered to indicate premalignancy. Thus "leukoplakia" would become solely a microscopic diagnosis. This would be a logical solution of the problem, but for the fact that just as not all white lesions are potentially malignant, so not all potentially malignant lesions appear as white patches. Indeed, lesions showing histological changes that are usually diagnosed as "pre-malignant" are frequently pinkish or red, or may be mottled (Pindborg and colleagues, 1963; Mashberg, Morrisey and Garfinkel, 1973). Then again, lesions that appear merely as white patches, with perhaps a minimal degree of ulceration or fissuring, and that could well be called leukoplakia, may be found on microscopic examination to be definite invasive carcinoma. It is clear, therefore, that the use of the term leukoplakia can be misleading; pathologists and clinicians should ensure that they have the same conceptions when employing it. It is now generally gaining acceptance that leukoplakia should be used as a macroscopic descriptive term only, although even so, two usages are possible. In the widest sense, the term may be employed for all mucosal white lesions, or it may be restricted to those white lesions that cannot be characterised clinically or pathologically as any other disease. Thus, conditions such as candidosis, lichen planus, white folded dysplasia and the like are referred to by their own specific designations and only those lesions that remain after all the known diagnostic entities have been separated off are referred to as leukoplakia

The designation of leukoplakia in the restricted sense just mentioned is recommended by the World Health Organization. Undoubtedly, the definition is a somewhat negative one, leaving for the entity only those white patches that cannot be diagnosed as anything else, but it does gather together a group of lesions (which may very well not all be of the same nature) and keeps them distinct from other definite diagnostic entities. Defined in this way, some leukoplakic lesions appear to be associated with tobacco. Others are due to trauma or irritation and some lesions are due to, or are associated with, some of the etiological factors that are discussed in connection with carcinoma of the mouth (p. 134).

The leukoplakic lesion may occur at any site in the oral mucous membrane. Some lesions are quite small and circumscribed, others can be extensive, involving large areas of mucosa. As already indicated, not all leukoplakic lesions are uniformly white; some are whitish-yellow or grey and others are mottled or speckled, with nodular white excrescences on an erythematous background. The surface of the plaque may be smooth or wrinkled. Smooth lesions sometimes show small cracks or fissures, the surface appearing like cracked mud.

Microscopically, the usual features are hyperkeratosis, acanthosis and often some chronic inflammatory infiltration in the corium, with lymphocytes predominating, but plasma cells are often also present. However, the appearances can be very variable; in some cases there is a thick layer of keratin and much acanthosis, in others there may be atrophy. In a small number of lesions dysplasia may be present, and it is in these cases that the question of possible future malignancy arises.

The prevalence of leukoplakia has not been widely investigated. Pindborg and colleagues (1967) cite Bruszt's (1962) Hungarian report as one of the few European studies on this subject: there was a 3·6 per cent prevalence. In India, Mehta and colleagues (1961) found a 3·5 per cent prevalence and again (1969) a prevalence ranging from 0·2 to 4·9 per cent. A similar figure was arrived at by Pindborg. The Indian studies have shown a striking correlation with tobacco usage and betel nut chewing.

The relationship of leukoplakia to carcinoma is not in doubt; malignancy does follow in a proportion of cases, as has of course been known for many years. What is in doubt, however, is the extent to which this occurs, both with regard to the incidence of coexisting leukoplakia in patients with carcinoma and to the incidence of leukoplakic lesions that subsequently become carcinomatous. So far as coexisting leukoplakia and carcinoma are concerned, the reported figures range from some 2 to 75 per cent. Thus Willis (1967) found that nearly one-third of cases of carcinoma of the lip have had leukoplakia, while in carcinoma of the tongue the figure was 10 per cent (Gibbel, Cross and Ariel, 1949). Moertel, Dockerty and Baggenstoss (1961) found leukoplakia in 75 per cent of patients with multiple cancers of the mouth, but Sharp, Bullock and Helsper (1961) found only one case of leukoplakia in 28 patients with multiple oral carcinomas. When the proportion of leukoplakic lesions that can reasonably be interpreted as precancerous is considered, again there is variation in the findings of different workers, but generally speaking the proportion tends to be low. Shafer and Waldron (1961) state that in the older literature an average incidence of 30 per cent malignant transformation in cases of leukoplakia has been found, but their own series and those of other recent authors show a much lower incidence (Cooke, 1956; Renstrup, 1958). The surveys of Pindborg and his colleagues (1968) indicate a malignant transformation rate in the region of 4 per cent. In Silverman and Rozen's (1968) series of 117 patients, there was a 6 per cent malignant transformation rate over a period of from 1 to 5 years. Bánóczy and Sugár (1972) found a 5·9 per cent rate in 520 patients followed for up to 25 years. Other European surveys, cited by Pindborg (1971), give similar figures. A recent Indian survey showed only one case of cancer occurring in 117 patients followed for 10 years. This very low rate is surprising, in view of the high incidence of oral cancer in India. However, special factors may be concerned (Mehta and colleagues, 1972).

In general, it is clear that the great majority of white lesions of the oral mucosa show no epithelial changes other than hyperkeratosis, parakeratosis or acanthosis. Only a minority show dysplasia.

EPITHELIAL DYSPLASIA AND ATYPIA

The changes in individual cells in those mucosal lesions that may in time become malignant are termed epithelial atypia. The general disturbance in the epithelium is designated dysplasia. Changes of this type have been studied most extensively in the uterine cervix and it is only in recent years that much attention has been given to the oral mucosa. However, it would appear that much of what is known with regard to the cervix will also be applicable to the oral mucous membrane. Epithelial dysplasia is diagnosed when there is disorderly maturation

such pseudoepitheliomatous hyperplasias as carcinoma (Fig. 50). On the other hand, the possibility of verrucous carcinoma must be kept in mind (p. 145).

The condition appears to be due to irritation and associated with chronic inflammation, rather than of neoplastic nature. Bhaskar, Beasley and Cutright (1970) have reviewed 341 cases and found that the lesion occurs ten times more frequently in patients who sleep with their dentures in situ than in those who do not. Also, it is five times more common in patients wearing acrylic dentures than in those with metallic dentures. In some cases replacement of the dentures has been followed by regression of the lesion but excision may also be required for extensive growths. It is possible that irritation due to amalgam fillings may also produce lesions of this type. A case in which regression occurred following removal of fillings has been reported by Bergenholtz (1965).

FOCAL EPITHELIAL HYPERPLASIA

Focal epithelial hyperplasia is a rare condition first described by Archard, Heck and Stanley (1965) in North American Indian children. Subsequently, the condition has been found in many areas in Central and South America. Although the condition occurs more often in American Indians, and in Eskimos, than in other ethnic groups, cases have been reported in Caucasians in America, Europe, the Middle East, in Negroes in Africa and in aborigines in Australia and Polynesia (see Clausen and colleagues (1969, 1970, 1973) and Praetorius-Clausen (1973) for review and references.

The focal lesions consist of small flat soft polypoid growths scattered over the oral mucosa, and particularly in the lower lip. Microscopically, there is acanthosis and cells with large nuclei and multinucleated cells are present. There is chronic inflammatory infiltration in the corium and often also ductal hyperplasia of the neighbouring minor salivary glands. The cause of this condition is unknown, though intranuclear inclusion bodies have been noted by Clausen, who postulates a possible virus etiology.

KERATOACANTHOMA

This benign lesion usually occurs on the exposed skin. It also occurs, although rarely, at mucocutaneous junctions and possibly in mucous membranes. The lesion was first fully described by McCormac and Scarff (1936) as molluscum sebaceum and by Rook and Whimster (1950) and others under its present name. It occurs as a small lump on the exposed areas of the skin and grows to its maximum size, 1 to 2 cm in diameter, in a few weeks, when it either remains stationary for an indefinite period or regresses. Microscopically, the lesion appears very similar to a well differentiated squamous cell carcinoma and in the absence of sufficient material for histological examination the distinction can be very difficult. However, when the lesion can be sectioned in its entirety, it shows a characteristic crater plugged with keratin and surrounded by hyperplastic epithelium (Fig. 50).

Keratoacanthoma probably originates in pilosebaceous follicles and this would account for its rare or indeed doubtful occurrence in the oral mucosa. Most lesions in the oral region have occurred in the lip, and although often largely situated on the vermilion border, they may well

Fig. 50 **a,** papillary hyperplasia of the palate. The mucosa shows numerous papillary projections over a wide area. × 7. **b,** higher magnification, showing the benign character of the epithelial proliferation. × 80. **c,** keratoacanthoma. The circumscribed nature of the lesion is seen in this low power view. × 4. **d,** higher magnification, showing the close similarity of the epithelial changes to squamous cell carcinoma. × 120.

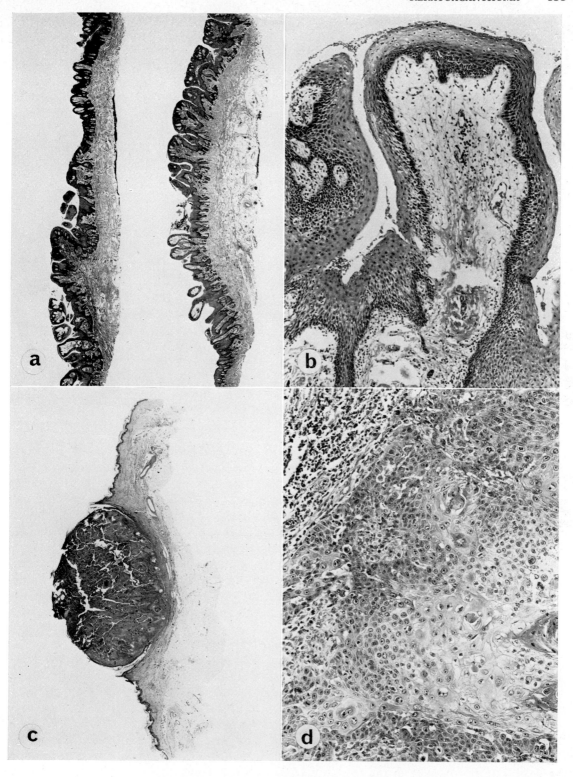

have arisen in adjacent skin. Lip lesions have been reviewed by Silberberg and colleagues (1962) and further cases have been reported by Pisanty (1966), Hardman (1971) and Kohn and Eversole (1972). An intraoral lesion has been reported by Helsham and Buchanan (1960). This was a fungating gingival tumour diagnosed clinically as squamous cell carcinoma. A palatal lesion has been reported by Scofield and colleagues (1974). The status of these rare solitary intraoral lesions is debatable; either keratoacanthoma must be regarded as, rarely, arising in mucosae from elements other than pilosebaceous follicles, or alternatively, mucosal lesions must be of different nature. Stevanovic (1960) reviewed lesions of mucous membranes.

As noted, keratoacanthoma is a benign and self-limiting lesion, but careful follow-up is required in all cases because of the difficulties in diagnosis. Even where the diagnosis seems quite definite, it is still possible for a lesion to turn out to be a squamous cell carcinoma, as Jackson (1969) points out in reporting four cases in which this occurred. Inverson and Vistnes (1973) make the same point, and indeed regard keratoacanthoma as a premalignant condition.

SQUAMOUS CELL CARCINOMA OF THE ORAL MUCOSA

Malignant tumours of the oral tissues constitute up to 5 per cent of malignant tumours in all sites, in most countries in the Western hemisphere. In England and Wales, for example, oral cancer accounts for about 2 per cent of all cancer registrations (Binnie and colleagues, 1972). In California, the figure is 4·6 per cent (Silverman and Galante, 1974). In Asiatic countries, however, oral cancer is very much commoner.

Ninety per cent of oral malignant tumours are squamous cell carcinomas, other forms of carcinoma together with the malignant mesenchymal tumours accounting for the remaining 10 per cent.

Etiology

Dental and oral infections. Many clinicians believe that oral cancer occurs more frequently in patients with a poor state of oral hygiene than in those whose mouths are properly cared for. However, it is difficult to obtain statistical proof of a significant relationship between the incidence of dental infections and other abnormalities and cancer. Conditions such as chronic infection following dental caries, the presence of sharp edges on broken-down teeth, badly fitting dentures and rough fillings are all quite common, so that the occurrence of carcinoma may be coincidental. For example, Lash, Erich and Dockerty (1961), among many others, state that oral sepsis was common in their series of patients with carcinoma of the tongue, and 96 per cent of 180 patients had leukoplakia. On the other hand Cade and Lee (1957) found that the oral mucosa was healthy in their 653 patients with the same disease. There is, too, a remarkable dearth of case reports of cancer following prolonged irritation, such as might be expected were this an important factor. Hobaek (1949) has reported four cases of squamous cell carcinoma occurring in relationship to the suction chamber of dentures but cases of this type are very uncommon. Even the carcinoma occurring in the epithelium over an area of fibrous proliferation caused by a denture that Persson and Wallenius (1961) have reported was not definitely due to the denture. And it is of interest to note that though fibrous proliferation due to pressure from dentures is common, malignant change either in the covering epithelium or in the fibrous tissue itself must be very rare. Furthermore, investigations such as those of Wynder, Bross and Feldman (1957) and Vogler, Lloyd and Milmore (1962) have failed to show that dental irritation and trauma are significant factors in oral cancer. On the other hand, there has been a pronounced decrease in the death rate from cancer of the mouth in recent years in Great Britain, which Wood (1961) considers might well be due to a rising standard of oral hygiene. Recent changes in smoking habits, however, may also be concerned.

Tobacco. There is a close connection between smoking and oral cancer, but unlike the association in cancer of the lung it has usually been considered that in oral cancer it is the pipe and the cigar that are the chief offenders rather than the cigarette.

For example, Wynder and Bross's (1957) survey has shown that the risk of cancer in all parts of the oral cavity is four times greater for pipe or cigar smokers than for non-smokers. This survey also brings out the fact that smokers of 35 or more cigarettes a day are only slightly less at risk than pipe or cigar smokers. Previously, it had been thought that there was no very close relationship between cigarette smoking and oral cancer (Sadowsky, Gilliam and Cornfield, 1953). The changing incidence in oral and respiratory cancers in recent years can also be correlated with a change in smoking habits. Thus within the past 30 years the death rate for oral cancer has halved, while that for lung cancer has increased five times. These changes correspond to the virtual replacement of the pipe by the cigarette which has taken place in this century. Another aspect of the effect of smoking has been brought out by Moore (1965), who has shown that approximately a third of patients who have been successfully treated for oral, pharyngeal or laryngeal cancer will develop new, second cancers if they continue smoking, whereas smokers who stop after getting their first cancer run only a small risk of developing another. Unfortunately, there is also some conflicting evidence, since Castigliano (1968) could not demonstrate any beneficial influence of the cessation of smoking on the incidence of second primary growths.

Tobacco chewing and snuff taking are also associated with an increased incidence of oral cancer. Vogler, Lloyd and Milmore (1962) found that the incidence was higher in white women in the Southern states than elsewhere in the United States. This was associated with the common practice amongst rural Southern women of holding snuff in the mouth ("snuff dipping").

The high incidence of oral cancer in India and Ceylon and other eastern countries has for many years been thought to be connected with betel-chewing (Orr, 1933). It is now believed that it is not the betel nut or leaf itself that is carcinogenic but the tobacco, slaked lime and other ingredients that are contained in the quid (Sanghvi, Rao and Khanolkar, 1955; Paymaster, 1957; Muir and Kirk, 1960; and others). However, Sobin (1969) has brought forward the seemingly rather anomalous finding of a relatively low frequency of oral cancer in Afghanistan, where tobacco chewing is common; and in New Guinea, where oral cancer is frequent, the betel nut quid does not contain tobacco. However, smoking is nearly universal (Atkinson and colleagues, 1964).

Alcohol. Alcohol has long been considered a factor in oral cancer, and studies in the United States would appear to confirm this view. Wynder and Bross have shown that heavy whisky drinkers are 15 times more liable to oral cancer than are occasional drinkers. The combination of heavy drinking and smoking appears to be particularly significant. It is of interest to note that in such cases it is the incidence of cancer of the floor of the mouth, pharynx and tonsil that is increased, and not cancer of the lip.

Trieger and colleagues (1958, 1959) have also shown that there is an association between spirit drinking and cirrhosis of the liver and cancer of the tongue and mouth. Vincent, Marchetta and Nigogosyan (1964) found evidence of cirrhosis in 28 per cent of 144 autopsies on patients with oral cancer, and clinical evidence of liver damage in 45 per cent of 106 patients.

The role of alcohol seems to be less definite in Britain. Although, as Binnie and colleagues (1972) point out, there has been a marked increase in alcoholism in the last thirty years, this cannot be related to any corresponding change in the statistics for oral cancer.

Syphilis. Syphilis is another of the factors which, with tobacco and alcohol, have been traditionally associated with oral cancer. Wynder and Bross found that there was in fact an

K

association between oral cancer and syphilis, but it was significant only for cancer of the lip and anterior two-thirds of the tongue. In Vogler, Lloyd and Milmore's series, syphilis did not appear to be a significant etiological factor. However, many investigations in the past have shown a definite correlation between syphilitic glossitis and cancer, though this is a causal relationship which has now become rare.

Other intraoral lesions. A proportion of white lesions of the oral mucosa are likely to become malignant (p. 120). Chronic ulceration and fissures are also common forerunners of overt cancer, particularly in the lip. So often has carcinoma of the lip been preceded by some sort of chronic lesion, an ulcer, a fissure or an acanthotic or hyperkeratotic area that it is standard practice to submit to excision biopsy all such lesions that persist for more than a short period in spite of treatment. The frequency with which lesions of this type precede or coexist with carcinoma indicates that there is often a widespread abnormality throughout the mucosa. Willis (1944, 1945) has shown that changes take place over fields of epithelium that are greater in extent than that of the growth itself, and that the potentially cancerous field is probably extensive. As Slaughter and colleagues (1953) have pointed out, this can explain the tendency to multicentric growths in the mucosa.

Herpes simplex is a common oral lesion and is not related to cancer in the vast majority of cases. However, it is possible that in old age it may occasionally be related to cancer in some way in a small number of cases. Wyburn-Mason (1957) has reported carcinoma of the lip following herpes simplex in old people.

Like herpes, *lichen planus* is not considered in the ordinary way as predisposing to cancer, though there have been reports of carcinoma supervening on the lichen lesion in a few cases, particularly those of the erosive or atrophic varieties of the disease. They have been reviewed by Andreasen (1968). In a recent investigation Silverman and Griffith (1974) found five associated cases of oral carcinoma in two hundred patients with oral lichen planus, a prevalence of 2·5 per cent. In a comparable age and sex-matched sample in the general population a 0·05 per cent occurrence would be expected. However in Fulling's (1973) follow-up study of 327 patients with oral lichen planus, only one patient developed carcinoma in a lichen lesion after a five-year observation period. Almost identical findings have been reported by Kövesi and Bánóczy (1973). As Shklar (1972) has pointed out, oral cancer is a relatively common condition and might be expected occasionally to co-exist with or follow lichen planus coincidentally. Moreover, when oral lesions only are present, it is possible that these might be misdiagnosed as lichen planus when they are in fact dysplastic lesions but not lichen (Reisman and colleagues, 1974).

Candidosis has been incriminated as a possible precursor of carcinoma by Cawson (1966, 1969). Candida infection is often associated with acanthosis and parakeratosis, and the hyphae can readily be demonstrated in the hyperplastic epithelium (Fig. 51). Cawson has found epithelial dysplasia in a number of cases of candidosis and suggests that such may go on to overt cancer. However, the candida infection in cases of this type may be simply a secondary infection of mucosa which is already abnormal, and there is certainly as yet no evidence that candidosis as such is carcinogenic.

Median rhomboid glossitis is another benign lesion that has exceptionally been followed by cancer. This condition has generally been considered as a developmental anomaly, due to failure of the tuberculum impar to withdraw when fusion of the two halves of the tongue occurs. There thus remains a slightly raised, or sometimes depressed, ovoid or rhomboid area devoid of filiform papillae, situated on the dorsum of the tongue anterior to the circumvallate papillae. More recently, there has been some evidence suggesting that the condition is infective, due to candidosis. It is usually symptomless. A case of squamous cell carcinoma developing in this condition has been reported by Sharp and Bullock (1958).

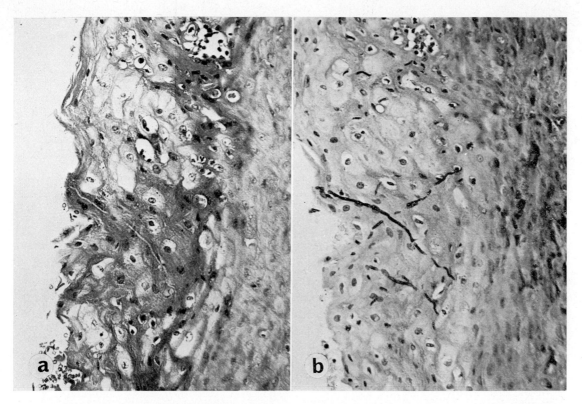

Fig. 51   Candidosis. **a,** the hyphae can be seen in the epithelium, although in sections stained by haematoxylin and eosin they are not so obvious as in PAS-stained sections. × 200. **b,** a consecutive section from the same block as the section in **a,** stained by the PAS technique. × 200.

The atrophic changes in the mucous membrane of the upper alimentary tract that occur in the *Plummer-Vinson syndrome* predispose to malignancy. Ahlbom (1936) found the syndrome to be present in 70 per cent of the women in his series of patients with carcinoma of the hypopharynx and upper portion of the oesophagus. The usual site for carcinoma in these cases is the junction of pharynx and oesophagus, but oral carcinoma also occurs. Wynder, Hultberg, Jacobsson and Bross (1957) have shown that the high incidence of upper alimentary tract and oral cancers in women in Sweden is correlated with the incidence of the Plummer-Vinson syndrome in that country.

The rare *epidermolysis bullosa dystrophica* is occasionally followed by carcinoma. In this condition, which usually appears in the newborn, bullae and ulcers appear on the skin and mucous membranes, usually induced by trauma. Healing is accompanied by much scarring. Dental anomalies may occur. The literature is reviewed by Kaslick and Brustein (1961).

A number of cases of carcinoma of the lip developing in the lesions of *discoid lupus erythematosus* have been reported. These are listed by Andreasen (1964).

In India, *submucous fibrosis* appears to be a precancerous lesion. In this condition there are areas of dense fibrosis of the hard and soft palate, the tonsillar fossa and also the buccal mucosa. The fibrosis is slowly progressive, with infiltration of the underlying muscles leading to trismus and to fixation of the palate. There is often also some anaemia and sometimes eosinophilia, and diminution of free hydrochloric acid in the gastric juice (Joshi, 1953; Sirsat and Khanolkar, 1957).

Paymaster (1957, 1962) found that in approximately one-third of his cases of submucous fibrosis a slow-growing squamous cell carcinoma developed, and the extensive investigations of

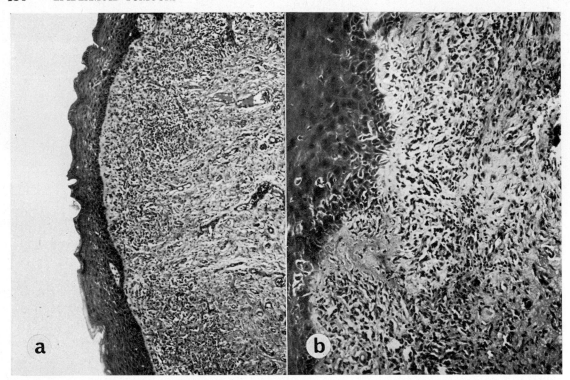

Fig. 52   Submucous fibrosis. **a,** the epithelium is atrophic, with loss of the rete processes. There is well marked chronic inflammatory infiltration in the subepithelial connective tissue. × 50. **b,** higher magnification, showing areas of degenerative change in the connective tissue, immediately subjacent to the epithelium. × 120.

Pindborg and his colleagues (1965, 1966, 1967, 1968) have confirmed the precancerous potentiality of the lesion. They believe that the thinning of the epithelium that occurs in the condition renders it more susceptible to carcinogens such as tobacco. The condition itself might represent a hypersensitivity reaction to chilli in the diet.

Microscopically the principal features are atrophy of the epithelium with the possible presence of dysplastic changes. The juxta-epithelial collagen shows degenerative changes and there is often well marked chronic inflammatory infiltration (Fig. 52).

Although submucous fibrosis occurs mainly in Indians living in India, cases have been reported from other parts of Asia and in Indians and Pakistans living in the United Kingdom (Rowell, 1967; Kennedy and MacDonald, 1968; Moos and Madan, 1968) and South Africa (Shear and Lemmer, 1967). It has also been reported in Europeans in India (Rao, 1962) and Simpson (1969) has reported the case of a European woman living in the United Kingdom and married to a Pakistani.

Oral melanosis also appears to be associated with oral cancer in India, since though present in 5 per cent of normal persons, it is seen in 20 per cent of patients with oral carcinomas.

Exposure to sunlight. The relationship between cancer of the lip and sunlight is well-known, the condition occurring particularly in farmers, sailors and other outdoor workers. Thus, lip cancer is more frequent in Newfoundland, where fishing is a major industry, than in other parts of Canada (Miller, 1974). Its incidence in Scotland is twice as high as in England and Wales, and this again may be related to outdoor occupations (Pogrel, 1974). Finland and Northern Ireland also have unusually high frequencies (Jones and Coyle, 1969). Cancer of the lip occurs more frequently in southern countries than in northern ones. On the other hand, negroes suffer much less from lip (and skin) cancer than white persons, probably the result of the protective effect of melanin pigmentation (Bernier and Clark, 1951; Schonland and Bradshaw, 1968; Shear, 1970).

Ionizing radiation. Carcinoma of the buccal mucosa may occur as a long-term complication of radiotherapy. Slaughter and Southwick (1957) have reported cases in which squamous cell carcinomas of the mucous membrane developed in areas treated by external irradiation from 9 to 25 years before the appearance of the tumours.

Occupation. Apart from outdoor workers, metal workers appear to suffer from an increased incidence of oral cancer.

Incidence

Carcinoma of the oral mucosa has a marked sex predilection, occurring more often in men than in women. The ratio varies from 8 to 10 males to one female in carcinoma of the lip to two to one in carcinoma of the gingiva. The ratio has gradually been diminishing over the past thirty to forty years; this is due to a decline in the incidence of oral cancer in men, while the incidence in women has shown little change. The peak age incidence is between 50 and 70 years, though not infrequently younger persons are affected. Figures for the distribution of tumours in the various sites are given in the table. These figures indicate the general trend; there is some variation in the different series reported in the literature (Lane-Claypon, 1930; Martin, 1941; Cross, Guralnick and Daland, 1948; Tiecke and Bernier, 1954, Binnie and colleagues, 1972), and there is a marked difference when non-European races are considered. Thus in those peoples who have distinctive smoking habits (e.g. the practice of smoking cigars with the lighted end in the mouth, as in some parts of India) or who chew betel, carcinoma of the palate, cheeks, tongue and floor of the mouth is relatively more frequent. In Western tobacco chewers, cancer most frequently develops in the cheek or buccal sulcus, where the quid is habitually held.

In addition to the differences in site distribution of oral cancers between East and West, there is also a striking difference in overall frequency. In Western countries oral cancer accounts for not more than 5 per cent of all cancers, while in some parts of India the figure is nearly 50 per cent, closely followed by Sri Lanka at over 40 per cent. The other countries of south-east Asia also show a high frequency of oral cancer. The global epidemiology of oral cancer is well discussed by Smith (1973), and Binnie and colleagues (1972) report on a national study of morbidity, mortality and other factors in England and Wales.

Table 1   Site distribution of carcinoma of the oral mucosa

	Percentage distribution	
Lip		
upper	4 ⎫ 100	25
lower	96 ⎭	
Floor of mouth		15
Gingiva		
upper	40 ⎫ 100	10
lower	60 ⎭	
Tongue		30
Cheek		10
Palate		10

Pathology

The earliest stages of carcinoma of the oral mucosa are often represented clinically by comparatively insignificant-appearing lesions, such as small areas of hyperkeratosis or of erythema, but in many cases the condition is more advanced when first seen and in most sites of the mucosa it usually presents as a papillary or as an ulcerative growth.

Microscopically, it may be possible to find in the early lesions the changes of carcinoma in situ. Presumably in such cases the sequence of changes commences with epithelial atypia, which becomes progressively more severe and eventually affects practically the whole thickness of the epithelium, when it is considered as carcinoma in situ. Finally, with penetration of epithelium into the surrounding tissues, the lesion becomes invasive carcinoma. However, as already indicated, the great majority of lesions are already invasive carcinomas when first seen, and whether or not they have passed through the stages just described is not known. They may well have been invasive carcinomas from the outset. In the invasive lesion strands and islands of epithelial cells, similar in general to prickle cells, penetrate the underlying connective tissue. In most oral growths the tumour is well differentiated and the neoplastic cells, though showing the stigmata of malignancy, such as hyperchromatism, pleomorphism, anisocytosis and the like, are still recognisably of prickle cell type, and indeed carry out the function of these cells by forming keratin. The keratin appears as circular or spherical masses or "pearls". The connective tissues through which the strands of epithelial cells are infiltrating generally show quite a well marked chronic inflammatory infiltration, consisting mainly of lymphocytes and plasma cells (Fig. 53).

Although the typical well differentiated squamous cell carcinoma, as just described, is a relatively easy neoplasm to diagnose microscopically, difficulty can arise when dealing with lesions at the extremes of the range of differentiation. On the one hand, there are a number of lesions that can be mistaken for well differentiated carcinoma, while on the other there are lesions that are so undifferentiated that there may be difficulty with their diagnosis even as carcinoma. Lesions in the former category include the overgrowth of epithelium that often occurs at the periphery of chronic ulcers, and these of course are frequently seen in the oral tissues. Tangential sectioning may cause areas of hyperplastic epithelium to look like detached invading masses of cells, and these may even show the presence of structures superficially similar to the keratin pearls of the carcinoma. However, detailed examination shows that the cells of the non-neoplastic proliferation are practically normal in size, shape, tinctorial qualities and the like; they do not display the attributes of neoplastic cells, even well differentiated ones. It is frequently stated that the basement membrane remains intact around cellular proliferations that are non-neoplastic, but is penetrated or disrupted by carcinoma. However, the basement membrane cannot be accurately identified in ordinary sections stained by haematoxylin and eosin; it seems probable that references to its integrity or discontinuity have often been based more on the architecture of the dermo-epidermal junction than on the examination of a distinctive subepidermal structure. Nevertheless, a band of material that stains more intensely with the PAS technique than does the adjacent connective tissue can be demonstrated immediately subjacent to the basal epithelial cells. Cahn, Eisenbud and Blake (1961) found that in frank squamous cell carcinoma this structure no longer stained heavily with PAS, and they considered that this change might be helpful in distinguishing potentially malignant epithelium from benign epithelium. However, Santis and Shklar (1964) and other workers have not been able to substantiate this. A number of attempts

---

Fig. 53   Examples of well differentiated squamous cell carcinoma. **a,** a tumour of the lip, showing invasion of the corium by strands of well differentiated cells. × 30. **b,** higher magnification, to show that the tumour cells are of recognisably prickle cell type and are forming keratin. × 300. **c,** a tumour of the gingiva, showing well marked keratinisation. × 30. **d,** a keratin pearl in a higher magnification from **c.** × 200.

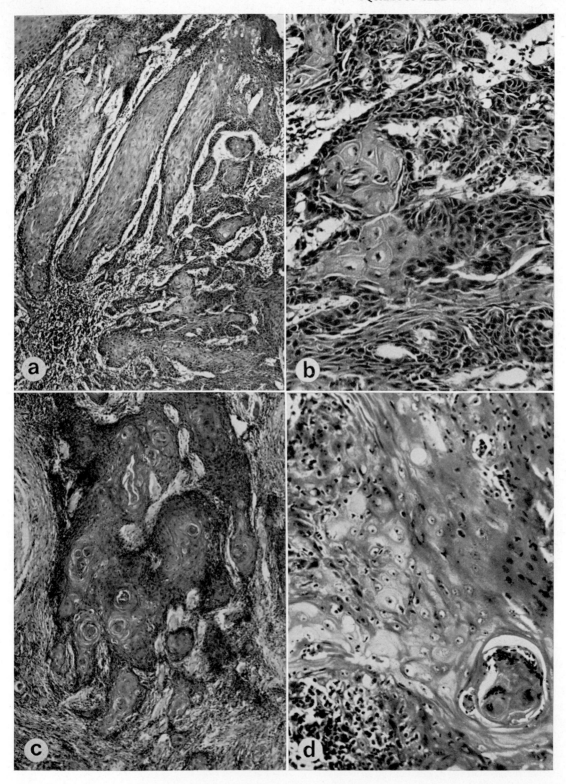

have been made to distinguish neoplastic from non-neoplastic epithelium by enzyme histo-chemistry, and though differences have been demonstrated between carcinomatous and normal epithelium these are not yet applicable to routine histological diagnosis (Santis and Shklar, 1964; Santis, Shklar and Chauncey, 1964; Shklar, 1966).

In addition to the type of non-neoplastic epithelial proliferation that has to be distinguished from squamous cell carcinoma and has just been described, carcinoma is closely resembled by keratoacanthoma (p. 132) and the pseudoepitheliomatous hyperplasia that occurs in connection with myoblastoma (p. 233). Verrucous carcinoma is a particularly well differentiated type of squamous cell carcinoma that is sufficiently distinctive as to warrant separate description (p. 145), as is spindle cell carcinoma (p. 147) and adenoid squamous cell carcinoma (p. 148).

At the other extreme of the range lie the poorly differentiated tumours. Anaplastic tumours are very rare in the oral mucosa. When they do occur they present the same problems of diagnosis as in other situations, with reticulum cell sarcoma, Ewing's tumour, neuroblastoma and metastatic deposit from a primary lesion elsewhere being amongst the possible diagnoses. More frequently, but still uncommonly, there occur tumours that are poorly differentiated but in which there is less doubt as to their nature and origin. In such tumours the cells have lost their resemblance to prickle cells, desmosomes being absent, and keratin is not formed. Hyperchromatism and pleomorphism are much in evidence. As might be expected, continuously varying degrees of differentiation between the very well differentiated and the completely anaplastic are encountered, but from the practical point of view it is sufficient to recognise, in addition to the separately described variants such as verrucous carcinoma and spindle cell carcinoma, well differentiated growths and poorly differentiated and anaplastic growths (Fig. 54).

Carcinoma of the lip. Carcinoma affects the lower lip much more commonly than the upper, commencing as a small warty growth, a fissure or a small area of ulceration on the ver-milion surface of the lip. As the lesion enlarges it takes a papillary or an ulcerative form. Papillary lesions grow slowly and infiltrate the deeper tissues relatively late whereas ulcerative growths, which are commoner, invade early. In the untreated case there is ultimately involvement and destruction of the entire lip and invasion of the cheek, the gums and the mandible. The first lymph nodes to be invaded are those of the submandibular and submental groups, with subsequent extension to the upper deep cervical nodes.

Histologically, the majority of tumours are well differentiated. Anaplastic growths are rare.

Carcinoma of the lip is the form of oral cancer with the most favourable prognosis, for this tumour metastasises to the regional nodes much less frequently, and at a later stage, than do tumours elsewhere in the oral tissues. Visceral metastases occur in the late stages. Carcinoma of the upper lip metastasises earlier and more frequently than carcinoma of the lower lip. Under the best conditions of treatment, and with early cases, five-year survival rates in the region of 80 to 85 per cent may be expected (Cross, Guralnick and Daland, 1948; Wood, 1961), the best results being obtained when the entire lip mucosal field is removed for early lesions, as this appears to prevent second primary growths appearing subsequently in the remaining lip ver-milion (Wilson and Kemble, 1972). When lymph node metastases are present the rate drops to the region of 40 per cent.

Carcinoma of the buccal mucosa. The term buccal mucosa is used to designate the

---

Fig. 54   Examples of poorly differentiated squamous cell carcinoma. **a,** a tumour of the fauces in a man of 74, which presented as a roughened white patch. × 80. **b,** detail from **a,** showing the lack of differentia-tion as evidenced by absence of intercellular bridges and keratin formation. Numerous mitoses are present. × 200. **c,** a tumour of the nasal mucosa. This very poorly differentiated tumour consists of masses of rather uniform cells. × 80. **d,** detail from **c.** × 300.

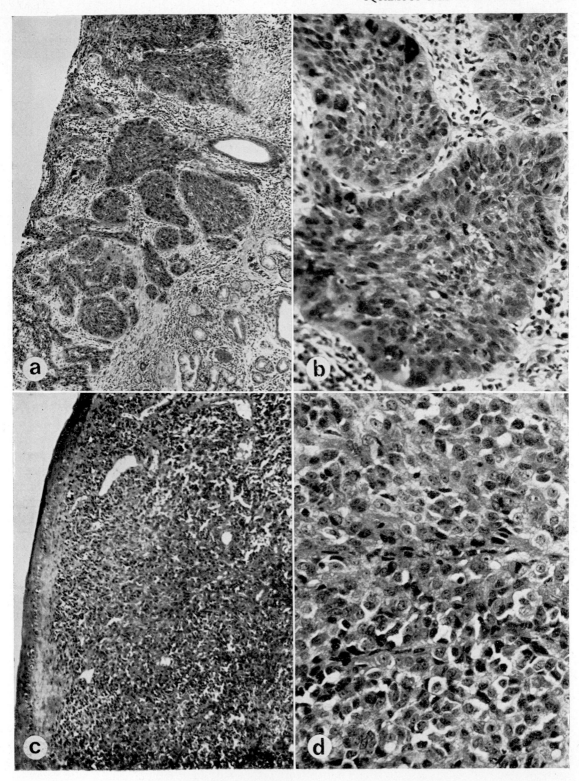

mucosa of the oral aspect of the cheek. Carcinoma in this site generally occurs in the area oppo-site the lower third molar tooth, very frequently on the basis of a long-standing leukoplakia. The tumour begins as a small nodule and enlarges to form a wart-like growth which ultimately ulcerates, or the lesion may be of ulcerating type from the outset. Extension occurs into the muscles of the cheek, the alveolar mucosa and ultimately the bone, or the soft palate.

Microscopically, the growth is well differentiated in the great majority of cases.

Metastases occur to the submandibular and upper cervical nodes in nearly one-half of the cases. However, if the case is early, with a small lesion and no metastases, the prognosis is better than for the other intraoral cancers. It is unfortunately not very common for patients to be treated at an early stage; generally the lesion is quite large when it is first seen. The five-year survival rate for early and late cases together is usually given as in the region of 25 per cent. However, like carcinoma in some other intraoral sites there has been some improvement in recent years; O'Brien and Catlin (1965) give a cure rate of 42 per cent at the Memorial Center, New York, as compared with 28 per cent 10 years previously. This corresponds with the change from radio-therapy to surgery in all resectable cases.

Carcinoma of the gingiva. Carcinoma of the gingiva occurs generally in the premolar and molar regions, the lower jaw being more often affected than the upper. Papillary and ulcerative types of growth occur. The papillary growths tend to remain relatively superficial longer than do the ulcerative forms, which invade the underlying tissues and bone at an early stage.

Microscopically, carcinoma of the gingiva is practically always a well differentiated growth.

Metastases occur to the submandibular nodes and then to the cervical nodes. They occur at an earlier stage and more frequently with growths of the lower gum than with those of the upper. Martin (1941) gave the five-year survival rate as about 27 per cent, but a figure of 50 per cent was subsequently achieved by Erich and Kragh by 1959. Recently Cady and Catlin (1969) have carried out a 20-year survey on some 600 patients with carcinoma of the gingiva and of the alveolar mucosa and have found some significant changes in the pattern of the disease. Although these changes are not individually large ones, the cumulative effect, together with improved treatment methods, has resulted in an absolute survival rate at the end of the survey period of 50 per cent. Localised lesions of under 3 cm in diameter were considered cured in 80 per cent of cases, but lesions over 5 cm in diameter had a poor outlook.

Carcinoma of the floor of the mouth. The growth generally occurs in the anterior portion of the floor of the mouth in the region of the junction with the tongue, to one or other side of the midline, or in the midline itself. Extension of the growth commonly occurs, to the tongue, mandible, lip or cheek. The tumour may take the form of a wart-like growth which tends to spread superficially rather than in depth, but more often it occurs as an ulcer or may be deeply placed in the submucosa, presenting only an ulcerated fissure to the oral cavity.

Histologically, most tumours are well differentiated.

Lymph node metastasis occurs in most cases of carcinoma of the floor of the mouth (70 per cent, in Cade's (1949) series), to the submandibular and then to the anterior jugular nodes. The five-year survival rate is 30 to 45 per cent (Cade, 1949; Dobbie, 1953; Windeyer, 1953; Erich and Kragh, 1959; Kolson and colleagues 1971).

Carcinoma of the palate. The soft palate is more frequently affected than the hard palate, the posterior border being the usual site. The uvula may be affected but this is rarer. The tumour appears as a papillary growth or as an ulcer and it may invade the underlying bone, with perfora-tion of the palate. It is usually well differentiated. Lymph node metastases occur in about 30 per cent of tumours of the hard palate and in 60 per cent of growths of the soft palate. The prognosis for carcinoma of the soft palate is poor, the five-year survival rate being about 5 per cent. The outlook for hard palate cases is much better, with a figure of about 50 per cent (Cade, 1949).

Carcinoma of the tongue. Lingual lesions are ulcerative or papillary and are often markedly infiltrative. The lateral border of the middle third of the tongue is the usual site, the posterior third being the next commonest. The tip or ventral surface or dorsum may be affected. Occasionally multiple tumours occur, which may coalesce to form a single large tumour. Most tumours are well differentiated; occasionally anaplastic growths are encountered, especially at the base of the tongue. Some of these tumours have the structural appearances described as lymphoepithelioma. Lymph node metastasis occurs early and often, to the upper cervical nodes, and the average five-year survival rate is relatively low (below 25 per cent). But if no metastases are present at the time of admission the rate is over 40 per cent, while if they are present, or develop later, it is below 5 per cent (Gibbel, Cross and Ariel, 1949; Beahrs, Devine and Henson, 1959). The prognosis for tumours of the anterior portion of the tongue is better than for tumours of the posterior third and base, since the anterior lesions are noticed earlier and, being in the mobile part of the tongue, are more easily treated. Survival rates for the two situations of about 45 per cent and 20 per cent have been recorded by Frazell and Lucas (1962). Dockerty and colleagues (1968) have shown that the degree of differentiation of the growth is also important in prognosis. With well differentiated growths the outlook is almost twice as good as for patients with anaplastic tumours (55 per cent and 29 per cent five-year survival respectively). In this respect it may be noted that the proportion of well differentiated tumours is higher in the anterior portion of the tongue than in the posterior.

VERRUCOUS CARCINOMA

This type of squamous cell carcinoma, noted in 1941 by Friedell and Rosenthal, was characterised by Ackerman (1948) as a special subvariety, on account of its typical clinical course and characteristic gross and microscopic findings.

The tumour occurs chiefly in elderly patients, nearly always over the age of 60 and more often males than females. The oral region is the commonest site, most tumours occurring in the cheek, alveolar or gingival mucosa, but any other site in the mouth may be affected. Similar tumours have also been found in the larynx, nasal mucosa, glans penis, vagina, scrotum and perineum. Characteristically the tumour presents as a warty growth that enlarges very slowly, and grows mainly in an exophytic manner, but it does in time invade adjoining tissues, including bone. Although the regional lymph nodes are often enlarged and tender this is nearly always due to associated infection and not to metastases, since the latter are very rare although they can occur (Duckworth, 1961). Other lesions may also be present; Jacobson and Shear (1972) and others have noted concurrent leukoplakic areas in a number of cases. Also, more than one carcinomatous lesion may be present.

There seems to be a striking relationship between tobacco chewing or snuff taking and verrucous carcinoma (Kraus and Perez-Mesa, 1966). In the form of snuff taking practised in some of the southern states of the U.S.A., the snuff is held in the buccal sulcus. Verrucous lesions are relatively common in "snuff dipper's" cancer.

The tumour has also been reported from India (Singh and van Essen, 1966) and Papua (Cooke, 1969), in association with tobacco-betel chewing. However, squamous cell carcinoma of the usual type also occurs in association with chewing as well as other tobacco habits and, as Shafer (1972) points out, we do not as yet know why some chewers should develop the usual type of carcinoma and others develop verrucous carcinoma.

Macroscopically, verrucous carcinoma presents as a papillary mass, composed of heaped-up folds of tissue with deep cleft-like spaces between them. Microscopically, the thickened epithelium

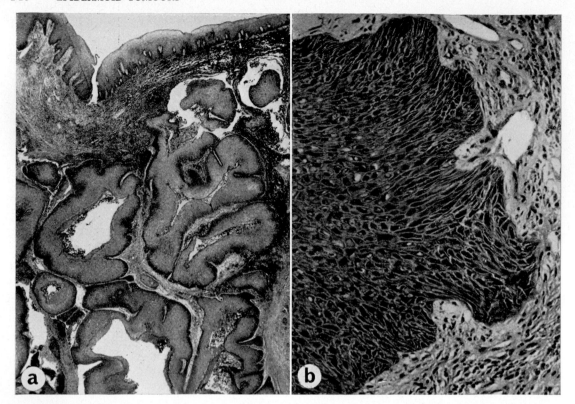

Fig. 55   **a,** verrucous carcinoma of the palate in a man aged 61. The lesion consists of convoluted and heaped-up folds of thickened squamous epithelium enclosing cleft-like spaces and small cystes. There is heavy chronic inflammatory infiltration in the surrounding connective tissue. × 13. **b,** higher magnification showing the well differentiated epithelium. × 200. This lesion was excised completely and the patient was well with no recurrence 18 months later.

is well differentiated. Epithelial pearls and small cysts are often seen but mitoses and cellular atypism tend to be rare. There is always heavy inflammatory infiltration in the adjacent connective tissue. The high degree of differentiation and the intact basement membrane make a diagnosis of carcinoma difficult, particularly if only superficial or small biopsy specimens are available. Deeper specimens will help to show the characteristic arrangement including, as Kraus and Perez-Mesa (1966) point out, the bulbous rete ridge pattern which serves to differentiate the lesion from pseudoepitheliomatous hyperplasia, in which the rete ridges are sharp-pointed and elongated. Moreover, the blunt processes all tend to infiltrate at more or less the same level, constituting the "pushing margin" described by Ackerman. Another feature, pointed out by Jacobson and Shear, is the manner in which the normal epithelium at the edge of the lesion is bent back upon itself by the continued growth of the tumour epithelium (Fig. 55).

Chronic hyperplastic candidosis may sometimes lead to appearances that are not dissimilar to verrucous carcinoma, but the epithelial hyperplasia is not so extensive as in the carcinoma and the cleft-like spaces often seen between the heaped-up masses of carcinomatous epithelium are not present in the hyperplastic condition. Chronic hyperplastic candidosis can of course be excluded if hyphae cannot be demonstrated, since they are abundantly present in the infection, but on the other hand their presence is not always discriminatory, since candidal infection of verrucous carcinoma is not uncommon.

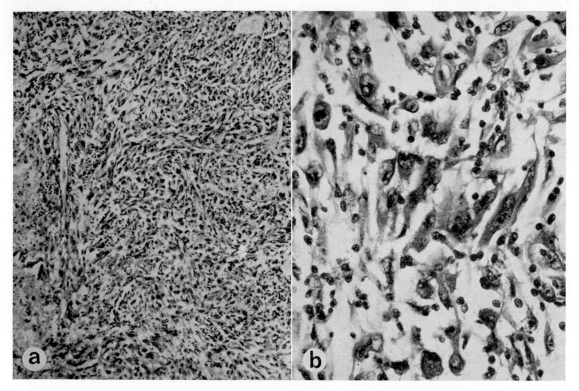

Fig. 56 **a, b,** spindle cell carcinoma of the antrum. × 80 and × 300.

In addition to pseudoepitheliomatous conditions, verrucous carcinoma must also be distinguished from well differentiated squamous cell carcinoma. The latter may resemble verrucous carcinoma very closely, but the presence of groups of cells showing less differentiated features should be sought. In such cases the usual course of development of squamous cell carcinoma is to be expected, with lymph node metastases.

The prognosis in verrucous carcinoma is very good, because of the absence, or very late appearance, of metastases. However, local recurrence is common in inadequately treated patients, so that excision must be sufficiently radical as to remove the entire lesion. Radiotherapy should not be used, since not only is local recurrence common but anaplastic changes may occur, with corresponding aggressive behaviour and metastasis (Perez and colleagues, 1966; Fonts and colleagues, 1969; Proffitt, Spooner and Kosek, 1970).

SPINDLE CELL CARCINOMA

Cells that are fusiform or spindle shaped are generally of mesodermal origin and accordingly neoplasms with spindle cells are usually either sarcomas or benign tumours of the mesodermal tissues. Very occasionally, however, carcinomas may be spindle celled, and tumours of this type have been reported in the breast, skin, oral mucosa, parotid, oesophagus, bronchus and cervix (Willis, 1967). These growths generally have a rather characteristic macroscopic appearance, since they are fleshy and polypoid. Microscopically, the immediate impression is of a sarcomatous tumour because of the dominance of spindle cells, often showing marked hyperchromatism, pleomorphism, increased and abnormal mitoses and tumour giant cells (Fig. 56). Areas showing the usual appearances of squamous cell carcinoma may be quite overshadowed by the exuberant mass of pseudosarcomatous tissue, and difficult to find.

The nature of the lesion is problematical. Martin and Stewart (1935) thought that the appearances could be due to radiation; many spindle cell tumours do occur in previously irradiated tissues but they can also occur in previously normal tissues. Lane (1957) reported a series of 10 cases in the upper respiratory tract, and considered that the pseudosarcomatous appearance was due to an exaggerated response in connective tissue and was not malignant. It was the associated squamous cell carcinoma, which might be quite inconspicuous, that was the important element. A similar line has been taken by Leake, Evans and Weisberger (1965) but Greene and Bernier (1959) believe that the spindle cell tissue can always be traced to continuity with the overlying epithelium if serial sections are examined. Sherwin, Strong and Vaugn (1963) also consider the pseudosarcomatous tissue to be epithelial. They believe that the polypoid nature of the growth is due to mucosal ulceration with granulation tissue overgrowth. Electron microscopy is also considered to support the epithelial nature of the spindle cells (Lichtiger, Mackay and Tessmer, 1970). On the other hand, Hudson and Winkelmann (1972) have reassessed 21 cases in which the original diagnosis was spindle cell carcinoma and considered 19 of them to be atypical fibroxanthomas.

In the oral tissues, lesions have been described in the lip (Greene and Bernier, 1959), floor of the mouth (Mittelman and colleagues, 1965; Snyder, Myers and Steinberg, 1974), tongue (Sherwin, Strong and Vaugn, 1963; Gelfman and Williams, 1969), and gingiva (Leake, Evans and Weisberger, 1965). Spindle cell carcinoma has a relatively good prognosis, because although metastases do occur, they are less frequent than in the usual type of squamous cell carcinoma.

ADENOID SQUAMOUS CELL CARCINOMA

This variant of squamous cell carcinoma generally occurs in the skin of the head and neck and occasionally the extremities. Recently, it has been described in the lip.

Most of the skin tumours have occurred in males over the age of 50, often of fair complexion and with an outdoor occupation, and there has frequently been a pre-existing senile keratosis or actinic keratosis. Tumours of the lip have been reported by Jacoway, Nelson and Boyers (1971), Tomich and Hutton (1972) and Weitzner (1974). As in the skin tumours, there was considered to be evidence of or susceptibility to solar damage in a number of patients with lip lesions. The lower lip is affected much more often than the upper and the tumour is always situated on the vermilion area, where it appears as an area of crusting or ulceration, or as a slightly elevated nodule. Microscopically, there is invasion of the corium by squamous cell carcinoma, but the proliferating tumour masses tend to undergo central acantholysis, so that cystic spaces containing desquamated cells are formed. The remaining tumour cells that border these spaces tend to be cuboidal and thus a pseudoglandular appearance results. There is heavy chronic inflammatory infiltration in the corium, which nearly always shows the basophilic degeneration typical of solar damage (Jacoway and colleagues).

Adenoid squamous cell carcinoma is a slowly growing neoplasm. From the small number of cases so far recorded, it would appear that the prognosis is good. No metastases have yet been reported.

INTRAEPIDERMAL CARCINOMA

Carcinoma in situ of the oral mucosa is characterised histologically by the changes of epithelial dysplasia affecting practically the whole thickness of the epithelium. Clinically, the condition may present as a white plaque that may not be in any way characteristic, revealing its potentialities only when examined microscopically. The significance of this condition is discussed on p. 122. In some cases the clinical appearances are those of a red patch on the mucosa, rather than a white one, and for this the term *erythroplakia* is used. Shear (1972) has extensively investigated this condition and recognises three clinical varieties; homogeneous erythroplakia, erythroplakia interspersed with patches of leukoplakia, and granular or speckled erythroplakia. Microscopically, erythroplakic patches, like the leukoplakias, may show a variety of changes. In some the epithelium shows no evidence of atypia, in others there are various grades of dysplasia, up to carcinoma in situ, and in some cases there is invasive carcinoma. Again, as with leukoplakia, some erythroplakic lesions may have nothing to do with cancer or pre-cancer, being purely inflammatory or of other non-neoplastic nature. Thus, there are many analogies with leukoplakia, but whereas only a small minority of leukoplakias are likely to show dysplasia, erythroplakias should be regarded with more suspicion, since the proportion of these lesions showing dysplastic changes is much greater. In Shafer and Waldron's (1975) series of 58 cases of homogeneous erythroplakia, no less than 91 per cent showed evidence of severe dysplasia, carcinoma in situ or invasive carcinoma.

Although now embraced in the general category of erythroplakia, *Queyrat's erythroplasia* is still sometimes used as the designation of certain mucosal lesions. In *Bowen's disease*, red lesions showing epithelial dysplasia occur in the skin; comparable lesions occur on the glans penis or in the mucosa of the clitoris or vulva. Oral lesions showing appearances similar to these skin lesions are rare, and have been reported under one or other of the designations. However, it would seem that both diseases are very similar, any differences being due mainly to differences in site, and Lever (1967) characterises Queyrat's erythroplasia as the term used for the lesions of Bowen's disease when these are situated either on the glans penis, the vulva or the oral mucosa. Gorlin (1950) has reviewed Bowen's disease of the oral tissues, where the lesions take the form of velvety erythematous patches which may be whitish if there has been keratinisation. The lesions may be flat or slightly raised, or they may be nodular, papillomatous or ulcerative. They occur anywhere in the oral mucosa, including the tongue and lips. Microscopically, the lesions show the same features as the commoner skin lesions. Further cases have been reported by Attenson and Kaufman (1966). Williamson (1964) reports cases of Queyrat's erythroplasia.

MULTICENTRIC ORAL CARCINOMA

Multiple primary tumours occur in about 10 per cent of patients with oral cancer, particularly in heavy smokers (Wynder, Bross and Feldman, 1957). This high proportion is probably due to the fact that the whole mucosa is so frequently in an abnormal state for long periods prior to the development of overt cancer, as Slaughter and colleagues (1946, 1953) have pointed out. In Sharp, Bullock and Helsper's (1961) 275 consecutive cases of oral cancer 28 patients (10 per cent) had multiple tumours and other lesions were frequently also present. The commonest finding was areas of atrophy, either adjacent to a carcinoma or randomly distributed. Acanthosis, hyperkeratosis, inflammation and fibrosis were also often found. Similarly, in Kraus and Perez-Mesa's (1966) series of 77 cases of verrucous carcinoma of the oral mucosa, 17 patients also had leukoplakia and 19 had additional neoplasms, in the mouth or elsewhere.

Oral carcinoma is also associated with primary carcinoma elsewhere in a proportion of cases. In Moertel, Dockerty and Baggenstoss's (1961) series of 723 patients with carcinoma in the oral cavity, 64 (8·7 per cent) had two or more discrete oral carcinomas and an additional 55 patients had independent carcinomas of the lip, pharynx or oesophagus, thus raising the overall occurrence rate of multiple lesions to 16·3 per cent. Multiple growths appear also to be associated with smoking. Wynder and colleagues (1969) have investigated 104 patients with multiple primary tumours of the upper alimentary and respiratory tracts and found that those patients who smoked heavily before developing cancer were more likely to develop second primary tumours. Silverman and Griffith (1972) report similar findings in their study of 174 patients.

Meyer and Shklar (1960) give a useful review of the literature of multiple growths. Horowitz and Chomet (1968) also review the subject and confirm that patients with intraoral carcinoma have more extraoral carcinomas than those without oral growths.

CARCINOMA IN THE JAWS

The great majority of carcinomas in the jaws are tumours that have arisen in adjacent structures such as gingiva, tongue or floor of mouth and have subsequently involved the bone by direct extension. Much less often, intraosseous carcinomas are metastatic deposits from distant sites such as the breast, thyroid, kidney or elsewhere. Rarely, intraosseous carcinomas are primary growths and they may remain as wholly intraosseous lesions, or they may in time perforate the bone and invade the adjoining soft tissues.

The possible sources of origin for primary intraosseous carcinomas are the lining of odontogenic cysts and epithelial rests (Fig. 57). Neoplasms of salivary tissue may also occur as intraosseous tumours; they are considered elsewhere (Ch. 30).

Carcinoma in odontogenic cysts

A number of cases have been reported in which a lesion diagnosed clinically and radiologically as an odontogenic cyst has proved to be carcinomatous on histological examination. Such a lesion may have been an originally non-neoplastic cyst in which carcinomatous change has subsequently developed or it might have been a neoplasm from the outset, in which secondary cystic degeneration has appeared. It is also possible that an adjacent carcinoma might involve an otherwise unrelated cyst. In many of the reported cases, especially the earlier ones, the purported demonstration of malignant change in a pre-existing non-neoplastic cyst is not convincing, but a number of recent case reports provide reasonable documentary and illustrative evidence of such change (Kay and Kramer, 1962; Ward and Cohen, 1963; Hankey and Pedler, 1957; Whitlock and Jones, 1967; Lee and Loke, 1967). Gardner (1969) reviews the literature; more recent reports include those by Chretien and colleagues (1970), Browne and Gough (1972), Hampl and Harrigan (1973) and Lapin and colleagues (1973).

Malignant change, when it does occur in odontogenic cysts, can presumably affect any of the cysts commonly found in the jaws. At the time of diagnosis, however, it is often difficult to be certain of the precise nature of the preexisting cystic lesion. Radicular, residual, dentigerous and primordial cysts have all been reported as undergoing malignant change. It has been suggested by Toller (1967) and others that the primordial cyst (odontogenic keratocyst) is more likely to develop malignancy than the other types of odontogenic cyst, although this requires substantiation.

Primary intra-alveolar carcinoma

Carcinomas arising as primary growths within the jaws, other than in connection with pre-existing cysts, are presumed to arise from cell rests of odontogenic epithelium or perhaps from enclaved epithelium at the sites of fusion of embryonic processes. Possible cases are reported by Aisenberg (1942), Campelia and Boyle (1943) and Jones and Whitlock (1968). Tumours of this type occur in children, grow rapidly and expand the jaw. The pulps of the developing teeth may

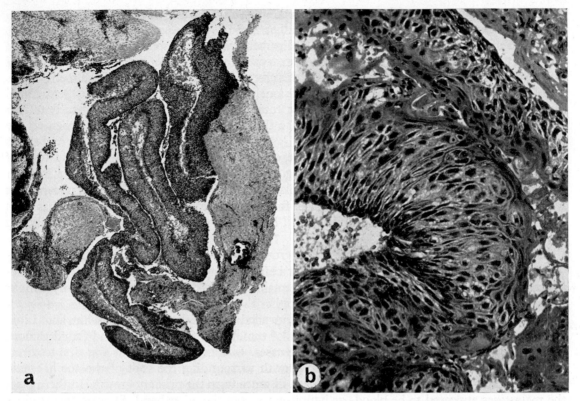

Fig. 57   Cystic carcinoma of the mandible in a woman of 45 years. A cyst had been removed from the canine-premolar region of the mandible 20 years previously; now there was swelling in the same area, of 3 months duration. At operation, a cyst was removed which showed changes in the lining suggestive of carcinoma. Nine months later the cyst had recurred and was again removed. The lining of the cyst consisted of keratinising squamous cell carcinoma, and a submandibular lymph node removed at the same time showed invasion by the tumour. Hemimandibulectomy was performed and the patient was alive and well 5 years later, **a, b,** the cyst wall consists of a regular layer of epithelium, but a higher power view shows this to be carcinomatous. × 25 and × 200.

be invaded. Cases in adults have been reported by Thoma (1938), Matheson (1951), Morrison and Deeley (1962), Willis (1967), Shear (1969) and De Lathouwer and Verhest (1974). The tumour appears to grow less rapidly than in children but eventually there may be widespread destruction. There is expansion of the jaw and ultimately perforation of the bone with ulceration of the tumour into the oral cavity. Pathological fracture may occur. Shear has recently reported six cases of intra-alveolar carcinoma and analyses 28 other cases from the literature. He points out that the histological appearances tend to be fairly characteristic, with features suggesting the origin of these growths from odontogenic epithelium. Thus, there is often an alveolar pattern or sometimes a plexiform arrangement, with palisading of the peripheral cells. Prickle cells are not seen in the majority of cases. However, these appearances cannot be regarded as specific, since they may sometimes be seen in carcinomas of the oral mucosa. Intra-alveolar carcinoma may also occur as typical squamous cell carcinoma (Sirsat, Sampat and Shrikhande, 1973).

Implication of the teeth by a neoplasm sometimes leads to the first clinical evidence of the presence of such a lesion. Loosening of the teeth is of course a very common occurrence, being due to periodontal disease in the great majority of cases. Occasionally, however, it is the result of invasion of the jaw by a neoplasm, with destruction of the alveolar bone around the roots of the

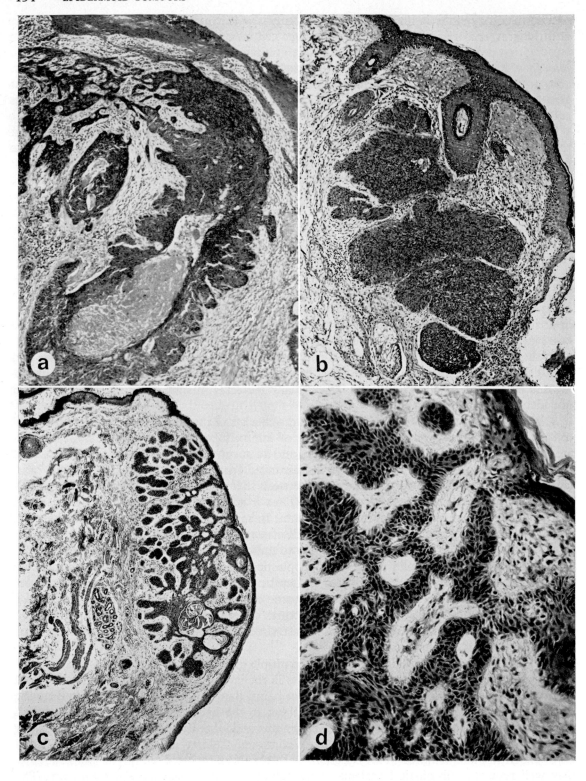

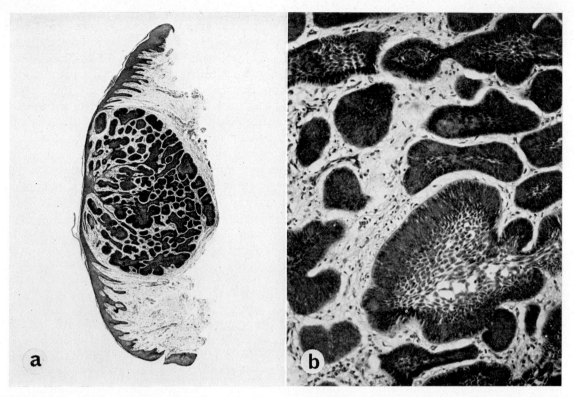

Fig. 59   Basal cell carcinoma of the lip. **a, b,** the general structure of the tumour is very similar to that of ameloblastoma. × 20 and × 120.

resemblances between basal cell carcinoma and ameloblastoma have already been mentioned (p. 46) On purely morphological grounds differential diagnosis between the two lesions may not be possible; the basal cell carcinoma of the skin of the lip illustrated in Fig. 59, for example, could very well be accepted as ameloblastoma were it an intraosseous tumour. The problems of histogenesis and taxonomy are discussed by Simpson (1974).

EXFOLIATIVE CYTOLOGY IN ORAL CANCER

Many investigators have claimed that oral cancer can be diagnosed by exfoliative cytology with a 95 per cent degree of accuracy (Pomeranz and Stahl, 1953; Silverman, Becks and Faber, 1958; Sandler and Stahl, 1958; Sandler, Freund and Stahl, 1959; Umiker and colleagues, 1960, Sandler, 1961). However, the results reported have not been consistent and more recently it has been shown that the false negative rate can be as high as 31 per cent (Hayes, Berg and Ross, 1969; Folsom and colleagues, 1972; Blozis, 1972; Reddy and colleagues, 1975). Similarly, the

Fig. 58   Various patterns of growth in basal cell carcinoma. **a,** a solid type of growth, with areas of squamous differentiation and keratin formation. × 50. **b,** another tumour of the solid type. × 50. **c,** a tumour of semi-cribriform type. × 30. **d,** detail from **c,** × 200.

diagnosis of precancerous lesions by exfoliative cytology is not a practicable procedure. Bánóczy (1969), Mehta and colleagues (1970), Dabelsteen and colleagues (1971) and others have shown that it is dangerous to rely on exfoliative cytology for this purpose, as there is very poor agreement between the cytological findings and the existence of epithelial dysplasia. While biopsy must therefore remain the only acceptable method for the definitive histological diagnosis of oral cancer, exfoliative cytology still has its uses. One application lies in deciding the site of biopsy in those cases in which a large area of the mucosa is abnormal. Leukoplakia may affect the mucosa extensively, but at the time of examination overt cancerous change may be confined to a relatively small area or areas and these are not obvious from naked-eye examination. It has been stated that sampling the exfoliated cells from a number of sites may give useful guidance as to the best site for biopsy. Another application has been indicated by Sandler and others, who have shown that cytological examination can demonstrate early evidence of recurrence of cancer after treatment, before macroscopic evidence has yet appeared, and can be used in distinguishing between a residual healing reaction or radionecrosis and carcinoma.

Apart from cancer diagnosis, exfoliative cytology can be useful in certain other lesions of the oral mucosa. These applications are discussed by Folsom and colleagues (1972).

REMOTE METASTASES OF ORAL CARCINOMA

It has often been said that cancer of the mouth does not metastasise below the clavicle but this generalisation is untrue, though visceral metastases from oral cancer are certainly uncommon in comparison with many other tumours and practically never occur in the early stages of the disease. Castigliano and Rominger (1954) have analysed a series of 752 cases of carcinoma in the oral cavity and have found that of the 321 patients known to have died of cancer, visceral metastases were present in 17, an incidence of 5·3 per cent. The organs chiefly involved were the lungs and bones. The incidence of visceral metastases, they consider, is probably increasing owing to improved treatment of the local lesion and its cervical metastases leading to a longer life span for these patients. Cade and Lee (1957) similarly note that remote metastases from carcinoma of the tongue are now more frequently observed. Willis (1967) found remote metastases in 8 of his 20 necropsies of cases of carcinoma of the tongue. The incidence of remote metastases in Topazian's (1961) series was 24 per cent of 83 cases. Carcinoma of the tonsil, floor of mouth, palate and tongue were the tumours that metastasised to distant sites with the greatest frequency. In another recent series (Hoye and colleagues, 1962) 55 per cent of 42 patients dying of carcinoma of the head and neck had distant metastases.

REFERENCES

Ackerman, L. V. (1948) Verrucous carcinoma of the oral cavity. *Surgery*, **23,** 670.
Adatia, D. K. (1968) Dental tissues and Burkitt's tumor. *Oral Surg.*, **25,** 221.
Ahlbom, H. E. (1936) Simple achlorhydric anaemia, Plummer-Vinson syndrome, and carcinoma of the mouth, pharynx and oesophagus in women. *Brit. med. J.*, **2,** 331.
Aisenberg, M. S. (1942) Malignant epithelial tumor in mandible of child aged 9. *Amer. J. Orthodont. (Oral Surg. Sect.)*, **28,** 736.
Andreasen, J. O. (1964) Oral manifestations in discoid and systemic lupus erythematosus. I. Clinical investigation. *Acta odont. scand.*, **22,** 298.
Andreasen, J. O. (1968) Oral lichen planus. I. A clinical evaluation of 115 cases. *Oral Surg.*, **25,** 31.
Andreasen, J. O. (1968) Oral lichen planus. II. A histologic evaluation of ninety-seven cases. *Oral Surg.*, **25,** 158.

Archard, H. O., Heck, J. W., and Stanley, H. R. (1965) Focal epithelial hyperplasia: an unusual oral mucosal lesion found in Indian children. *Oral Surg.*, **20**, 201.

Atkinson, L., Chester, I. C., Smyth, F. G., and ten Seldam, R. E. J. (1964) Oral cancer in New Guinea. A study in demography and etiology. *Cancer*, **17**, 1289.

Attenson, M., and Kaufman, M. (1966) Bowen's disease: evaluation of malignancy and report of two cases. *J. oral Surg.*, **24**, 258.

Baker, R., Cherry, J., Lott, S., and Bischofberger, W. B. (1966) Carcinoma of the maxillary sinus. *Arch. Otolaryngol.*, **84**, 201.

Bánóczy, J. (1969) Exfoliative cytologic changes in oral leukoplakia. *J. dent. Res.*, **48**, 17.

Beahrs, O. H., Devine, K. D., and Henson, S. W. (1959) Treatment of carcinoma of the tongue. End-results in 168 cases. *Arch. Surg.*, **79**, 399.

Bergenholtz, A. (1965) Multiple polypous hyperplasias of the oral mucosa with regression after removal of amalgam fillings. *Acta odont. scand.*, **23**, 111.

Bernier, J. L., and Clark, M. L. (1951) Squamous cell carcinoma of lip: critical statistical and morphological analysis of 835 cases. *Mil. Surgeon*, **109**, 379.

Bhaskar, S. N., Beasley, J. D., and Cutright, D. E. (1970) Inflammatory papillary hyperplasia of the oral mucosa: report of 341 cases. *J. amer. dent. Ass.*, **81**, 949.

Binnie, W. H., Cawson, R. A., Hill, G. B., and Soaper, A. E. (1972) *Oral Cancer in England and Wales. A National Study of Morbidity, Mortality, Curability and Related Factors.* Studies on Medical and Population Subjects No. 23. London. H.M.S.O.

Blozis, G. G. (1972) The value of exfoliative cytology in the diagnosis of oral cancer. *Internat. dent. J.*, **22**, 481.

Brown, H., and Gorlin, R. J. (1960) Oral mucosal involvement in nevus unius lateris (icthyosis hystrix). *Arch. Dermatol.*, **81**, 509.

Browne, R. M., and Gough, N. G. (1972) Malignant change in the epithelium lining odontogenic cysts. *Cancer*, **29**, 1199.

Cade, S. (1949) Malignant disease of the mouth. *Ann. roy. Coll. Surg. Engl.*, **4**, 381.

Cade, S., and Lee, E. S. (1957) Cancer of the tongue. A study based on 653 patients. *Brit. J. Surg.*, **44**, 433.

Cady, B., and Catlin, D. (1969) Epidermoid carcinoma of the gum. A 20-year survey. *Cancer*, **23**, 551.

Cahn, L., Eisenbud, L., and Blake, M. M. (1961) Histochemical analysis of white lesions of the mouth. I. The basement membranes. *Oral Surg.*, **14**, 596.

Campelia, C. M., and Boyle, P. E. (1943) Embryonal carcinoma primary in the mandible of a child with involvement of tooth pulp. *Amer. J. Orthodont. (Oral Surg. Sect.)*, **29**, 299.

Castigliano, S. G. (1968) Influence of continued smoking on the incidence of second primary cancers involving mouth, pharynx, and larynx. *J. amer. dent. Ass.*, **77**, 580.

Castigliano, S. G., and Rominger, C. J. (1954) Distant metastasis from carcinoma of the oral cavity. *Amer. J. Roentgenol.*, **71**, 997.

Cawson, R. A. (1966) Chronic oral candidiasis and leukoplakia. *Oral Surg.*, **22**, 582.

Cawson, R. A. (1969) Leukoplakia and oral cancer. *Proc. roy. Soc. Med.*, **62**, 610.

Chretien, P. B., Carpenter, D. F., White, N. S., Harrah, J. D., and Lightbody, P. H. (1970) Squamous cell carcinoma arising in a dentigerous cyst. Presentation of a fatal case and review of four previously reported cases. *Oral Surg.*, **30**, 809.

Clausen, F. P. (1969) Histopathology of focal epithelial hyperplasia. *Tandlaegebl.*, **73**, 1013.

Clausen, F. P., and Emmersten, M. (1973) Occurrence of focal epithelial hyperplasia among Amerindians in Ecuador. *Internat. J. oral Surg.*, **2**, 45.

Clausen, F. P., Møgeltoft, M., Roed-Petersen, B., and Pindborg, J. J. (1970) Focal epithelial hyperplasia of the oral mucosa in a South-West Greenlandic population. *Scand. J. dent. Res.*, **78**, 287.

Colman, R. S. (1951) Multiple polyps of the buccal mucous membrane. *Oral Surg.*, **4**, 466.

Cooke, R. A. (1969) Verrucous carcinoma of the oral mucosa in Papua-New Guinea. *Cancer*, **24**, 397.

Cranmer, L. R. (1953) Malignant neoplasms of the paranasal sinuses. *Arch. Otolaryngol.*, **58**, 704.

Cross, J. E., Guralnick, E., and Daland, E. M. (1948) Carcinoma of the lip. A review of 563 case records of carcinoma of the lip at the Pondville hospital. *Surg. Gynec. Obstet.*, **87**, 153.

Dabelsteen, E., Roed-Petersen, B., Smith, C. J., and Pindborg, J. J. (1971) The limitations of exfoliative cytology for the detection of epithelial atypia in oral leukoplakias. *Brit. J. Cancer* **25**, 21.

De Lathouwer, C., and Verhest, A. (1974) Malignant primary intraosseous carcinoma of the mandible. *Oral Surg.*, **37**, 77.

Dobbie, J. L. (1953) Carcinoma of the floor of the mouth. *Brit. J. Surg.*, **41**, 250.

often a moderate degree of chronic inflammatory infiltration in the sub-epithelial connective tissue, but this is rarely heavy. The range of microscopic appearances in these lesions is well described by Cutright (1974).

Behaviour

Fibrous overgrowths of the soft tissues are readily dealt with by simple excision but recurrence is not unusual if the whole lesion is not removed, together with any causal factor. The pregnancy tumour may regress spontaneously after childbirth. If it does not so do it may be excised. This is curative, though further lesions may appear in the same area in a subsequent pregnancy.

FIBROMATOSES

Overgrowths of fibrous tissue occur not only as true neoplasms or as circumscribed tumour-like though essentially non-neoplastic hyperplasias, but also as more diffuse lesions that may be ill-defined and that may even infiltrate adjacent normal tissues. These lesions, grouped together as the fibromatoses, often present problems both in diagnosis and in treatment. From the diagnostic aspect their infiltrative propensities may suggest a diagnosis of fibrosarcoma, and such a view may be strengthened by the microscopic appearances, which again are often very like those of fibrosarcoma. However, metastases do not occur, though in some types recurrences are frequent if the lesions are not completely excised.

Fibromatoses may be congenital or appear in later life.

Congenital Fibromatosis. Lesions consisting of rather diffuse overgrowths of fibrous tissue occur in infants, usually as solitary growths but sometimes multiple, and after the vascular tumours are the most common congenital tumours or tumour-like lesions. They occur most frequently in the head and neck region. Kauffman and Stout (1965) give a general account of these congenital fibromatous lesions, including lesions in the tongue and in the mandibular and submandibular regions. In one of their cases the infant had an infiltrating growth around the neck and jaw, with invasion of the mandible. A lesion of the floor of the mouth has been reported by Takagi and Ishikawa (1973).

Nodular Fasciitis. Lesions of the fibromatosis type occur in older children and adults in a variety of situations and some are quite well-known entities, for example, Dupuytren's fibromatosis of the palms of the hands and abdominal fibromatosis (abdominal desmoid). In the oral region such lesions are rare, though the variety known as nodular or pseudosarcomatous fasciitis has been reported in the mandibular region (Stokke, 1967; Henny and colleagues, 1969; Rakower, 1971; Miller, Cheris and Stratigos, 1975) and in the cheek (Lumerman, Bodner and Zambito, 1972; Solomon, Rosen and Delman, 1974). This condition usually occurs in the upper limb (about half the cases), trunk, lower limb or head and neck region. Appearing as a small lump, which may be painful, the lesion often enlarges rapidly, but only to a maximum size of some 4 cm, when it may remain stationary or regress. Microscopically the appearances may be very

---

Fig. 62   **a,** bony metaplasia is common in fibrous lesions of the oral mucosa. The photomicrograph shows osteoid and bone forming directly from the fibrous tissue. × 80. **b,** a more mature specimen, in which numerous bony trabeculae are present. × 30. **c,** pyogenic granuloma, showing the numerous dilated capillaries and inflammatory infiltration that are characteristic of this lesion. × 200. **d,** gingival hyperplasia in an epileptic patient under treatment with diphenylhydantoin. There is pronounced increase in the fibrous tissue of the gingiva and the epithelium is acanthotic, with long slender, often thread-like or branched, interpapillary processes. × 30.

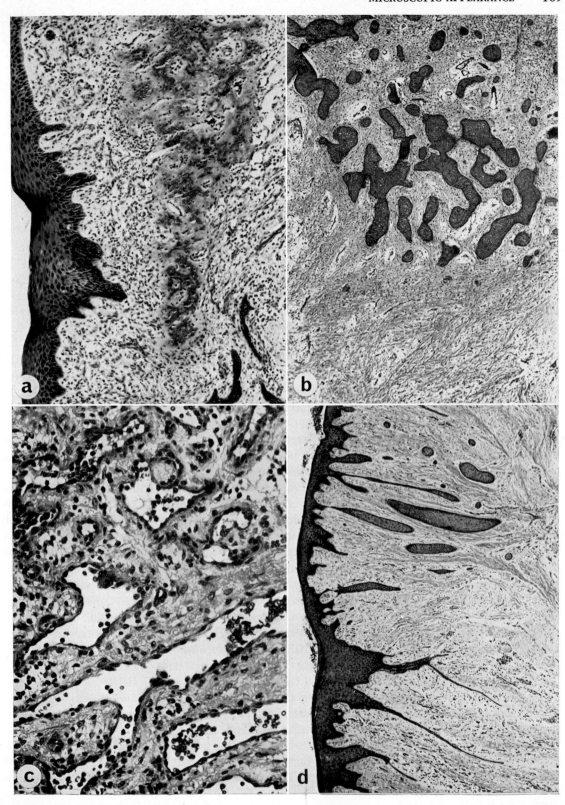

associated with unerupted teeth and is composed of fibroblastic tissue with, usually, relatively little collagen. The differentiation is not, however, of great practical importance for both lesions are benign, though there may be recurrence following incomplete removal.

The important differential diagnosis is from a well differentiated fibrosarcoma. That tumour may on cursory examination show a similar general pattern to fibroma but at least some mitotic figures and nuclear variation will be evident. Even when these features are absent, in very well differentiated tumours, the fibroblasts are always larger and plumper than in fibroma.

Odontogenic Fibroma. This tumour is considered to arise from mesenchymal dental tissue —periodontal ligament, dental papilla or dental follicle—on the grounds of its proximity to the teeth and its structural appearance. Generally, the tumour is situated in close relation to the root of a tooth or to the crown of an unerupted tooth, or a tooth may be congenitally missing from the area.

The tumour forms a circumscribed mass that may be enucleated complete, with an associated tooth or teeth. Tumours that are mainly fibroblastic are moderately firm and the cut surface is pinkish-white. Those in which there is much myxomatous tissue are soft, and when sectioned show a characteristic mucoid appearance. Microscopically, the tumour consists of rather primitive-appearing fibroblastic connective tissue, similar to that seen in the developing dental pulp. Between the evenly distributed plump fibroblasts there is a ground substance in which there is a variable quantity of collagen. In some cases collagen fibres may form quite a noticeable proportion of the tumour, but there is not usually as much collagenisation as in non-odontogenic fibroma. Small groups of epithelial cells, representing rests of dental epithelium, may be seen scattered about the tumour and serve to emphasise the odontogenic origin of the growth (Fig. 63). Epithelial elements of this type are not constantly present, however. An unusual gingival lesion reported by Baden and colleagues (1968) as gingival hamartoma may be of similar nature to the odontogenic fibroma, but occurring extraosseously. Similar lesions have also been reported by Gardner (1973) and Farman (1975).

The odontogenic fibroma is probably closely related to myxoma of the jaws. It grows slowly and painlessly and follows a benign course. Complete removal effects a cure.

MYXOMA

Tumours consisting either partly or wholly of myxomatous tissue may occur both in the soft tissues and in bone, but there is much difference of opinion as to whether such lesions are in fact distinct pathological entities. Some pathologists (Stout, 1948; Dutz and Stout, 1961; Evans, 1966) regard the myxoma as a tumour of primitive mesenchyme, whereas for others such a tumour does not exist. Thus Willis (1967) considers that there is no such cell as a "myxoblast", as distinct from a fibroblast, and that therefore the myxoma is not a specific tumour. According to this author, tumours of myxomatous appearance are in most cases nothing but fibromas or fibrosarcomas in which much mucin has developed. Also, intercellular mucin may appear in other mesenchymal tumours, particularly those originating from fat or cartilage.

Myxomatous tumours are not very common. The most frequent sites of occurrence are skin and subcutaneous tissue and striated muscle, and tumours may also occur in bone. In most cases myxoma is a solitary tumour; occasionally multiple tumours may occur and in such cases there may also be present fibrous dysplasia of bone. Therefore, skeletal survey should be undertaken in such cases. The association of multiple myxomas and fibrous dysplasia may be due to an underlying connective tissue dysplasia that predisposes to both conditions (Wirth and colleagues, 1971).

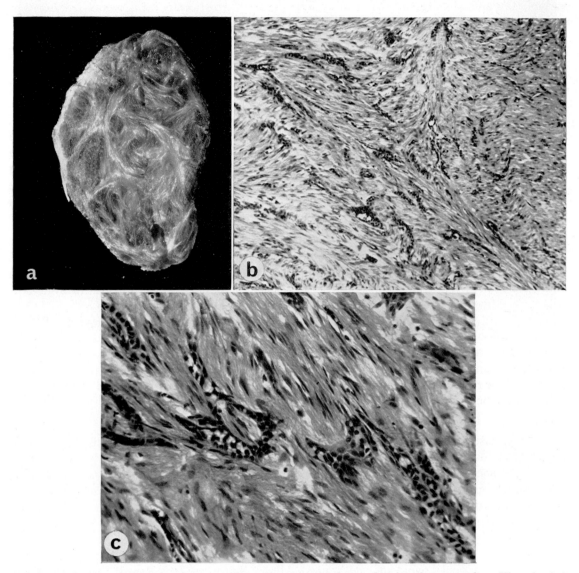

Fig. 63 Odontogenic fibroma of the maxilia. **a,** the gross specimen, showing the cut surface. The whorled, interlacing bands of fibrous tissue are well seen. Natural size. **b,** numerous strands of epithelial cells are interspersed between the bundles of fibrous tissue. × 80. **c,** higher magnification showing the groups of odontogenic epithelial cells. × 200.

case reports describing such lesions may be mentioned those of Harbert, Gerry and Dimette (1949), Hovnanian (1953), Brewer and Johnston (1955) and Miglani and Ballantyne (1959). Dutz and Stout (1961) include examples of myxoma of the jaws in their paper on the myxoma in childhood.

More frequently, a variable amount of collagen is present and a number of cases appear in the literature under the designation of fibromyxoma. Strands or nests of epithelial cells of odontogenic type may be scattered here and there throughout the myxomatous or fibromyxomatous tissue (Fig. 64). Bone may be present, rarely, as in the two cases seen by Large, Niebel and Fredericks (1960). Publications that include reviews of the literature are those of Bruce and Royer (1952), Astaff (1953), Sirsat (1954), Schultz and Vazirani (1957), Lund and Waite (1966) and Harrison and Eggleston (1973). Zimmerman and Dahlin (1958) give a very useful account of 26 cases and Barros, Dominguez and Cabrini (1969) review in detail 95 cases.

Zimmerman and Dahlin (1958) have attempted to divide myxomatous tumours into benign and malignant types, using as criteria the numbers of binucleate cells and mitotic figures, the degree of cellularity and the presence of nuclear hyperchromatism. However, typing of this kind does not appear to yield useful results.

Histogenesis

The association of the tumour with unerupted or missing teeth, its occurrence in younger persons and the presence on occasion of odontogenic epithelium indicate that in most cases it arises from dental tissues. A possible origin from non-dental mesenchyme must also be considered but cases of this type are probably very rare.

Although it is now generally believed that myxomatous tumours in other parts of the body are basically fibromas or other neoplasms in which there has been an accumulation of intercellular mucin, this argument almost certainly does not apply in comparable terms to myxoma of the jaw. The considerations just mentioned indicate that this tumour arises from dental mesenchyme, which it closely resembles, and hence the myxomatous appearance is in fact a resemblance to the tissue of origin and not the result of secondary changes in some other tissue. It is of course possible that myxomatous change may occur in an odontogenic fibroma, but that tumour also arises from dental mesenchyme. Bernier (1959) suggested that the myxoma is the less differentiated tumour and that myxofibroma and fibroma are the result of further differentiation with collagen production. On the other hand, Cahn (in Radden and Reade, 1962) believes that the myxoma of the jaws is a dysplastic condition akin to fibrous dysplasia, being a myxoid variant of that condition. Hodson and Prout (1968) believe that the tumour is a genuine neoplasm derived from the myxoblast, which they consider to be a mesenchymal cell that is metabolically different from the sulphated mucopolysaccharide-collagen-producing fibroblast; the myxoblast is an active mucopolysaccharide-secreting cell and the mucin in the tumour is not derived from degenerating fibroblasts or collagen. Harrison (1973) has investigated the histochemistry and ultrastructure of the tumour and found that many of the cells in the myxomatous tissue have prominent rough endoplasmic reticulum and seem to be actively secretory. Cells containing collagen fibrils were also seen. White and colleagues (1975) also concluded that the tumour cells were metabolically active, and responsible for secreting the myxomatous element of the lesion, and Simes and colleagues (1975) considered the jaw tumour to be distinct from other connective tissue tumours. Westwood and colleagues (1974), however, who have also studied the histochemistry and ultrastructure, believe the proliferating cell of the neoplasm to be a fibroblast. There is, therefore, a considerable amount of uncertainty about the basic nature of the tumour. However, it does seem that myxomatous tumours in the jaws are lesions peculiar to these bones, not directly comparable with myxomatous lesions elsewhere.

Behaviour

Myxoma of the jaws is generally a slowly growing lesion, but occasional tumours behave more aggressively or take on accelerated growth (Hayward, 1955; Dutz and Stout, 1961). Infiltrative growth is often a feature of the tumour, as noted, and probably accounts for the appreciable proportion of recurrences in some series (e.g., Sonesson, 1950; Zimmerman and Dahlin, 1958; Barros and colleagues, 1969). Cawson (1972) reports a patient with a mandibular tumour, followed for 35 years. There were recurrences after attempted excisions over a prolonged period.

Although extensive resections are not indicated (Kangur, Dahlin and Turlington, 1975), complete removal of all tumour tissue must be ensured, and when this has been done the prognosis is good. There should then be no recurrences, and metastases do not occur. Myxomatous tumours in other parts of the body seem much more prone to recur than the jaw tumour, as Thoma and Goldman (1947) have noted. Doubtless this is due to the fact that some of these tumours are sarcomas with secondary myxomatous change. This again points to the distinct nature of the jaw tumour.

Myxoma of the Soft Tissues

Very few examples of myxomatous tumours of the oral soft tissues have been recorded. These include tumours of the soft tissues over the mandible (Daniels, 1908), the palatal soft tissues (Tholen, 1936; Babbitt and Pfeiffer, 1937), the cheek (Spengos and Schow, 1965), lip (Traiger and Lawson, 1969). Fibromyxoma of the palate has been reported by Sealey (1948) and Salama and Hilmy (1951) and gingiva (Tashinoğlu and colleagues, 1975). Bernier (1960) illustrates a myxoma of the interdental soft tissues extending into the adjacent bone.

It is hardly possible to discuss the nature of these growths on the basis of the scanty and incomplete reports available. They may well fall into the same category as myxomatous tumours elsewhere, with reason for regarding them as fibromas with intercellular mucinous changes (Fig. 65).

FIBROSARCOMA

Some of the problems attached to the diagnosis of fibrous tumours have already been mentioned (p. 163); it is clear that this is in an area where a change of emphasis and outlook has been taking place over the years. In a recent report from the Mayo Clinic, for example, Pritchard and colleagues (1974) reviewed the records and material from 330 patients whose soft tissue tumours had been diagnosed as fibrosarcoma between the years 1910 and 1968. In 113 cases they revised the diagnosis, to other types of sarcoma or to other entities. So far as tumours of the oral tissues are concerned, many of the reported cases are rather poorly documented and illustrated; taking also into account changing ideas, it is difficult to be sure how many of the reported cases of fibrosarcoma of the soft tissues or of the jaws would survive as such if they could be reassessed.

Fibrosarcoma may occur anywhere in the oral cavity. Sometimes these lesions resemble at first the familiar benign fibrous overgrowths, since at the outset they may be relatively circumscribed, but they grow more rapidly than the benign lesions, produce a larger tumour and are prone to ulceration. In Fletcher and Crabb's (1961) case the tumour, a gingival growth, presented in just the same way as an ordinary fibrous epulis. Metastatic growth was present in a regional node. Eversole, Schwartz and Sabes (1973) have tabulated from the literature 20 reports of soft tissue fibrosarcoma; they point out that some of these tumours may well have been lesions that would now be classified under designations such as histiocytoma, fibromatosis, fasciitis or the like. However, taking the cases on their reported assessment as fibrosarcoma, they found that they occurred equally in the sexes, in both adults and children. There was a 69 per cent 5-year survival rate.

Postradiation fibrosarcoma has occurred in the oral tissues, usually in the tongue, following radiotherapy for carcinoma (Castigliano, 1968). Other cases of fibrosarcoma of the tongue are cited by Nagy (1973).

Fibrosarcoma of the jaws usually occurs in the mandible. Only three histologically documented cases have been reported in the maxilla (Richardson, Fine and Goldman, 1972). In some cases implication of bone is the result of invasion, but in others the tumour arises intraosseously, from the outset (Fig. 65). The cases in the literature are tabulated by Eversole and colleagues and by MacFarlane (1972), who reports a patient with a mandibular tumour and pulmonary metastases. Males have been affected more often than females, in the small number of cases so far reported. Ages have ranged from infancy up to 73 years. The symptoms include pain and swelling and loosening of teeth, with an ill-defined radiolucent bone defect. Most of the reported tumours had not metastasised; however, local recurrence is a distinct danger, although it may be long delayed, as in Hamilton's (1945) patient, who died from recurrent fibrosarcoma of the mandible 16 years after the tumour was first noticed. The prognosis for jaw tumours has appeared to be rather better than is the case for other bones. Dahlin and Ivins (1969) reviewed 114 cases of fibrosarcoma of bone, including 13 tumours of the mandible. The 5-year survival rate of 28·7 per cent was better than that for osteosarcoma, and the 5- and 10-year rates for the mandibular tumours were 40 per cent and 25 per cent as against 28·7 per cent and 21·6 per cent for the whole series. However, Eversole has calculated only a 27 per cent 5-year survival rate for the published jaw tumours that have the requisite information. Van Blarcom, Masson and Dahlin (1971) also stress the propensity for local recurrence. Since metastasising growths are very rare, it does seem that the long term prognosis could be considerably improved by sufficiently radical surgery.

Amongst the single case reports are those of Hamilton (1945), Stuteville (1955), Vazirani and Bolden (1958), Gingrass and Hinz (1961), Hoggins and Brady (1962), Van Wyk and Jonck (1964) and Reade and Radden (1966).

REFERENCES

Angelopoulos, A. P. (1971) Pyogenic granuloma of the oral cavity; statistical analysis of its clinical features. *J. oral Surg.*, **29**, 840.

Angelopoulos, A. P., and Goaz, P. W. (1972) Incidence of diphenylhydantoin gingival hyperplasia. *Oral Surg.*, **34**, 898.

Agazzi, C., and Belloni, L. (1951) Non-osteogenic fibroma of the jaw. *Ann. Otol.*, **60**, 365.

Astaff, A. (1953) Myxofibroma. *Oral Surg.*, **6**, 247.

Babbitt, J. A., and Pfeiffer, D. B. (1937) Myxoma of the palate and pharynx. *Arch. Otolaryngol.*, **26**, 453.

Babcock, J. R., Commiskey, L. V., and White, G. O. (1966) Oral bilateral symmetrical fibromas. Report of a case. *Oral Surg.*, **21**, 4.

Baden, E., Moskow, B. S., and Moskow, R. (1968) Odontogenic gingival epithelial hamartoma. *J. oral Surg.*, **26**, 702.

Fig. 65   **a**, myxoma of the palate. This small tumour presented as a pedunculated mass, slightly flattened against the palate by the tongue. × 11. **b**, showing the myxomatous appearance of the tumour tissue. × 200. **c**, fibrosarcoma of the mandible in a woman of 30 years. The mandible was resected and the patient was well with no recurrence 12 years later. The radiograph shows an osteolytic lesion destroying the alveolar ridge and invading the anterior half of the ascending ramus. **d**, showing well differentiated fibrosarcoma. × 200.

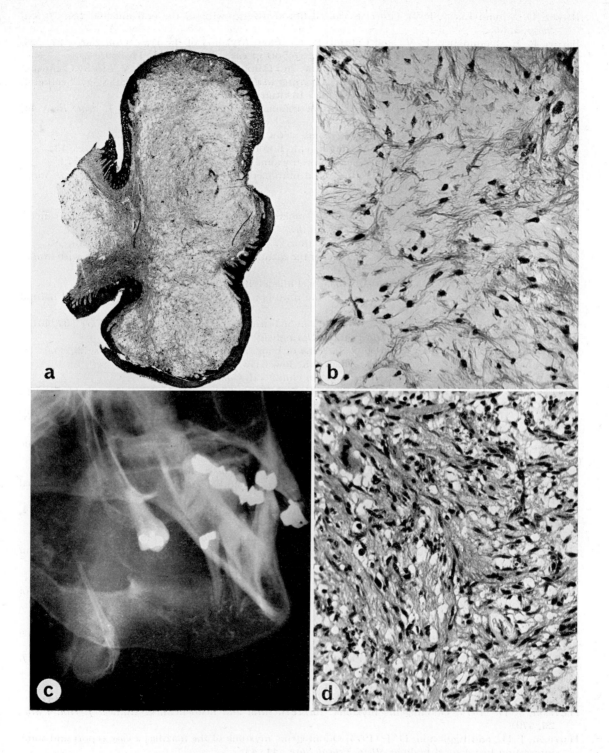

Barker, D. S., and Lucas, R. B. (1967) Localised fibrous overgrowths of the oral mucosa. *Brit. J. oral Surg.*, **5**, 86.

Barros, R. E., Dominguez, F. V., and Cabrini, R. L. (1969) Myxoma of the jaws. *Oral Surg.*, **27**, 225.

Beers, M. D. (1953) Bilateral fibroma of the palate: report of case. *J. oral Surg.*, **11**, 330.

Bernier, J. L. (1959) *The Management of Oral Disease.* 2nd Edition. St. Louis. The C. V. Mosby Company.

Bernier, J. L. (1960) *Tumors of the Odontogenic Apparatus and Jaws.* Atlas of Tumor Pathology. Section 4. Fascicle 10a. Washington, D.C. Armed Forces Institute of Pathology.

Bhaskar, S. N., and Lilly, G. E. (1962) Effect of traumatic injuries on rat tongue. *J. dent. Res.*, **40**, 64.

Brewer, A. C., and Johnston, J. H. (1955) Myxoma of the mandible. *Brit. J. Surg.*, **43**, 325.

Bruce, K. W., and Devine, K. D. (1955) Odontogenic fibroma: report of a case. *J. oral Surg.*, **13**, 73.

Bruce, K. W., and Royer, R. Q. (1952) Central fibromyxoma of the maxilla. *Oral Surg.*, **5**, 1277.

Burch, R. J., and Woodward, H. W. (1960) Central fibroma of mandible: report of a case. *J. oral Surg.*, **18**, 432.

Cahn, L. R. (1962) See Radden and Reade.

Castigliano, S. G. (1968) Influence of continued smoking on the incidence of second primary cancers involving mouth, pharynx and larynx. *J. amer. dent. Ass.*, **77**, 580.

Cawson, R. A. (1972) Myxoma of the mandible with a 35 year follow-up. *Brit. J. oral Surg.*, **10**, 59.

Colburn, J. F., and Epker, B. N. (1975) Myxoma of the mandibular condyle—surgical excision with immediate reconstruction. *J. oral Surg.*, **33**, 351.

Colby, R. A. (1956) *Color Atlas of Oral Pathology.* Philadelphia. Lippincott.

Cooke, B. E. D. (1952) The fibrous epulis and the fibro-epithelial polyp: their histogenesis and natural history. *Brit. dent. J.*, **93**, 305.

Cutright, D. E. (1974) The histopathologic findings in 583 cases of epulis fissuratum. *Oral Surg.*, **37**, 401.

Dahlin, D. C. (1967) *Bone Tumors.* 2nd Edition. Springfield, Ill. Charles C. Thomas.

Dahlin, D. C., and Ivins, J. C. (1969) Fibrosarcoma of bone. A study of 114 cases. *Cancer*, **23**, 35.

Daniels, D. W. (1908) A case of pure myxoma of the lower jaw. *Lancet*, **2**, 1747.

Dutz, W., and Stout, A. P. (1961) The myxoma in childhood. *Cancer*, **14**, 629.

Emerson, T. G. (1965) Hereditary gingival hyperplasia. A family pedigree of four generations. *Oral Surg.*, **19**, 1.

Evans, R. W. (1966) *Histological Appearances of Tumours.* 2nd Edition. London and Edinburgh. E. & S. Livingstone Ltd.

Eversole, L. R., Schwartz, W. D., and Sabes, W. R. (1973) Central and peripheral fibrogenic and neurogenic sarcoma of the oral regions. *Oral Surg.*, **36**, 49.

Farman, A. G. (1975) The peripheral odontogenic fibroma. *Oral Surg.*, **40**, 82.

Farrer-Brown, G., Lucas, R. B., and Winstock, D. (1972) Familial gingival fibromatosis: an unusual pathology. *J. oral Path.*, **1**, 76.

Fletcher, J. P., and Crabb, H. S. M. (1961) Fibrosarcomatous epulis. Report of a case. *Oral Surg.*, **14**, 1091.

Fogh-Andersen, P. (1943) Fibroma symmetrica gingivalis. *Tandlaegebladet*, **47**, 145.

Gardner, D. G. (1973) An ameloblastoma and a hamartoma of the dental lamina in two siblings. *J. oral Surg.*, **31**, 697.

Giansanti, J. S., McKenzie, W. T., and Owens, F. C. (1973) Gingival fibromatosis, hypertelorism, anti-mongoloid obliquity, multiple telangiectases and cafe au lait pigmentation; a unique combination of developmental anomalies. *J. Perio.*, **44**, 299.

Gingrass, R. P., and Hinz, L. E. (1961) Fibrosarcoma of the mandible. *J. oral Surg.*, **19**, 241.

Griffith, J. G., and Irby, W. B. (1965) Desmoplastic fibroma. Report of a rare tumor of the oral structures. *Oral Surg.*, **20**, 269.

Gusterson, B. A., and Greenspan, J. S. (1974) Multiple polypoid conditions of the oral mucosa. *Brit. J. oral Surg.*, **12**, 91.

Hamilton, I. (1945) Fibro-sarcoma of the lower jaw. *Aust. & N.Z.J. Surg.*, **15**, 54.

Harbert, F., Gerry, R. G., and Dimette, R. M. (1949) Myxoma of the mandible. *Oral Surg.*, **2**, 1414.

Harrison, J. D. (1973) Odontogenic myxoma: ultrastructural and histochemical studies. *J. clin. Path.*, **26**, 570.

Harrison, J. D., and Eggleston, D. J. (1973) Odontogenic myxoma of the maxilla; a case report and some interesting histological findings. *Brit. J. oral Surg.*, **11**, 43.

Hayward, J. R. (1955) Odontogenic myxofibroma of the mandible: report of a case. *J. oral Surg.*, **13**, 149.

Hayward, J. R. (1973) Multiple recurrent fibro-osseous epulides. *Int. J. oral Surg.*, **2**, 115.

Henny, F. A., Catone, G. A., Walker, R. V., and Epker, B. N. (1969) Pseudosarcomatous fasciitis: report of three cases. *J. oral Surg.*, **27**, 196.

Hiebert, A. E., and Brooks, H. W. (1950) Fibroma of the palate. *Plast. reconstr. Surg.*, **5**, 532.

Hinds, E. C., Kent, J. N., and Fechner, R. E. (1969) Desmoplastic fibroma of the mandible: report of case. *J. oral Surg.*, **27**, 271.

Hodson, J. J., and Prout, R. E. S. (1968) Chemical and histochemical characterization of mucopolysaccharides in a jaw myxoma. *J. clin. Path.*, **21**, 582.

Hoggins, G. S., and Brady, C. L. (1962) Fibrosarcoma of maxilla. Report of a case. *Oral Surg.*, **15**, 34.

Hora, J. F., and Weller, W. A. (1961) Extranasopharyngeal juvenile angiofibroma. *Ann. Otol. Rhinol. Laryngol.*, **70**, 164.

Hovnanian, A. P. (1953) Myxoma of the maxilla. Report of two cases. *Oral Surg.*, **6**, 927.

Jaffe, H. L. (1958) *Tumors and Tumorous Conditions of the Bones and Joints.* London, Henry Kimpton.

Kangur, T. T., Dahlin, D. C., and Turlington, G. (1975) Myxomatous tumors of the jaws. *J. oral Surg.*, **33**, 523.

Kauffman, S. L., and Stout, A. P. (1965) Congenital mesenchymal tumors. *Cancer*, **18**, 460.

Large, N. D., Niebel, H. H., and Fredericks, W. H. (1960) Myxoma of the jaws. Report of two cases. *Oral Surg.*, **13**, 1462.

Lee, K. W. (1968) The fibrous epulis and related lesions. Granuloma pyogenicum, "pregnancy tumour", fibro-epithelial polyp and calcifying fibroblastic granuloma. A clinico-pathological study. *Periodontics*, **6**, 277.

Lichtenstein, L. (1972) *Bone Tumors.* 4th Edition. St. Louis. The C. V. Mosby Company.

Lumerman, H., Bodner, B., and Zambito, R. (1972) Intraoral (submucosal) pseudosarcomatous nodular fasciitis. Report of a case. *Oral Surg.*, **34**, 239.

Lund, B. A., and Waite, D. B. (1966) Mandibular myxoma: report of case. *J. oral Surg.*, **24**, 454.

MacFarlane, W. I. (1972) Fibrosarcoma of the mandible with pulmonary metastases: a case report. *Brit. J. oral Surg.*, **10**, 168.

McIndoe, A., and Smith, B. O. (1958) *Brit. J. plastic Surg.*, **11**, 62.

Mackenzie, D. H. (1964) Fibroma: a dangerous diagnosis. A review of 205 cases of fibrosarcoma of soft tissues. *Brit. J. Surg.*, **51**, 607.

Mark, H. I. (1955) Central fibroma of the mandible. Case report with a brief review of the literature. *Oral Surg.*, **8**, 366.

Miglani, D. C., and Ballantyne, A. J. (1959) Myxoma of the mandible, followed by resection and prosthetic repair. Report of a case. *Oral Surg.*, **12**, 1032.

Miller, R., Cheris, L., and Stratigos, G. T. (1975) Nodular fasciitis. *Oral Surg.*, **40**, 399.

Nagy, L. T. (1973) Fibrosarcoma of the tongue. *Int. J. oral Surg.*, **2**, 303.

Perko, M., Uehlinger, E., and Hjørting-Hansen, E. (1969) Nasopharyngeal angiofibroma of the maxilla: report of case. *J. oral Surg.*, **27**, 645.

Pritchard, D. J., Soule, E. H., Taylor, W. F., and Ivins, J. C. (1974) Fibrosarcoma—a clinicopathologic and statistical study of 199 tumors of the soft tissues of the extremities and trunk. *Cancer*, **33**, 888.

Rabhan, W. N., and Rosai, J. (1968) Desmoplastic fibroma. Report of ten cases and review of the literature. *J. Bone Jt. Surg.*, **50A**, 487.

Radden, B. G., and Reade, P. C. (1962) Odontogenic myxoma of the jaw. *Oral Surg.*, **15**, 355.

Rakower, W. (1971) Fasciitis, an unusual diagnosis, and the clinician's dilemma: report of case. *J. oral Surg.*, **29**, 503.

Ramon, Y., Berman, W., and Bubis, J. J. (1967) Gingival fibromatosis combined with cherubism. *Oral Surg.*, **24**, 435.

Reade, P. C., and Radden, B. G. (1966) Oral fibrosarcoma. *Oral Surg.*, **22**, 217.

Richardson, J. F., Fine, M. A., and Goldman, H. M. (1972) Fibrosarcoma of the mandible: a clinicopathologic controversy: report of case. *J. oral Surg.*, **30**, 664.

Rushton, M. A. (1957) Hereditary or idiopathic hyperplasia of the gums. *Dent. Practit.*, **7**, 136.

Salama, N., and Hilmy, A. (1951) Cases from the clinic of the Cairo dental school. *Oral Surg.*, **4**, 966.

Schultz, L. W., and Vazirani, S. J. (1957) Central odontogenic fibromyxoma of the mandible. Report of a case. *Oral Surg.*, **10**, 690.

Sealey, V. T. (1948) An unusual tumour on the palate. *Aust. J. Dent.*, **52**, 177.

Shafer, W. G., Hine, M. K., and Levy, B. M. (1974) *A Textbook of Oral Pathology.* 3rd Edition. Philadelphia and London. W. B. Saunders Company.

Silverman, L. M. (1958) Odontogenic fibroma of the maxilla. Report of a case. *Oral Surg.*, **11**, 128.

Simes, R. J., Barros, R. E., Klein-Szanto, A. J. P., and Cabrini, R. L. (1975) Ultrastructure of an odontogenic myxoma. *Oral Surg.*, **39**, 640.

Sirsat, M. V. (1954) Central myxoma of the jaw. Report of a case. *Ind. J. med. Sci.*, **8**, 639.

Solomon, M. P., Rosen, Y., and Delman, A. (1974) Intraoral submucosal pseudosarcomatous fibromatosis. *Oral Surg.*, **38**, 264.

Sonesson, A. (1950) Odontogenic cysts and cystic tumours of the jaws. *Acta radiol.*, Suppl. 81.

Southam, J. C., and Venkataraman, B. K. (1973) Calcification and ossification in epulides in man (excluding giant cell epulides). *Arch. oral Biol.*, **18**, 1243.

Spengos, M. N., and Schow, C. E. (1965) Myxomas of the soft tissues. Report of a case of myxoma in the cheek. *J. oral Surg.*, **23**, 140.

Stewart, D. J., and O'Brien, F. V. (1973) Juvenile angiofibroma. Report of a case occurring within the mouth. *J. Dent.* **1**, 150.

Stokke, T. (1967) Pseudosarcomatous fibromatosis of the jaw. A case report. *Norske tannlaegef. Tid.*, **77**, 85.

Stones, H. H. (1962) *Oral and Dental Diseases*. 4th Edition. Edinburgh and London. E. & S. Livingstone Ltd.

Stout, A. P. (1948) Fibrosarcoma. The malignant tumor of fibroblasts. *Cancer*, **1**, 30.

Stout, A. P. (1948) Myxoma, the tumor of primitive mesenchyme. *Ann. Surg.*, **127**, 706.

Stout, A. P. (1953) *Tumors of the Soft Tissues*. Atlas of Tumor Pathology. Section 2. Fascicle 5. Washington, D.C. Armed Forces Institute of Pathology.

Stuteville, O. H. (1955) Fibrosarcoma of the mandible. Report of a case. *Quart. Bull. Northwestern Univ. med. School*, **29**, 400.

Tahsinoğlu, M., Çöloğlu, A. S., and Kuralay, T. (1975) Myxoma of the gingiva: a case report. *Brit. J. oral Surg.*, **13**, 95.

Takagi, M., and Ishikawa, G. (1973) Fibrous tumor of infancy—report of a case originating in the oral cavity. *J. oral Path.*, **2**, 293.

Tholen, E. F. (1936) Myxomata of the jaw and pharynx. *Trans. amer. laryng. rhin. otol. Soc.*, 608.

Thoma, K. H., and Goldman, H. M. (1947) Central myxoma of the jaw. *Amer. J. Orthont. (Oral Surg. Sect.)*, **33**, 532.

Thoma, K. H., and Goldman, H. M. (1960) *Oral Pathology*. 5th Edition. London. Henry Kimpton.

Thoma, K. H., Holland, D. J., and Rounds, C. E. (1947) Tumors of the mandibular condyle: report of two cases. *Amer. J. Orthodont.*, **33**, 597.

Traiger, J., and Lawson, W. (1969) Soft-tissue myxoma of the oral cavity. Report of a case. *Oral Surg.*, **27**, 247.

Vazirani, S. J., and Bolden, T. E. (1958) Oral fibromyxosarcoma of the maxilla. Report of a case. *Oral Surg.*, **11**, 227.

Van Blarcom, C. W., Masson, J. K., and Dahlin, D. C. (1971) Fibrosarcoma of the mandible. A clinicopathologic study. *Oral Surg.*, **32**, 428.

Van Wyk, C. W., and Jonck, L. M. (1964) A peripheral fibrosarcoma of the upper jaw and a central fibrosarcomatous tumour of the lower jaw. *J. dent. Ass. S. Africa*, **19**, 18.

Wesley, R. K., Wysocki, G. P., and Mintz, S. M. (1975) The central odontogenic fibroma. Clinical and morphologic studies. *Oral Surg.*, **40**, 235.

Westwood, R. M., Alexander, R. W., and Bennett, D. E. (1974) Giant odontogenic myxofibroma. Report of a case with histochemical and ultrastructural studies and a review of the literature. *Oral Surg.*, **37**, 83.

White, D. K., Chen, S.-Y., Mohnac, A. M., and Miller, A. S. (1975) Odontogenic myxoma. A clinical and ultrastructural study. *Oral Surg.*, **39**, 901.

Whitlock, R. I. H. (1961) Angiofibroma of cheek. *Brit. dent. J.*, **111**, 372.

Willis, R. A. (1967) *Pathology of Tumours*. 4th Edition. London. Butterworth & Co. (Publishers) Ltd.

Winstock, D. (1965) Hereditary gingivo-fibromatosis. *Brit. J. oral Surg.*, **2**, 59.

Wirth, W. A., Leavitt, D., and Enzinger, F. N. (1971) Multiple intramuscular myxomas. Another extraskeletal manifestation of fibrous dysplasia. *Cancer*, **27**, 1167.

Zimmerman, D. C., and Dahlin, D. C. (1958) Myxomatous tumors of the jaws. *Oral Surg.*, **11**, 1069.

Liposarcoma is very rar
in the cheek and tumours h
and colleagues, 1960), soft

The term osteoma is us
that increase in size by
ultimate complete ossif
known causes such as
membrane bones and i
growths in different bc

Clinical Features

In the jaws, the os
from the bone, or as a
involved than the max
age of 40 than in you
from producing facial
Gross and Miller (197

Radiologically, the
truding from the bone

Pathology

The subperiosteal t
smooth surface that is
or by quite a slender
of bone that is preser
perhaps some thicker
appears whitish-yellov
within the bone, whic

Microscopically, th
intervening fatty or fi
bone with very few m

Histogenesis

Many authors expl
designation of osteom
different conditions l
pletely ossified osteo
fibrous dysplasia lesio
which do have some

Traditionally, oste
according to anatomic
lesions fell into one
of osteoma in these
with radiographic ev

Brooke, R. I., and MacGreg
    28, 223.
Browne, W. G. (1970) Herni
Bruce, K. W., and Royer, R
    930.
Cameron, A. L. (1921) Lipoi
    case. *J. amer. med. Ass.*,
Clawson, J. R., Kline, K. K
    pad into the mouth: rep
Correia, P. de C. (1956) Rec
Csiba, A. (1967) Buccal lipor
Desmond, A. M. (1947) A c
Dutescu, N., Georgescu, L.,
    plasia. *Oral Surg.*, **35**, 6
Duvoir, M., Pollet, L., and
    symétrique. *Bull. Soc. n*
Enterline, H. T., Culberson
    and pathological study c
Greer, R. O., and Richardson
    A review and report of c
Hart, J. A. L. (1973) Intraos
Hatziotis, J. C. (1971) Lipor
Horton, J. E. (1968) Lipoma
Hughes, C. L. (1966). Intrac
Johnson, E. C. (1969) Intrac
Lawson, H. P. (1942) Lipom
MacGregor, A. J., and Dysc
    new cases. *Oral Surg.*,
Newman, C. W. (1957) Fibr
Oringer, M. J. (1948) Lipom
Panders, A. K., and Scherpe
Ransohoff, J. (1917) Congen
Salzer, M., and Salzer-Kunt
    path. Anat., **132**, 365.
Samuels, H. S., and Oatis,
Sauk, J. J. (1971) Liposarcol
Seldin, H. M., Seldin, S. L
    J. oral Surg., **25**, 270.
Shapiro, D. N. (1969) Lipor
Shear, M. (1967) Lipoblasto
Stout, A. P. (1944). Liposar
Vellios, F., Baez, J., and S
    from hibernoma. Repor
    Amer. J. Path., **34**, 114
Wehrle, D. P., Emmings, F.
    Oral Surg., **20**, 138.

17. Tumours of Adipose Tissue

Although tumours of adipose tissue are the commonest benign neoplasms, until quite recently they have been considered very unusual growths in the mouth. However, in the last few years there have been published appreciable numbers of case reports and also some larger series. These are reviewed by Hatziotis (1971) and subsequent reports are cited by Greer and Richardson (1973).

Generally, the lipoma is a solitary lesion occurring in an adult, usually in the subcutaneous tissue, particularly of the upper part of the trunk, neck and arms, though it may occur anywhere. Much less commonly lipomas occur in internal organs or tissues, for instance the kidney, adrenal, mesentery or retroperitoneal tissues. Sometimes lipomas are multiple, but very often multiple and sometimes symmetrically disposed deposits of fat are not true neoplasms but are congenital anomalies or are due to endocrine or other abnormalities. Conditions of such nature, referred to as lipomatoses, include the symmetrical masses of fat that sometimes occur around the neck in middle-aged men, and the painful deposits of fat in women in Dercum's disease. Congenital lesions in infants may consist of mature fat, as in adults, or sometimes of immature adipose tissue.

In the oral tissues, the lipoma generally occurs as a solitary tumour though it may also occur as part of a multiple lipomatosis. The tumour usually originates in the submucous fat and grows out into the oral cavity as a round or ovoid mass with a smooth surface. The tumour may be lobulated and may be broadly based or it may have a relatively narrow pedicle. Owing to the thinness of the overlying epithelium the yellow coloration of the fat can often be seen through the mucosa. The tumour has a characteristic soft yet elastic consistency and on section the cut surface shows the usual appearance of adipose tissue. Microscopically, the tumour consists of large cells, often so filled with fat that the nucleus is flattened against the cell wall. The tumour cells are arranged in lobules with an intervening connective tissue stroma. Often this is quite delicate and of minimal quantity, but this is very variable and in some tumours there may be an appreciable fibrous tissue element (Fig. 66). Osseous metaplasia may rarely occur (Hughes, 1966; Dutescu and colleagues, 1973).

The lipoma may occur almost anywhere in the soft tissues of the mouth. The cheek and tongue account for about one-half of the published cases, the floor of mouth being the next most frequent site. Lingual tumours are often more deeply situated than tumours of the other oral tissues, since they tend to occur well within the substance of the tongue, and the muscle fibres may be intimately intermingled with the tumour tissue. Multiple lingual tumours have been recorded (Duvoir, Pollet and Herrenschmidt, 1937; Desmond, 1947; Wehrle, Emmings and Koepf, 1965). Lipoma also occurs in the lip, palate, and gingiva. The literature is reviewed by Bruce and Royer (1954), and MacGregor and Dyson (1966) have published a comprehensive review of 57 cases. Subsequent cases have been reported by Panders and Scherpenisse (1967), Csiba (1967), Horton (1968), Shapiro (1969) and Samuels and Oatis (1969) among others. Seldin and colleagues (1967) report a series of 26 cases.

Ransohoff (1917) and Cameron (1921) have reported congenital fatty lesions in the cheek in infants. These appear to be overgrowths, or possibly true neoplasms, of the buccal sucking pad. This normal fatty structure is situated between the buccinator and masseter muscles in infants and sometimes persists throughout life. Willis (1967) has recorded a lipomatous growth below the angle of the mandible in an infant aged 5 months. The adipose tissue contained salivary tissue,

Fig. 66 Lipoma
culated lump in t
fat-containing cel

which had been in
Yoshimura and col
lipoblastomatosis.
pointed out that
However, in certa
may still persist at
mass, the conditio
Shear (1967).

The possibility
noted by Brooke
pedunculated fatty
ately preceding th
through both the
fat. Similar cases
(1970).

Lipoma of bor
reported over a
Oringer (1948), N
(1942) and Salzer

Miles, A. E. W. (1
Mohnac, A. M. (1
Offer, O., and Bac
    Rev. Stomat.,
Paddison, G. M.,
    supervoltage
Paterson, W. (195
Pincus, P. (1938)
Pittman, M. R., a
    443.
Potdar, G. G., an
Ramon, Y., Lern
    of a case. Or
Richter, K. J., Fr
    report of cas
Ringertz, N. (193
    Acta otolaryi
Robinson, H. B.
    (Oral Surg.
Roper-Hall, H. 1
Rosen, M. D. (1
Rowe, N. L. (19
    two cases. B
Salvador, A. H.,
    on 30 new c
Sandler, H. C. (
Schutt, P. G., a
Shackelford, R.
    Surg. Gynec
Shackelford, R.
    process. J.
Spjut, H. J., Do
    Atlas of Tu
    Pathology.
Strang, C., and
    Jt. Surg., 3
Thoma, K. H.
    mas. Int. J.
Vassar, P. S. (1
Willis, R. A. (1
Yoel, J., and Pt

gene is involved (Krahl, 1949), and Suzuki and Sakai (1960) have found that where both parents had either palatal or mandibular tori, the prevalence in the children was 63·9 per cent and 58·6 per cent respectively.

Torus palatinus occurs as a flat, lobulated or nodular ridge of bone, sometimes with a median groove, extending anteroposteriorly in the midline of the palate. The mandibular torus forms a bony ledge on the inner aspect of the mandible, extending towards the midline from the pre-molar region. It is often present bilaterally. Microscopically, tori consist of lamellae of compact bone of normal structure. An inner core of cancellous bone may be present in the larger speci-mens.

Although often discovered quite late in life, it is thought that torus palatinus originates about puberty and undergoes its period of most active growth in early adult life. Even so, its general rate of growth is very slow. Torus mandibularis is also of very slow growth. These lesions are not usually treated actively unless interfering with dentures.

OSTEOMATOSIS

Multiple osteomas may occur, rarely, in the oral tissues, usually as a feature of Gardner's syndrome (Fitzgerald, 1943; Gardner, 1951; Gardner and Richards, 1953; Plenk and Gardner, 1954; Gorlin, Chaudhry and Kelln, 1960). In this condition, which is familial, bony tumours appear in the maxilla, mandible, and other cranial bones. The tumours consist of dense mature cortical bone with normal haversian systems, no cartilage being present. In addition to the cranial osteomas, diffuse cortical thickenings of long bones may occur. Multiple fibromas of the skin and epidermal and sebaceous cysts also form part of the syndrome, as does polyposis coli. Multiple impacted supernumerary and permanent teeth have been found in both jaws (Fader and colleagues, 1962). The colonic polypi in cases of osteomatosis show a pronounced tendency to malignant change. This is in contrast to the polypi in the Peutz-Jeghers syndrome (Peutz, 1921; Jeghers, McKusick and Katz, 1949), which is characterised by the occurrence of polypi in the small intestine and melanosis of the buccal mucosa, lips and perioral region. Here, the polypi very seldom become malignant (see also p. 284). Recent illustrative case reports of Gardner's syndrome include those of Rayne (1968), Amato and Small (1970), Davies (1970) and Halse, Roed-Petersen and Lund (1975).

Multiple osteomas can also occur in the absence of other abnormalities. MacLennan and Brown (1974) report a patient with three osteomas of the mandible; none of the other features of Gardner's syndrome were present.

Multiple osteomas may occur, rarely, in the soft tissues. Meskin, Peterson and Gorlin (1964) report a case in which there were lesions in the skin of the scalp, deltoid, gluteal and cervical regions, together with lesions in the palate, gingiva and buccal mucosa.

OSTEOID OSTEOMA AND OSTEOBLASTOMA

Osteoid osteoma was first characterised by Jaffe and Mayer (1932) and Jaffe (1935); previously, the condition was probably diagnosed as chronic osteomyelitis, non-suppurative osteomyelitis, chronic bone abscess, or the like. Osteoid osteoma occurs most frequently between the ages of 10 and 25 years, affects males at least twice as commonly as females, and lesions of the femur and the tibia together account for about one-half of all cases. In the remaining cases, the lesion occurs in other limb bones, ribs or vertebrae. It is rare in the jaws.

Pain is a very characteristic feature of osteoid osteoma, and this is relieved by aspirin (though the same is also true of some other bone lesions). The radiological appearances are also characteristic, showing a central radiolucent area, generally referred to as the nidus, surrounded by a zone of sclerosis. The nidus is round or ovoid, and may show evidence of spotty calcification. The surrounding sclerosis may vary from a narrow zone to a more extensive area of several centimetres.

These lesions are generally excised complete, and histological examination shows the nidus of osteoid tissue surrounded by, and quite sharply demarcated from, the adjacent zone of reactive sclerotic bone. The nidus itself measures up to 1 cm in diameter and consists of an interlacing meshwork of osteoid trabeculae, with an intervening vascular connective tissue stroma. Numerous osteoblasts are usually present, and also osteoclasts in some areas.

With regard to lesions in the jaws, Jaffe (1958) considered that most of the reported cases represent a focus of osteocementum occurring around a tooth, and not the genuine lesion. However, Foss, Dockerty and Good (1955) have reported a case of osteoid osteoma of the mandible in a woman age 26, the lesion being situated close to the lower border of the bone away from the roots of the teeth. The clinical, radiological and pathological features were typical of osteoid osteoma as seen in the usual sites. Another mandibular lesion has been reported by Jurgens (1968), but although the clinical and radiological features are consistent with osteoid osteoma, the photomicrographs are not conclusive. A maxillary lesion has been reported by Brynolf (1969).

After its initial growth, to a diameter not exceeding 1 cm, the lesion becomes stationary, but continues to be painful. The treatment is excision, which relieves the pain immediately and is curative.

Osteoblastoma (giant osteoid osteoma) was first described by Lichtenstein (1951) as osteogenic fibroma and subsequently by Dahlin and Johnson (1954) as giant osteoid osteoma and by Jaffe (1956) and Lichtenstein (1956) as benign osteoblastoma. This condition was considered to differ from osteoid osteoma in being a progressive lesion with a greater tendency to cause local expansion of bone and less painful than osteoid osteoma, and histologically showing marked vascularity, a more orderly pattern of the osteoid trabeculae and more osteoblasts, but no surrounding zone of reactive bone formation. However, there is now a growing body of opinion that there are no definitive histological differences between the two lesions, except for size. One centimetre is taken as the arbitrary upper limit of size for osteoid osteoma, larger lesions being considered as osteoblastomas (Flaherty, Pugh and Dockerty, 1956; Lichtenstein, 1964; Byers, 1968). Like osteoid osteoma, osteoblastoma is rare in the jaws. Maxillary tumours have been reported by Borello and Sedano (1967), Kent, Castro and Girotti (1969) and Yip and Lee (1974). Mandibular lesions have been reported by Kramer (1967), Anand, Davey and Cohen (1967), Byers (1968), Brady and Browne (1972), Smith (1972) and Remagen and Prein (1975). A mandibular tumour in the coronoid processes has been recorded by Kopp (1969).

OSTEOSARCOMA

Although osteosarcoma is the commonest of the primary malignant neoplasms of bone it is still a comparatively rare tumour and is less common in the jaws than in many other bones. In New and Cabot's (1935) series of 295 tumours of the maxilla and antrum, 9 were fibrosarcomas or osteosarcomas. Seventeen of Geschickter's (1935) 323 jaw tumours were osteosarcomas. Richards and Coleman (1957) surveyed the literature and found 50 cases reported as osteosarcoma, but only 17 were sufficiently documented to permit confirmation of the diagnosis. Later case reports and series (Garrington and colleagues, 1967; Potdar, 1970) indicate that appreciably more examples of jaw tumours have been recognised in recent years.

Clinical Features

Osteosarcoma in general occurs in young persons, usually between the ages of 10 and 30 years, though sometimes older patients are affected, up to the age of 50 or 60 years or over. Kragh, Dahlin and Erich (1958) found a higher age incidence in their series of 44 tumours of the jaws and facial bones, the average age being just over 33 years. Garrington and colleagues (1967) in their analysis of 56 cases of osteosarcoma of the jaws found the average age incidence to be about a decade later than for osteosarcoma in other bones and this was also so in Potdar's series and in Roca, Smith and Jing's (1970) twenty cases.

Osteosarcoma occurs most frequently in the lower end of the femur, other common sites being the upper ends of the tibia, humerus and fibula. However, any bone may be affected. In the jaws, mandibular tumours are commoner than maxillary growths. The tumour presents as a swelling that enlarges fairly rapidly and may be accompanied by pain, numbness of the lip and chin due to involvement of the inferior alveolar nerve by mandibular tumours, limitation of movement, displacement and loosening of teeth and, in the case of maxillary tumours, nasal obstruction and pressure on the eye. Ulceration of the skin or oral mucosa occurs only in the late stages. A history of antecedent trauma is often obtained, but here as in other sites the question of a causal relationship remains open.

The radiological appearances of osteosarcoma are variable. In the so-called sclerosing types of growth much tumour bone is formed and the radiograph shows evidence of excessive bone formation, sometimes with a "sun-ray" appearance. This is due to the formation of laminae of bone, deposited in a radiating manner around the periphery of the lesion. Although this radiological sign is well known, it is not always present in osteosarcoma and may indeed be seen in other conditions. In growths that are predominantly osteolytic the appearances are almost entirely those of an area of bone destruction. However, a combination of these appearances is often noted, areas of radiolucency and radiopacity being interspersed. The cortical plates of bone are at first expanded and later perforated (Fig. 73). Garrington and colleagues (1967) have noted that symmetrical widening of the periodontal ligament about one or more teeth may be an early sign of osteosarcoma, appearing before any other radiographic changes are evident.

Pathology

Osteosarcoma has traditionally been classified as medullary or periosteal, depending upon the site of origin within the affected bone. However, it is usually impossible to make such a distinction in pathological material, since by the time of operative treatment the growth has generally infiltrated the affected area of bone, including the periosteum, and invaded the soft tissues. Microscopically, sclerosing and osteolytic types of growth have been recognised, according to the degree of new bone formation or destruction, and fibroblastic, telangiectatic, osteoblastic and chondroblastic types have also been described. The value of such histological subdivision is problematic, since there is little correlation with prognosis, but it indicates the variability of the cellular pattern that may be encountered. What does emerge from the many clinico-pathological studies and attempts to correlate the histological picture with clinical course and prognosis, is that despite all the cellular variability the one essential feature of osteosarcoma is the formation of tumour bone by malignant osteoblasts (Fig. 73). These neoplastic osteoblasts are spindle-shaped or polyhedral, are generally larger than normal osteoblasts and show nuclear hyper-chromatism and pleomorphism. Mitoses may or may not be frequent. The number of tumour cells is very variable. They may more or less rim the trabeculae of newly formed bone, much as

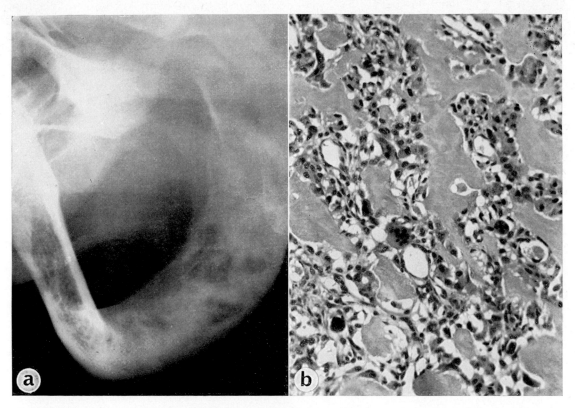

Fig. 73   Osteosarcoma of the mandible in a man of 63 years. There was a swelling of the jaw of some weeks duration. **a,** the radiograph shows loss of the normal bony pattern of the mandible, with numerous irregular areas of radiolucency interspersed with areas of osteosclerosis. This type of radiological picture could also be caused by Paget's disease. **b,** microscopic examination shows osteoblasts of varying size and shape, many having hyperchomatic nuclei and mitoses. Osteoid and coarse immature bone is being formed. × 200. A year after excision there was a recurrence in the submandibular region.

normal osteoblasts relate to normal bony trabeculae, though this is uncommon, or they may be so numerous as to make the tumour almost entirely cellular. In such cases, where the tumour cells tend to be spindle-shaped, fibrosarcoma may be closely simulated, but there can usually be found some tumour bone formation, even if only in very small quantity. The newly formed tumour bone is very variable in quantity and in structure, forming masses of osteoid and osseous tissue, with the osteoblasts irregularly distributed throughout. In the so-called chondroblastic growths much cartilage may be present, but here again at least some malignant bone formation will be found. In the telangiectatic types of growth numerous large and poorly formed blood vessels are present.

Apart from fibrosarcoma and chondrosarcoma, fibrous dysplasia is the other condition that has to be kept in mind in the histological diagnosis of osteosarcoma. Sometimes these lesions are very cellular, especially in young patients, but the fibrous tissue of the lesion, despite the cellularity, and the osteoid and bone that develop from it, do not show any of the histological signs of malignancy. Sarcoma has developed in connection with fibrous dysplasia and other lesions in various bones, including the jaws, usually following radiotherapy (Arlen and colleagues, 1971).

The serum alkaline phosphatase level may be raised in patients with osteosarcoma, and the tumour tissue itself may be shown to have a high alkaline phosphatase content.

Parosteal osteosarcoma. This is a rare but special type of osteosarcoma that warrants separate consideration, since the prognosis is much better than for osteosarcoma of the usual type.

As the name implies, the tumour grows from the external surface of a bone, and consists of well formed bony trabeculae in a fibrocellular stroma. This fibroblastic stroma is also well differentiated but does contain cells showing nuclear hyperchromatism and mitoses, though these are not always numerous. Parosteal osteosarcoma grows slowly and metastasises late. Mandibular tumours have been reported by Som and Peimer (1961), Hofmann (1966) and Roca, Smith and Jing (1970).

Extraskeletal osteosarcoma. Osteosarcoma may, very rarely, develop in the soft tissues as an extraosseous growth. A tumour of this type in the lip has been reported by Parsons and Henthorne (1944).

Relationship to Pre-existing Bone Disease

Pre-existing Paget's disease accounts for a number of cases of osteosarcoma in older patients. According to Willis (1967), between 5 and 10 per cent of patients with this condition ultimately develop osteosarcoma or other sarcomas in bone. However, Porretta, Dahlin and Janes (1957) found an incidence of only 0·9 per cent of sarcoma supervening on Paget's disease in the Mayo Clinic cases. Though Paget's disease affects the jaws not infrequently osteosarcoma developing in jaw lesions is very rare, and the few reported cases have involved the mandible (Karpawich, 1958; Wilner and Sherman, 1965; Rosenmertz and Schare, 1969).

Postradiation osteosarcoma may occur in the jaws. The bone may have been normal at the outset of treatment, the radiation having been given for a soft tissue lesion such as carcinoma of the gingiva (Cruz, Coley and Stewart, 1957), cervico-facial actinomycosis (Jones, 1953) or keloids (Sabanas and colleagues, 1956; Kragh and colleagues, 1958), or there may have been a lesion in the bone itself. Thus osteosarcoma has followed radiation treatment of fibrous dysplasia, giant cell granuloma (Cahan and colleagues, 1948; Sabanas and colleagues, 1956) and other tumours (Arlen and colleagues, 1971). The interval between radiation and the appearance of osteosarcoma has varied between 6 and 21 years.

These few cases indicate that the incidence of postradiation sarcoma is very low in the jaws (as it is in other bones), considering the extent to which radiation has been used in the treatment both of bone lesions and of soft tissue lesions which involve the incidental radiation of adjacent normal bone. Perhaps, as Cahan and colleagues point out, few patients with cancer of the mouth, jaws and neck survive long enough for postradiation sarcomas to develop. It is clear that radiotherapy should not ordinarily be used for benign lesions.

It may be noted here that though a case of fibrosarcoma of the mandible following irradiation of a carcinoma of the gingiva has been reported by Kaae and Glahn (1949), no other types of neoplasm, apart from the osteosarcomas, have been recorded in the jaws following radiation. It is of interest to note in this connection that Rushton and colleagues (1961) were able to produce osteosarcomas in the jaws of rabbits by administration of ^{90}Sr, but no tumours arose from the dental tissues.

Behaviour

Osteosarcoma is a highly malignant growth. Metastases occur at an early stage and the five-year survival rate is only between 10 and 20 per cent. Metastases generally occur in the lungs, but may be found in other organs, including the brain, and in other bones.

In the jaws, the prognosis is better than in other bones. Kragh, Dahlin and Erich found a five-year survival rate of at least 25 per cent, as compared with 19 per cent in a series of osteosarcomas that excluded the jaws (Coventry and Dahlin, 1957). They thought that this better prognosis might be due to the later systemic spread shown by jaw tumours, and a relatively low average degree of histological malignancy. A better prognosis for jaw tumours has also been noted by Garrington and colleagues, who found a 35 per cent five-year survival rate in 34 patients.

The prognosis for mandibular growths has been found in all series to be better than for maxillary tumours. This may be due to the more accessible situation of the former (Gomez, Youmans and Chambers, 1960). Chambers and Mahoney (1970) report good results from the use of intensive local irradiation followed by wide surgical resection.

REFERENCES

Amato, A. E., and Small, E. W. (1970) Oral manifestations of Gardner's syndrome: report of case. *J. oral Surg.*, **28**, 458.

Anand, S. V., Davey, W. W., and Cohen, B. (1967) Tumours of the jaws in West Africa. *Brit. J. Surg.*, **54**, 901.

Arlen, M., Higinbotham, N. L., Huvos, A. G., Marcove, R. C., Miller, T., and Shah, I. C. (1971) Radiation-induced sarcoma of bone. *Cancer*, **28**, 1087.

Borello, E. D., and Sedano, H. O. (1967) Giant osteoid osteoma of the maxilla. Report of a case. *Oral Surg.*, **23**, 563.

Brady, C. L., and Browne, R. M. (1972) Benign osteoblastoma of the mandible. *Cancer*, **30**, 329.

Brynolf, I. (1969) Osteoid osteoma and fibrous dysplasia in the periapical region of maxillary incisors. Report of three cases. *Oral Surg.*, **28**, 243.

Byers, P. D. (1968) Solitary benign osteoblastic lesions of bone. Osteoid osteoma and benign osteoblastoma. *Cancer*, **22**, 43.

Cahan, W. G., Woodward, H. Q., Higinbotham, N. L., Stewart, F. W., and Coley, B. L. (1948) Sarcoma arising in irradiated bone; report of eleven cases. *Cancer*, **1**, 3.

Chambers, R. G., and Mahoney, W. D. (1970) Osteogenic sarcoma of the mandible: current management. *Amer. Surg.*, **8**, 463.

Coventry, M. B., and Dahlin, D. C. (1957) Osteogenic sarcoma. A critical analysis of 430 cases. *J. Bone Jt. Surg.*, **39A**, 741.

Cruz, M., Coley, B. L., and Stewart, F. W. (1957) Postradiation bone sarcoma. Report of eleven cases. *Cancer*, **10**, 72.

Dahlin, D. C., and Johnson, E. W. (1954) Giant osteoid osteoma. *J. Bone Jt. Surg.*, **36A**, 559.

Davies, A. S. (1970) Gardner's syndrome—a case report. *Brit. J. oral Surg.*, **8**, 51.

Drennan, M. R. (1938) The torus mandibularis in the Bushman. *J. Anat.*, **72**, 66.

Fader, M., Kline, S. N., Spatz, S. S., and Zubrow, H. J. (1962) Gardner's syndrome (intestinal polyposis, osteomas, sebaceous cysts) and a new dental discovery. *Oral Surg.*, **15**, 153.

Fitzgerald, G. M. (1943) Multiple composite odontomes coincidental with other tumorous conditions: report of a case. *J. amer. dent. Ass.*, **30**, 1408.

Flaherty, R. A., Pugh, D. G., and Dockerty, M. B. (1956) Osteoid osteoma. *Amer. J. Roentgenol.*, **76**, 1041.

Foss, E. L., Dockerty, M. B., and Good, C. A. (1955) Osteoid osteoma of the mandible. Report of a case. *Cancer*, **8**, 592.

Gardner, E. J. (1951) A genetic and clinical study of intestinal polyposis, a predisposing factor for carcinoma of the colon and rectum. *Amer. J. hum. Genet.*, **3**, 167.

Gardner, E. J., and Richards, R. C. (1953) Multiple cutaneous and subcutaneous lesions occurring simultaneously with hereditary polyposis and osteomatosis. *Amer. J. hum. Genet.*, **5**, 139.

Garrington, G. E., Scofield, H. H., Cornyn, J., and Hooker, S. P. (1967) Osteosarcoma of the jaws. Analysis of 56 cases. *Cancer*, **20**, 377.

Geschickter, C. F. (1935) Tumors of the jaws. *Amer. J. Cancer*, **26**, 90.

Gomez, A. C., Youmans, R. D., and Chambers, R. G. (1960) Osteogenic sarcoma of the mandible. A method of treatment. *Amer. J. Surg.*, **100**, 613.

Gorlin, R. J., Chaudhry, A. P., and Kelln, E. E. (1960) Oral manifestations of the Fitzgerald–Gardner, Pringle–Bourneville, Robin, adrenogenital, and Hurler–Pfaundler syndromes. *Oral Surg.*, **13**, 1233.

Green, A. E., and Bowerman, J. E. (1974) An osteoma of the mandible. *Brit. J. oral Surg.*, **12**, 225.

Halse, A., Roed-Petersen, B., and Lund, K. (1975) Gardner's syndrome. *J. oral Surg.*, **33**, 673.

Hofmann, W. B. (1966) Osteogenic sarcoma of the mandible. *Arch. Otolaryngol.*, **84**, 439.

Jaffe, H. L. (1935) "Osteoid-osteoma." A benign osteoblastic tumor composed of osteoid and atypical bone. *Arch. Surg.*, **31**, 709.

Jaffe, H. L. (1956) Benign osteoblastoma. *Bull. Hosp. Jt. Dis.*, **17**, 141.

Jaffe, H. L. (1958) *Tumors and Tumorous Conditions of the Bones and Joints.* London. Henry Kimpton.

Jaffe, H. L. and Mayer, L. (1932) An osteoblastic osteoid tissue forming tumor of a metacarpal bone. *Arch. Surg.*, **24**, 550.

Jeghers, H., McKusick, V. A., and Katz, K. H. (1949) Generalized intestinal polyposis and melanin spots of the oral mucosa, lips and digits. A syndrome of diagnostic significance. *New Engl. J. Med.*, **241**, 993, 1031.

Jones, A. (1953) Irradiation sarcoma. *Brit. J. Radiol.*, **26**, 273.

Jurgens, P. E. (1968) Osteoid osteoma of the mandible: report of case. *J. oral Surg.*, **26**, 129.

Kaae, S., and Glahn, M. (1949) Case of sarcoma in irradiated mandible. *Acta Radiol.*, **31**, 431.

Karpawich, A. J. (1958) Paget's disease with osteogenic sarcoma of maxilla. *Oral Surg.*, **11**, 827.

Kent, J. N., Castro, H. F., and Girotti, W. R. (1969) Benign osteoblastoma of the maxilla. Case report and review of the literature. *Oral Surg.*, **27**, 209.

Kolas, S., Halperin, V., Jefferis, K., Huddleston, S., and Robinson, H. B. G. (1953) The occurrence of torus palatinus and torus mandibularis in 2,478 dental patients. *Oral Surg.*, **6**, 1134.

Kopp, W. K. (1969) Benign osteoblastoma of the coronoid process of the mandible. *J. oral Surg.*, **27**, 653.

Kragh, L. V., Dahlin, D. C., and Erich, J. B. (1958) Osteogenic sarcoma of the jaws and facial bones. *Amer. J. Surg.*, **96**, 496.

Krahl, V. E. (1949) A familial study of the palatine and mandibular tori. *Anat. Rec.*, **103**, 477.

Kramer, H. S. (1967) Benign osteoblastoma of the mandible. Report of a case. *Oral Surg.*, **24**, 842.

Krolls, S. O., Jacoway, J. R., and Alexander, W. N. (1971) Osseous choristomas (osteomas) of intraoral soft tissues. *Oral Surg.*, **32**, 588.

Leopard, P. J. (1972) Osteoma of the maxillary antrum. *Brit. J. oral Surg.*, **10**, 73.

Lichtenstein, L. (1951) Classification of primary tumors of bone. *Cancer*, **4**, 335.

Lichtenstein, L. (1956) Benign osteoblastoma—a category of osteoid and bone-forming tumors other than classical osteoid osteoma, which may be mistaken for giant-cell tumor or osteogenic sarcoma. *Cancer*, **9**, 1044.

Lichtenstein, L. (1964) Benign osteoblastoma. Further observations and report of 20 additional cases. *J. Bone Jt. Surg.*, **46A**, 755.

MacLennan, W. D., and Brown, R. D. (1974) Osteoma of the mandible. *Brit. J. oral Surg.*, **12**, 219.

Meskin, L. H., Peterson, W. C., and Gorlin, R. J. (1964) Multiple primary osteomas of oral mucous membrane: report of case. *J. oral Surg.*, **22**, 365.

Miller, S. C., and Roth, H. (1940) Torus palatinus: a statistical study. *J. amer. dent. Ass.*, **27**, 1950.

Moorrees, C. F. A. (1951) The dentition as a criterion of race with special reference to the Aleut. *J. dent. Res.*, **30**, 815.

Nelson, D. F., Gross, B. D., and Miller, F. E. (1972) Osteoma of the mandibular condyle: report of case. *J. oral Surg.*, **30**, 761.

New, G. B., and Cabot, C. M. (1935) The curability of malignant tumors of the upper jaw and antrum. *Surg. Gynec. Obstet.*, **60**, 971.

Parsons, W. H., and Henthorne, J. C. (1944) Extraskeletal osteogenic sarcoma. *Ann. Surg.*, **119**, 595.

Peutz, J. L. A. (1921) Cited by Jeghers, McKusick and Katz.

Plenk, H. P., and Gardner, E. J. (1954) Osteomatosis (leontiasis ossea). Hereditary disease of membranous bone formation associated in one family with polyposis of the colon. *Radiology*, **62**, 830.

Porretta, C. A., Dahlin, D. C., and Janes, J. M. (1957) Sarcoma in Paget's disease of bone. *J. Bone Jt. Surg.*, **39A**, 1314.

Potdar, G. G. (1970) Osteogenic sarcoma of the jaws. *Oral Surg.*, **30**, 381.

Rayne, J. (1968) Gardner's syndrome. *Brit. J. oral Surg.*, **6**, 11.

Remagen, W., and Prein, J. (1975) Benign osteoblastoma. *Oral Surg.*, **40**, 279.

Richards, W. G., and Coleman, F. C. (1957) Osteogenic sarcoma of the jaw. *Oral Surg.*, **10**, 1156.

Roca, A. N., Smith, L. J., and Jing, B.-S. (1970) Osteosarcoma and parosteal osteogenic sarcoma of the maxilla and mandible. Study of 20 cases. *Amer. J. clin. Path.*, **54**, 625.

Rosenmertz, S. K., and Schare, H. J. (1969) Osteogenic sarcoma arising in Paget's disease of the mandible. Review of the literature and report of a case. *Oral Surg.*, **28**, 304.

Rushton, M. A., Owen, M., Holgate, W., and Vaughan, J. (1961) The relation of radiation dose to radiation damage in the mandible of weanling rabbits. *Arch. oral Biol.*, **3**, 235.

Sabanas, A. O., Dahlin, D. C., Childs, D. S., and Ivins, J. C. (1956) Postradiation sarcoma of bone. *Cancer*, **9,** 528.

Smith, N. H. H. (1972) Benign osteoblastoma of the mandible: report of case. *J. oral Surg.*, **30,** 288.

Som, M., and Peimer, R. (1961) Juxtacortical osteogenic sarcoma of the mandible. *Arch. Otolaryngol.*, **74,** 532.

Suzuki, M., and Sakai, T. (1960) A familial study of torus palatinus and torus mandibularis. *Amer. J. phys. Anthropol.*, **18,** 263.

Willis, R. A. (1967) *Pathology of Tumours.* 4th Edition. London. Butterworth & Co. (Publishers) Ltd.

Wilner, D., and Sherman, R. S. (1965) Bone sarcoma associated with Paget's disease. *CA*, **16,** 238.

Yip, W.-K., and Lee, H. T. L. (1974) Benign osteoblastoma of the maxilla. *Oral Surg.*, **38,** 259.

loosening of the teeth and anaesthesia of the skin and mucous membrane in the areas supplied by the mental or infraorbital nerves. In some cases, where there are also vascular anomalies in other parts of the body, the cumulative effect may be sufficient to give an increased pulse pressure. Radiologically, there is an irregular osteolytic defect that may appear multicystic. There may be a "soap bubble" appearance as a result of fine fibrillary trabeculation within the loculi, but in general there are no specific appearances.

Macroscopically, the lesion may be diffuse or circumscribed. Related teeth may be loose, with bleeding from them, and extraction of such teeth, even though loose, has given rise to severe and even fatal haemorrhage in some cases (Macansh and Owen, 1972). In one of Broderick and Round's (1933) cases death occurred following extraction of loose teeth, despite ligation of the common carotid artery. Microscopically, the lesion generally consists of large cavernous blood spaces, though tumours of capillary type also occur. There is often an abundance of connective tissue between the vascular spaces and osteoid and bone may also be present.

In some cases, the lesion may take the form of arteriovenous aneurysm. Cases of this type have been reported by Clay and Blalock (1950), Hayton-Williams (1955) and Cook and Zbar (1962). These rare lesions produce a small area of radiolucency which, if situated at the root of a tooth, leads to the clinical diagnosis of a cyst. There is copious haemorrhage on extraction of the tooth and the friable material that can be curetted from the affected area shows the presence of numerous arteries and veins with walls of varying thickness. Communications between arterial and venous channels may be noted.

An arteriovenous aneurysm of the traumatic type has been reported by Howe and Wilson (1964).

Salivary Gland. See Chap. 30.

ANGIOMATOUS SYNDROMES

Haemangiomas may occur with other lesions in recognisable symptom complexes. Oral lesions occur in a number of these syndromes, which though rather uncommon or even in some cases rare, are nevertheless important because the oral or skin lesions may be the first pointers to more widespread disease. Comprehensive descriptions of those syndromes in which oral lesions may occur are given by Gorlin and Pindborg (1964).

Hereditary haemorrhagic telangiectasia (Osler-Rendu-Weber syndrome) is a familial disease characterised by multiple capillary telangiectases in the skin and mucous membranes, including the oral mucosa, and in internal organs. The telangiectases are localised areas of dilatation of existing capillary vessels, and not proliferative growths. They bleed very readily, epistaxis being the commonest symptom, even in childhood before the cutaneous telangiectases appear, which they do about the age of 30 or later. Haemorrhage from oral lesions is also common and should suggest the possibility of the diagnosis if widespread lesions do not already make it obvious. Cases with oral lesions have been reported by Bird and colleagues (1957), Syrop (1957), Scoop and Quart (1958), Durocher and colleagues (1961), Harrison (1964), Caldwell, Schweber and Lucchesi (1970), Killey and Kay (1970) and Soudah and Tilson (1971).

Fig. 74 Examples of oral haemangiomas, **a,** a common type of haemangioma of the gingiva. The lesion presented as a dark red mass, 0·5 cm in diameter. It consists of dilated capillaries with proliferated endothelium. Small solid masses of endothelium are also present. × 80. **b,** a haemangioma of the gingiva, consisting of large numbers of small capillaries. × 80. **c,** a small haemangioma of the gingiva of the angiokeratoma type. Blood-containing spaces lined by endothelium are present both in the subepithelial connective tissue and in the epithelium itself. × 20. **d,** a small thrombosed vessel close to a gingival haemangioma. Calcification may occur in such thrombi. × 30.

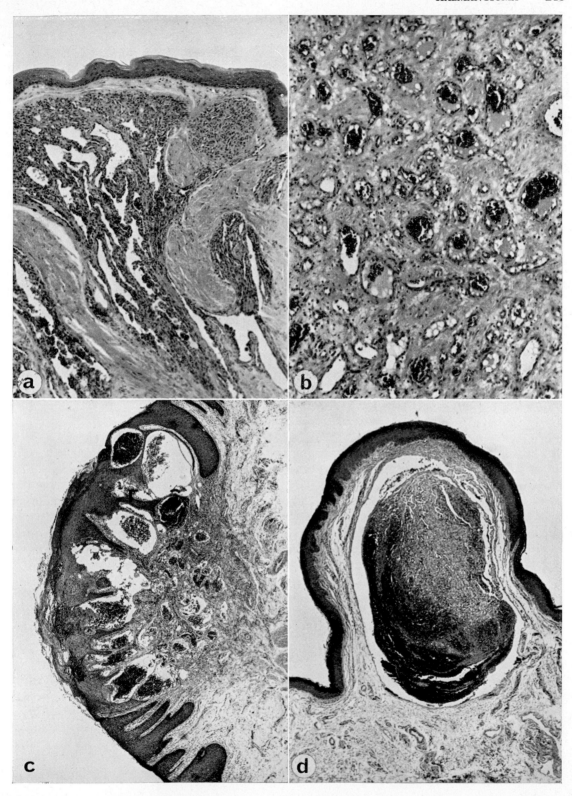

In the **Sturge-Weber syndrome** the characteristic triad of symptoms is naevus flammeus in the distribution of one or more branches of the trigeminal nerve, evidence of intracerebral angioma and calcification on the same side as the facial naevus and convulsions affecting the opposite side. Angiomas may also occur in the oral and other mucosae, elsewhere in the skin and in internal organs. In the mouth, haemangiomas may occur in the buccal mucosa, lips, tongue or palate. Gingival lesions, when fully developed, have a rather characteristic appearance, since they present as diffuse enlargements that may practically obscure the teeth. These soft, purple masses consist of collagen and numerous capillaries and show heavy chronic inflammatory infiltration. Cases of this type have been reported by Protzel (1957), Gyarmati (1960) and Royle, Lapp and Ferrara (1966).

The association of arteriovenous angioma of the mandible with similar lesions in the face, orbit, retina and brain has been reported by Bower and colleagues (1942), Krayenbühl and Yaçargil (1958), La Dow, Henefer and McFall (1964) and Hoyt and Cameron (1968).

In **Maffucci's syndrome** there are multiple chondromas and multiple haemangiomas, usually of the skin but sometimes also of the oral mucosa. The cases in which oral lesions have been reported are reviewed by Kennedy (1973).

Apart from their occurrence in well defined syndromes, haemangiomas may also be associated with other abnormalities, though not sufficiently consistently to form recognisable clinical complexes. For example, Castleman (1956) and Weinstein, Yamanaka and Fuchihata (1963) have reported haemangioma of the mandible associated with fibrous dysplasia. In Pusey's (1967) patient a mandibular haemangioma was associated with a cutaneous haemangioma.

It is clear, therefore, that although oral haemangiomas, either of bone or of the soft tissues, often occur as isolated lesions, they can also be associated with other abnormalities.

HAEMANGIOPERICYTOMA

This tumour arises from pericytes, the contractile cells that form with their interlacing processes a network around the outer aspect of the basement membrane of capillary vessels. On the inner side of the basement membrane lies only the capillary endothelium. Thus the network of pericytes embraces the capillary and is thought to subserve the functions of contraction and dilatation.

Tumours of the pericytes, first characterised by Stout and Murray (1942), are uncommon, but they may occur in a wide variety of tissues, very often in the head and neck, in the extremities, in the uterus and elsewhere.

The haemangiopericytoma occurs at any age and in both sexes, as a rather slowly growing circumscribed tumour. It is generally painless. Microscopically, the tumour reproduces the normal arrangement of capillary endothelial channels surrounded by pericytes, although in the tumour these cells are present in large numbers. Thus the tumour is very vascular, with the capillaries, which are more or less normal in structure, surrounded by the ovoid or elongated pericytes forming interlacing patterns or large masses. When the typical structure is present it is readily recognised, but there is a good deal of variability in the cellular pattern of this tumour and microscopic diagnosis is not always easy. However, the demonstration of the capillary basement membrane by silver staining shows that the tumour cells lie outside this structure and this helps to differentiate the tumour from other vascular growths in which the endothelial cells themselves are proliferating. A further difficulty is that little guide to prognosis can be obtained from the microscopic appearances of the tumour. An appreciable proportion of tumours recur locally and metastasise, but the likely behaviour of any given tumour is very difficult to forecast.

Backwinkel and Diddams (1970) have collected 224 cases from the literature, and show that the tumour has a rather poor prognosis, not so much in a five-year period, but over a lifetime. Prognosis is related more to the system involved than to any other factor. There were 21 cases in the series from the orbit, oral and nasal cavity and sinuses; these had a recurrence rate of 33 per cent after 5 years.

In the oral region, where tumours have been described by Stout (1956), Small and Bloom (1959), Das and Gans (1965), Itkin and Lapeyrolerie (1967), Stenhouse and Mason (1968), Sage and Salman (1968) and Orlian (1973), among others, the lesion appears as a small, generally painless, circumscribed swelling. The examples so far reported have not behaved unusually, except for Sage and Salman's case, in which the tumour appeared at the site from which an ameloblastoma had been removed 4 years previously. The haemangiopericytoma grew rapidly and the patient died, probably with pulmonary metastases.

GLOMUS TUMOUR

The glomus tumour is thought to be closely related to the haemangiopericytoma. The glomera are arteriovenous anastomoses that control the blood supply and temperature of the skin and certain deeper tissues. These functions appear to be mediated in some way by the rich nerve supply and by certain epithelioid cells that ensheath the arteriole of the glomus. These epithelioid cells are thought to be comparable to pericytes. Glomus tumours probably arise from these specialised glomus cells and occur most frequently under the nails and also elsewhere on the body surface. Though they are very small lesions, rarely exceeding a centimetre in diameter, they often give rise to attacks of very severe pain and are exquisitely tender. Histologically, the picture is variable. The tumour consists of glomus cells, and these may reproduce to some extent the structure of the normal glomus. In other cases, the glomus cells may be arranged around blood vessels in a manner suggesting haemangiopericytoma, or the blood vessels may be so prominent as to resemble cavernous haemangioma.

The glomus tumour is benign and removal effects a cure.

ANGIOSARCOMA

Malignant tumours of vascular tissue are rare in all sites, including the oral tissues. In the mouth, these tumours occur in the soft tissues, having been reported in the lip, palate, tongue and gingivae, and in the maxilla and mandible. Representative reports include those of Berger (1942), Cheyne and Silberstein (1942), Henny (1949), Blake and Blake (1956), Toto and Lavieri (1959), Pindborg and Philipsen (1960), and Gandhi and colleagues (1966). Wesley, Mintz and Wertheimer (1975) review the literature.

In general, angiosarcomas appear as rather rapidly growing lesions that tend to ulcerate. Regional lymph node and visceral metastases are common, so the prognosis is usually poor, but in well differentiated growths metastasis may be delayed for some time. Microscopically, the vascular origin of the tumour is usually obvious, since the picture is that of irregular vascular channels lined by endothelial cells that are often pleomorphic and may show numerous mitoses. Giant cell types may also be present. Some growths, however, tend to be more solid.

Metastatic angiosarcoma of the tongue, probably from a primary tumour of the lung, has been reported by Crymes and Taylor (1966).

P

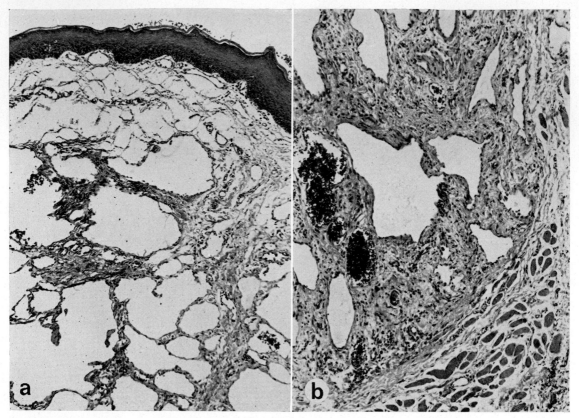

Fig. 75. Lymphangioma of the cheek. **a,** the dilated lymph channels in the corium extend up to the epithelium. **b,** more deeply, the lesion encroaches upon adjacent muscle. × 80.

KAPOSI'S DISEASE

Oral lesions are occasionally seen in this condition. The characteristic manifestations of Kaposi's disease are multiple dark blue or purple vascular lesions of the skin, particularly of the extremities, and of lymph nodes and internal organs, especially the gastrointestinal tract. Microscopically, the lesions show vascular channels lined by endothelial cells and spindle cells. The spindle cell element gives to the lesion its sarcomatous appearance. Chronic inflammatory infiltration is often also present, and it may be difficult to make a histological diagnosis particularly in early cases, since the picture may be practically indistinguishable from a non-specific granulomatous lesion. However, in the course of time the development of the clinical picture and the maturation of the lesions to show the characteristic vascular-sarcomatous appearance point to the diagnosis.

The course of Kaposi's disease is variable, but very often patients may live for many years. Representaive reports of oral lesions include those by Pearce and Valker (1936), Levin (1957), Shklar and Meyer (1965), Howland, Armbrecht and Miller (1966) and Gambardella (1974). Oral lesions are usually part of the disseminated condition, but they may be the first to appear. Farman and Uys (1975) have found eight such cases in the literature, which they review. Oral lesions occur most frequently in the palate, then in the lips and tongue, and they are commonly multiple. The lesions show no special diagnostic features macroscopically, being similar to an ordinary haemangioma or pyogenic granuloma.

LYMPHANGIOMA

The lips, cheek, palate and particularly the tongue are the usual sites for oral lymphangioma. Some lesions are circumscribed but often the growth forms a rather diffuse ill-defined mass. The surface of the lesion may be smooth or nodular. Sometimes the lymph spaces may be so superficial that the mucous membrane over the lesion appears to be covered in vesicles or bullae. Lymphangioma of the tongue is the usual cause of macroglossia. Lymphangioma of the soft tissues of the neck may take the form of a circumscribed lesion or it may ramify in a complex manner in the musculature and may even extend into the axilla. In this situation the lesion is often termed cystic hygroma.

Microscopically, lymphangiomas consist of a mass of dilated, intercommunicating lymph channels (Fig. 75). In the oral tissues, they are particularly liable to suffer trauma. Because of this, these lesions are subject to periodic attacks of inflammation which cause the swelling to become larger and tender for the time being. Suppuration does not usually occur, however, and when the attack subsides fibrosis occurs. Longstanding lesions are therefore likely to feel rather knotty or nodular, and to show microscopic evidence of scarring. Calcification may also occur.

REFERENCES

Allen, P. W., and Enziger, F. M. (1972) Hemangioma of skeletal muscle. An analysis of 89 cases. *Cancer*, **29,** 9.

Andersen, D. H. (1951) Tumors of infancy and childhood. I. A Survey of those seen in the pathology laboratory of the Babies Hospital during the years 1935–1950. *Cancer*, **4,** 890.

Backwinkel, K. D., and Diddams, J. A. (1970) Hemangiopericytoma. Report of a case and comprehensive review of the literature. *Cancer*, **25,** 896.

Baum, S. M., Pochaczevsky, R., Sussman, R., and Stoopack, J. C. (1972) Central hemangioma of the maxilla. *J. oral Surg.*, **30,** 885.

Berger, A. (1942) Hemangiosarcoma of the mandible (metastatic?). *Ann. Den.*, **1,** 15.

Bird, R. M., Hammarsten, J. F., Marshall, R. A., and Robinson, R. R. (1957) A family reunion: a study of hereditary hemorrhagic telangiectasia. *New Engl. J. Med.*, **257,** 105.

Blake, H., and Blake, F. S. (1956) Angiosarcoma. Report of a case. *Oral Surg.*, **9,** 821.

Bower, L. E., Ditkowsky, S. P., Klein, B. A., and Bronstein, I. P. (1942) Arteriovenous angioma of mandible and retina with pronounced hematemesis and epistaxis. *Amer. J. Dis. Child.*, **64,** 1023.

Broderick, R. A., and Round, H. (1933). Cavernous angioma of the maxilla. Fatal haemorrhage after teeth extraction. *Lancet*, **2,** 13.

Brodsky, R. H. (1934) Mandibular cavernous hemangioma. *Dent. Digest*, **40,** 60.

Bucy, P. C., and Capp, S. (1930) Primary hemangioma of bone with special reference to roentgenologic diagnosis. *Amer. J. Roentgenol.*, **23,** 1.

Caldwell, T. A., Schweber, S. J., and Lucchesi, F. J. (1970) Resection of tongue lesion associated with hereditary telangiectasia (Osler-Weber-Rendu disease): report of case. *J. oral. Surg.*, **28,** 299.

Castleman, B. (1956) Case record. *New Engl. J. Med.*, **254,** 70.

Cheyne, V. D., and Silberstein, H. E. (1942) Hemangioendothelioma. A discussion of differential criteria with a report of three oral cases. *Amer. J. Orthodont. (Oral Surg. Sect.)*, **28,** 703.

Chipps, J. E., and Weiler, T. J. (1950) Erectile cavernous hemangioma of the masseter muscle. Report of a case. *Oral Surg.*, **3,** 1509.

Clay, R. C., and Blalock, A. (1950) Congenital arteriovenous fistulas in the mandible. *Surg. Gynec. Obstet.*, **90,** 543.

Cook, T. J., and Zbar, M. J. (1962) Arteriovenous aneurysm of the mandible. *Oral Surg.*, **15,** 442.

Crymes, T., and Taylor, R. G. (1966) Angiosarcoma metastatic to the tongue: report of case. *J. oral Surg.*, **24,** 63.

21. Tumours of Neural Tissues

Tumours of neural tissue arise in connection with the sheaths of peripheral nerves, the neuroglia and the nerve cells themselves. The tumours of the nerve sheath are the neurilemmoma and the neurofibroma. The tumours of neuroglia, the gliomas, are found only in the central nervous system. Tumours of the neurones, the neuroblastoma and ganglioneuroma, occur in the ganglia of the sympathetic system and in the adrenal medulla.

NEURILEMMOMA AND NEUROFIBROMA

The axons of peripheral nerves are ensheathed by the nucleated membrane of Schwann, a structure of neuro-ectodermal origin. Thus enveloped, the axons are grouped in bundles and the bundles are held together to form the nerve trunk by the mesodermal fibroblastic membranes, the endoneurium, perineurium and epineurium. Two types of tumour arise in connection with these membranes; the neurilemmoma, which is believed to arise from the Schwann cells, and the neurofibroma, which is probably composed of elements from the connective tissue of the sheath of Schwann and of the other membranes, as well as the Schwann cells themselves.

The neurilemmoma occurs at any age and in connection with both the intracranial and the peripheral nerves, usually as a solitary tumour. Intracranially, the acoustic nerve is the usual site. Tumours of the peripheral nerves can occur anywhere, but the head and neck area is frequently affected. The tumours usually occur in the subcutaneous tissue, but internal organs like the stomach and other parts of the gastrointestinal tract may be affected. Uncommonly, neurilemmomas may be multiple, sometimes as a feature of neurofibromatosis.

The neurofibroma, on the other hand, occurs only rarely as a solitary tumour. Much more often there are multiple tumours (neurofibromatosis) occurring in connection with the nerves of the skin and subcutaneous tissues and also those of internal organs.

Clinical Features

In the oral region, these tumours occur both in the soft tissues and in the mandible and maxilla. There are few symptoms, other than those due to the size and location of the tumour. There may be complaint simply of a lump in the mouth, or swelling of the jaw with intra-osseous tumours, but there is usually no pain and tumours of this type are generally of slow growth.

Soft tissue tumours occur as smooth, convex swellings beneath the mucosa. They are soft on palpation and may be tender. They have been described in the submucosa of the palate (Schroff, 1945; Hitchin, 1952; Hayton-Williams, 1953), the floor of the mouth (Schroff, 1945; Couch, 1954; Swanson and White, 1960) and the tongue. The literature on tongue tumours has been listed by Robertson (1952) and further cases have been reported by Crowe (1959) and Cameron (1959). In Stout's (1935) series there are examples of tumours of the palate, tongue, lip, angle of mouth, cheek and submaxillary region. Tumours of the facial nerve have been described by Loeliger (1947) and Lundgren (1947). Small tumours of the gingiva may present clinically in the same way as the common fibrous epulis (McMillan, 1963).

Hatziotis and Asprides (1967) have listed the reports in the literature of soft tissue tumours and find the following incidence: tongue, 59; palate, 11; floor of mouth, 10; buccal mucosa, 9;

gingiva, 6; lip, 6; vestibule, 5. Cherrick and Eversole (1971) report on a series of 37 cases, finding much the same distribution.

The jaws appear to be a favoured site for nerve sheath tumours. In Fawcett and Dahlin's (1967) review of neurilemmoma of bone, 17 out of 31 tumours (including neurofibromas) occurred in the jaws. Bone tumours may originate intraosseously or may arise from a nerve outside the bone and subsequently lead to bony involvement as they grow. Thus, in Baetz and Shackelford's (1951) case, a tumour of the inferior alveolar nerve in the region of the mental foramen formed a large soft mass over the angle of the mandible and also resorbed the buccal plate of bone. Other cases of bone involvement of this type have been reported by Rushton (1944) and Wilson and Walsh (1948). Intraosseous tumours cause enlargement of the jaw with expansion of the cortex that may lead to perforation. Maxillary tumours, examples of which have been reported by Goldman (1944), Stillman (1952) and Friedman (1964) are very much rarer than mandibular tumours. Radiologically, there is an area of translucency such as might be produced by some other tumours or cysts, but in mandibular lesions the bony defect is the result of enlargement of the mandibular canal by the growth on the mandibular nerve. If the tumour is not so large as to obliterate it completely, the canal may still be seen on either side of the area of translucency and in continuity with it (Fig. 76). Mandibular tumours have been reported by Zilkens (1937), Goldman (1944), Schroff (1945), Blackwood and Lucas (1951), Spilka (1953), Cornell and Vargas (1955), Johnson and colleagues (1959), Gutman and colleagues (1964), Shimura and colleagues (1973) and others. Those tumours that appear to have been solitary neurofibromas are listed by Eversole (1969) and Prescott and White (1970). In Hodson's (1961) unusual case a mandibular tumour was associated with and apparently invaded by an ameloblastoma.

Pathology

The neurilemmoma is generally a round or ovoid tumour that is well circumscribed and encapsulated. The related nerve may often be seen on one side of the tumour or spread out over the capsule. The cut surface is white, yellowish or pink and may be firm or fibrous-appearing, but often it has a rather mucinous or gelatinous texture and cysts are not infrequently present.

Microscopically the tumour shows two distinct cellular patterns designated as Antoni type A and Antoni type B. Antoni type A tissue consists of cells like fibrocytes together with intercellular collagenous tissue, the cells and fibres often being arranged in a parallel manner that gives rise to the very characteristic appearance described as palisading or regimentation of the nuclei. However, in some cases palisading may be inconspicuous or even absent. Antoni type B tissue is described as reticular, since it consists of a rather loose meshwork of fibrils enclosing microcysts, the coalescence of which produces the cysts that are sometimes noted macroscopically. The two types of tissue are generally seen in most tumours, though some may consist entirely of the one or the other (Fig. 76).

It seems probable that the neurofibroma is a developmental anomaly rather than a true neoplasm. As already noted, the lesions are multiple and involve nerves in any part of the body. Although some lesions, particularly the smaller ones, may appear to be well circumscribed and encapsulated, larger tumours are not infrequently rather ill-defined and tend to merge into the surrounding tissues. Microscopically, the neurofibroma consists of collagenous tissue and of nerve fibres, the latter running throughout the lesion rather than over the surface of it, as in neurilemmoma. Moreover, the characteristic cellular pattern of neurilemmoma is not seen, although very occasionally there may be some nuclear palisading or structures resembling tactile corpuscles may be evident. The proportion of collagenous tissue varies very considerably. Some lesions appear very similar to ordinary fibromas, consisting mainly of collagenous tissue and being

and colleagues, 1944), maxillary tumours (Kawabe and colleagues, 1969; Takagi and Ishikawa, 1972), a tongue tumour (Goldberg and colleagues, 1970) and a palatal tumour (Phillips and Brown, 1971).

The microscopic diagnosis can often be difficult. In Takagi and Ishikawa's case the initial diagnosis was fibrosarcoma, but electronmicroscopy showed the presence of myofilaments. There is no close correlation between rate of growth and liability to metastasise and the histological appearances.

RHABDOMYOMA AND RHABDOMYOSARCOMA

Benign tumours of striated muscle are very rare. So-called rhabdomyomas occur as congenital lesions in the heart, but these are almost certainly developmental anomalies and not neoplasms. True benign neoplasms occur mostly in the tongue, and in infants or young children, though a tumour of the tongue in a woman of 21 has been reported by Misch (1958). This author also reviews the few previously recorded cases, all in infants and children. Subsequent reports are those of Sirsat and Vakil (1962), who describe a palatal tumour in a woman of 42 years, Goldman (1963), Tsukada and Pickren (1965) (sublingual region), and Kay, Gerszten and Dennison (1969) (floor of mouth).

Malignant tumours of striated muscle, though not so rare as the benign ones, are not common. They are generally classified as of the following types: pleomorphic, alveolar, embryonal, botryoid (Horn and Enterline, 1958). The pleomorphic types of tumour occur in skeletal muscle, chiefly of the extremities, and adults are mainly affected. As the name implies, tumours of this variety show a very varied cellular picture. Strap-like, racquet-shaped and tadpole-shaped cells are frequently present, together with rounded, oval and spindle-shaped cells. The nuclei of these cells are often hyperchromatic and numerous mitoses are seen. Multinucleated giant cells are also often seen. The presence of cross-striations in the tumour cells is conclusive proof of striated muscle origin, but it is often impossible to demonstrate these structures. However, the pleomorphism of the tumour with its peculiarly shaped cells is rather characteristic, and the diagnosis is frequently made on the general appearances (Fig. 78).

The alveolar type of growth occurs principally in children though sometimes in adults, and again it is commonest in the muscles of the extremities. Here the histological picture is one of groups of round or oval cells arranged with some resemblance to glandular alveoli, though sometimes the cells may form more diffuse masses. The racquet or tadpole cells of the pleomorphic type of growth are sometimes also to be seen, but again it is difficult to demonstrate cross-striations.

The embryonal type of tumour occurs in children under the age of 5 years, and is found particularly in the genito-urinary tract and in the nasopharynx. Some of these tumours, both in

Fig. 78 **a,** leiomyoma in a boy of 12 years. The tumour presented as a purple swelling of the gingiva, 1·0 cm in diameter. Microscopically, it consists of fasciculi of smooth muscle fibres. × 200. This patient was well 2 years after local excision of the lesion. **b,** myosarcoma of cheek in a man of 25 years. The lesion appeared as a soft lobulated swelling, of rather haemorrhagic appearance. The tumour was excised widely but it was later learned that it recurred and the patient had died of pneumonia. No metastases were detected clinically, but no autopsy was performed. Microscopic examination shows the general configuration of a malignant neoplasm of muscle. × 500. **c,** rhabdomyosarcoma of the soft palate in a girl of 8 years. The tumour was excised locally and radiotherapy was given. The patient was well 6 years later. × 200. **d,** higher magnification, showing cross-striation in a tumour cell. × 820.

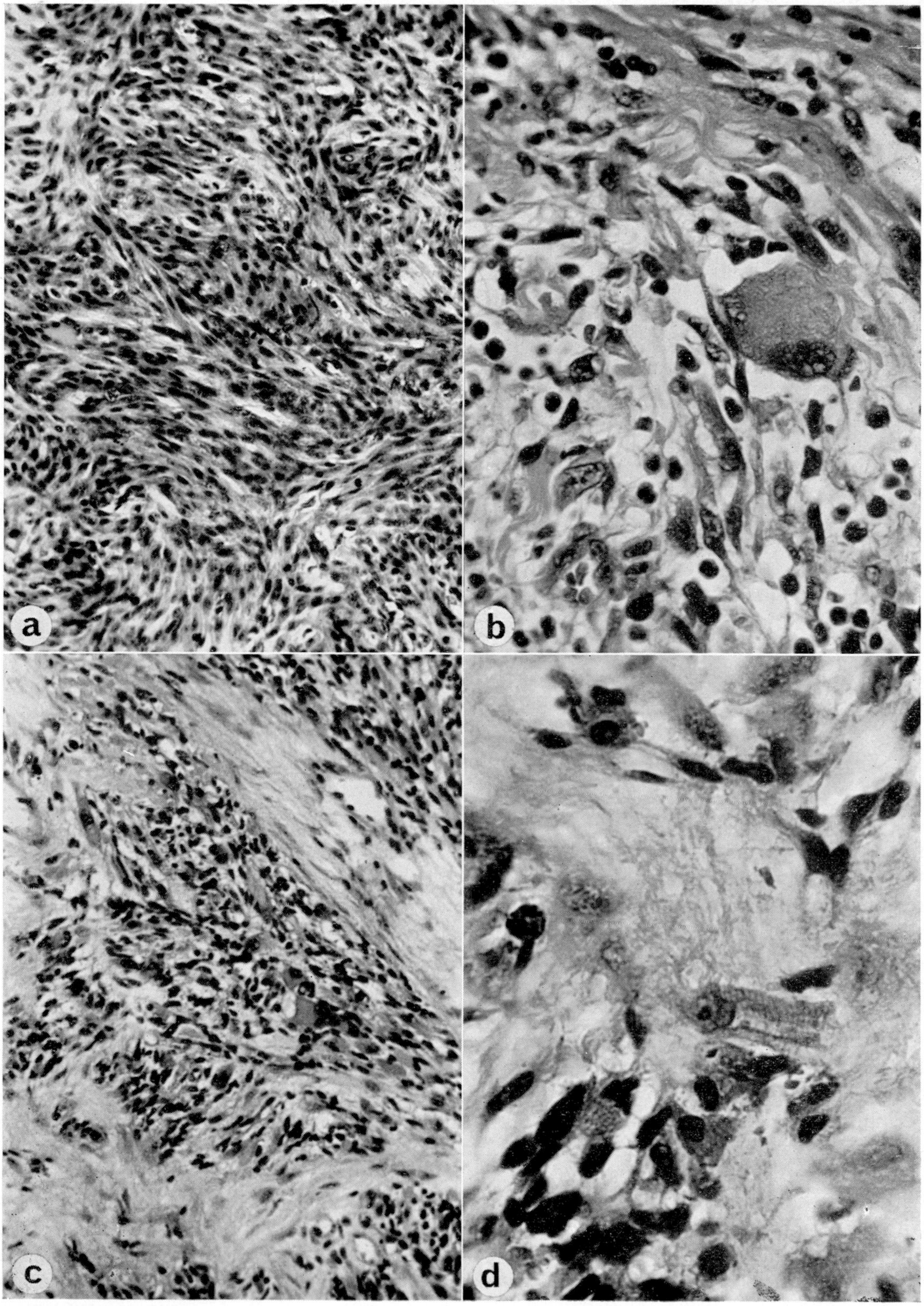

have be
line (1

Kauf
mouth

Rhal
Batsak
their o
progn
excisi
as is e
be tho
contr
sensit
Chen
unde

T
as
brea
(194
exa
196
450
tur

Cl

cir
th
ha
ne

li
o

P

n
a
a
t

electron microscopy and histochemistry. They found that the granular cells were morpho-logically and enzymically similar to the Schwann cells observed in severed nerve and were dissimilar to damaged and fetal skeletal muscle. They consider that the lesion arises from Schwann cells, as do Garancis, Komorowski and Kuzma (1970), also on the basis of fine structure studies. This view is now accepted by many workers.

Another detailed electron microscopic and histochemical investigation has been made by Aparicio and Lumsden (1969). These workers conclude that apparent transitions between the granular cells and normal striated muscle fibres are an illusory feature that is noted at the level of light microscopy; the electron microscope shows that the tumour cells are separated from normal muscle by basement membranes. Histochemically, the granules are non-lipid and are composed of a muco- or glycoprotein. They believe that the cell of origin is a primitive fibroblast-like stem cell. This view is also supported by Sobel, Schwarz and Marquet (1973). Thus, even the more recent methods of studying fine structure have failed to resolve the question of the histo-genesis of the granular cell myoblastoma, which still remains controversial.

The rare occurrence of tumours reported as malignant myoblastoma does not afford much aid in resolving the question of the origin and nature of the lesion, for there is no consensus of opinion that these malignant growths really are the malignant counterparts of the benign myo-blastoma. Gamboa (1955) and Cadotte (1974) have reviewed the reported cases.

Behaviour

Although the nature of the myoblastoma remains obscure, there is no doubt as to its behaviour. The lesion is entirely benign and local excision effects a cure. The characteristic pseudo-epitheliomatous hyperplasia of the epithelium overlying many tumours does not proceed to carcinoma.

REFERENCES

Abrikossoff, A. (1926) Über Myome, ausgehend von der quergestreiften willkürlichen Muskulatur. *Virchows Arch.*, **260**, 215.

Abrikossoff, A. I. (1931) Weitere Untersuchungen über Myoblastenmyome. *Virchows Arch.*, **280**, 723.

Aparicio, S. R., and Lumsden, C. E. (1969) Light- and electron-microscope studies on the granular cell myoblastoma of the tongue. *J. Path.*, **97**, 339.

Ashburn, L. L., and Rodger, R. C. (1952) Myoblastomas, neural origin. Report of six cases, one with multiple tumors. *Amer. J. clin. Path.*, **22**, 440.

Azzopardi, J. G. (1956) Histogenesis of the granular-cell "myoblastoma." *J. Path. Bact.*, **71**, 85.

Bangle, R. (1952) A morphological and histochemical study of the granular-cell myoblastoma. *Cancer*, **5**, 950.

Bangle, R. (1953) An early granular-cell myoblastoma confined within a small peripheral myelinated nerve. *Cancer*, **6**, 790.

Bardwil, J. M., and MacComb, W. S. (1964) Sarcomas of the head and neck. With special references to rhabdomyosarcomas. *Amer. J. Surg.*, **108**, 476.

Bernier, J. L., and Thompson, H. C. (1946) Myoblastoma. *J. dent. Res.*, **25**, 253.

Beyer, T. E., and Blair, J. R. (1948) Sublingual rhabdomyoma. *Arch. Otolaryngol.*, **47**, 678.

Burford, W. N., Ackerman, L. V., and Robinson, H. B. G. (1944) Leiomyoma of the tongue. *Amer. J. Orthodont. (Oral Surg. Sect.)*, **30**, 395.

Cadotte, M. (1974) Malignant granular-cell myoblastoma. *Cancer*, **33**, 1417.

Cappell, D. F., and Montgomery, G. L. (1937) On rhabdomyoma and myoblastoma. *J. Path. Bact.*, **44**, 517.

Carmody, T. E., Janney, H. M., and Huseman, A. L. (1944) Leiomyosarcoma of the mandible. Report of case. *J. Amer. dent. Ass.*, **31**, 1110.

Cherrick, H. M., Dunlap, C. L., and King, O. H. (1973) Leiomyomas of the oral cavity. Review of the literature and clinicopathologic study of seven new cases. *Oral Surg.*, **35**, 54.

Christopherson, W. M., Foote, F. W., and Stewart, F. W. (1952) Alveolar soft-part sarcomas. Structurally characteristic tumors of uncertain histogenesis. *Cancer*, **5**, 100.

Cove, P. (1974) An unusual presentation of rhabdomyosarcoma: a case report. *Brit. J. oral Surg.*, **12**, 240.

Crane, A. R., and Tremblay, R. G. (1945) Myoblastoma (granular cell myoblastoma or myoblastic myoma). *Amer. J. Path.*, **21**, 357.

Dito, W. R., and Batsakis, J. G. (1962) Rhabdomyosarcoma of the head and neck. An appraisal of the biologic behaviour in 170 cases. *Arch. Surg.*, **84**, 162.

Fisher, E. R., and Wechsler, H. (1962) Granular cell myoblastoma—a misnomer. Electron microscopic and histochemical evidence concerning its Schwann cell derivation and nature (granular cell schwannoma). *Cancer*, **15**, 936.

Fust, J. A., and Custer, R. P. (1949) On the neurogenesis of so-called granular cell myoblastoma. *Amer. J. clin. Path.*, **19**, 522.

Gamboa, L. G. (1955) Malignant granular-cell myoblastoma. *Arch. Path.*, **60**, 663.

Garancis, J. C., Komorowski, R. A., and Kuzma, J. F. (1970) Granular cell myoblastoma. *Cancer*, **25**, 542.

Garrett, J. R. (1969) Angiomyoma of the palate. Report of a case. *Oral Surg.*, **27**, 103.

Goldberg, M. H., Polivy, C., and Saltzman, S. (1970) Leiomyosarcoma of the tongue: report of case. *J. oral Surg.*, **28**, 608.

Goldman, R. L. (1963) Multicentric benign rhabdomyoma of skeletal muscle. *Cancer*, **16**, 1609.

Gray, S. H., and Gruenfeld, G. E. (1937) Myoblastoma. *Amer. J. Cancer*, **30**, 699.

Gutmann, J., Cifuentes, C., Balzarini, M. A., Sobarzo, V., and Vicuña, R. (1974) Angiomyoma of the oral cavity. *Oral Surg.*, **38**, 269.

Hagen, J. O., Soule, E. H., and Gores, R. J. (1961) Granular-cell myoblastoma of the oral cavity. *Oral Surg.*, **14**, 454.

Hagy, D. M., Halperin, V., and Wood, C. (1964) Leiomyoma of the oral cavity. Review of the literature and report of a case. *Oral Surg.*, **17**, 748.

Henny, F. A., and Downs, J. R. (1968) Treatment of embryonal rhabdomyosarcoma of the maxilla with combined therapy. *J. oral Surg.*, **26**, 316.

Herschfus, L., and Wolter, J. G. (1970) Granular-cell myoblastoma of the oral cavity. *Oral Surg.*, **29**, 341.

Horn, R. C., and Enterline, H. T. (1958) Rhabdomyosarcoma: a clinicopathological study and classification of 39 cases. *Cancer*, **11**, 181.

Horn, R. C., and Stout, A. P. (1943) Granular cell myoblastoma. *Surg. Gynec. Obstet.*, **76**, 315.

Kauffman, S. L., and Stout, A. P. (1965) Congenital mesenchymal tumors. *Cancer*, **18**, 460.

Kawabe, Y., Kondo, T., and Hosoda, S. (1969) Two cases of leiomyosarcoma of the maxillary sinuses. *Arch. Otolaryngol.*, **90**, 492.

Kay, S., Gerszten, E., and Dennison, S. M. (1969) Light and electron microscopic study of a rhabdomyoma arising in the floor of the mouth. *Cancer*, **23**, 708.

Kerr, D. A. (1949) Myoblastic myoma. *Oral Surg.*, **2**, 41.

Klemperer, P. (1934) Myoblastoma of the striated muscle. *Amer. J. Cancer*, **20**, 324.

Leroux, R., and Delarue, J. (1939) Sur trois cas de tumeurs à cellules granuleuses de la cavité buccale. *Bull. Assoc. franç. Cancer*, **28**, 427.

MacDonald, D. G. (1969) Smooth muscle tumours of the mouth. *Brit. J. oral Surg.*, **6**, 207.

McGowan, D. Λ., and Jones, J. H. (1969) Angioma (vascular leiomyoma) of the oral cavity. *Oral Surg.*, **27**, 649.

Mann, J. B., Ash, J. E., and Bernier, J. L. (1944) *Atlas of Dental and Oral Pathology*. 3rd Edition. Chicago. American Dental Association.

Merrill, R. G., and Downs, J. R. (1967) Oral leiomyomas. Report of two cases. *Oral Surg.*, **23**, 438.

Miles, A. E. W., and Waterhouse, J. P. (1962) A leiomyosarcoma of the oral cavity with metastasis to lymph-glands. *J. Path. Bact.*, **83**, 551.

Misch, K. A. (1958) Rhabdomyoma purum: a benign rhabdomyoma of tongue. *J. Path. Bact.*, **75**, 105.

Moore, O., and Grossi, C. (1959) Embryonal rhabdomyosarcoma of the head and neck. *Cancer*, **12**, 69.

Moscovic, E. A., and Azar, H. A. (1969) Multiple granular cell tumors ("myoblastomas"). Case report with electron microscopic observations and review of the literature. *Cancer*, **20**, 2032.

Murray, M. R. (1951) Cultural characteristics of three granular-cell myoblastomas. *Cancer*, **4**, 857.

O'Day, R. A., Soule, E. H., and Gores, R. J. (1965) Embryonal rhabdomyosarcoma of the oral soft tissues. *Oral Surg.*, **20**, 85.

Pearse, A. G. E. (1950) The histogenesis of granular-cell myoblastoma (? granular-cell perineural fibroblastoma). *J. Path. Bact.*, **62**, 351.

Phillips, H., and Brown, A. (1971) Leiomyosarcoma: report of case. *J. oral Surg.*, **29**, 194.

Ringertz, N. (1942) Über das sog. Myoblastenmyom mit beschreibung 7 neuer Fälle. *Acta path. microbiol. scand.*, **19**, 112.

and in fact various viruses have since been isolated from tumour tissue. However, such viruses are common in other parts of the world and, moreover, the disease does occur in some areas where insect vectors are not likely to operate. It is now thought possible that more than one factor is implicated. It may be that virus infection, acting on a reticuloendothelial system already widely affected by chronic malarial infection, which is endemic in Africa, accounts for the neoplastic change.

HODGKIN'S DISEASE

Hodgkin's disease, like the lymphomas already discussed, is a multicentric condition that affects lymph nodes and other tissues, particularly the spleen and the liver. The cervical nodes are frequently affected and are often the presenting sign, so that the possibility of the condition has always to be considered in patients with cervical lymphadenopathy. Moreover, Hodgkin's disease is the commonest type of lymphoma, and although it occurs at all ages it is seen particularly in patients below middle age and also in children. It is surprising, therefore, that lesions are rare in the oral tissues, particularly since the incidence of skeletal lesions giving rise to symptoms is in the region of 10 to 20 per cent and autopsy findings indicate that bony involvement occurs in up to 78 per cent of cases (Steiner, 1943; Jackson and Parker, 1944, 1945). One would therefore have expected to find records of more lesions in the jaws, but very few indeed have been reported. In Meyer, Roswit and Unger's (1959) case there was a lesion of the mucous membrane of the retromolar area. This patient already had lesions in the cervical lymph nodes. Eisenbud and Kotch (1954) have reported the case of a man of 55 with a lesion in the cheek that presented as an indurated mass the size of a walnut in the region of the opening of Stenson's duct. Involvement of the mandible has been reported by Forman and Wesson (1970). Other reports in the literature are summarised by Greer and Richardson (1974).

In this condition the lesions consist of pleomorphic cellular tissue containing reticulum cells, lymphoid cells, plasma cells, polymorphonuclear and eosinophil leucocytes (Fig. 85). The microscopic picture is thus very varied but this in itself is rather characteristic, particularly when contrasted with the uniformity of the cellular picture in lymphosarcoma and, often, in reticulum cell sarcoma. A well known feature of the histological picture, and essential for diagnosis, is the presence of Sternberg-Reed giant cells. These are reticulum-like cells that characteristically have two nuclei in a mirror-image pattern, although on occasion there may be up to eight or ten nuclei. In some cases the cellular tissue is subdivided by bands of fibrous tissue and in the later stages diffuse fibrosis may develop, either following on the band-like fibrosis or occurring in lesions in which there had been no previous fibrosis. The predominance or otherwise of the various features is the basis for the subdivision of Hodgkin's disease into lymphocyte-predominant, nodular sclerosing, mixed cellularity and lymphocyte-depleted types.

Hodgkin's disease was formerly inevitably fatal, in most cases within some three to five years, but cures are now being increasingly claimed for patients energetically treated at an early stage. In general, the prognosis is best for the lymphocyte-predominant and nodular sclerosing types.

Fig. 85. **a,** lymph node in Hodgkin's disease. The architecture of the node is destroyed by a pleomorphic infiltrate. × 200. **b,** fibrous bands may be a feature in some cases. × 200. **c,** the characteristic Sternberg-Reed giant cells often have mirror-image nuclei. × 300. **d,** mycosis fungoides. A facial skin lesion, showing the infiltrate in the dermis. × 80. **e,** detail from **d.** The cellular infiltrate is pleomorphic, resembling that in Hodgkin's disease. × 500.

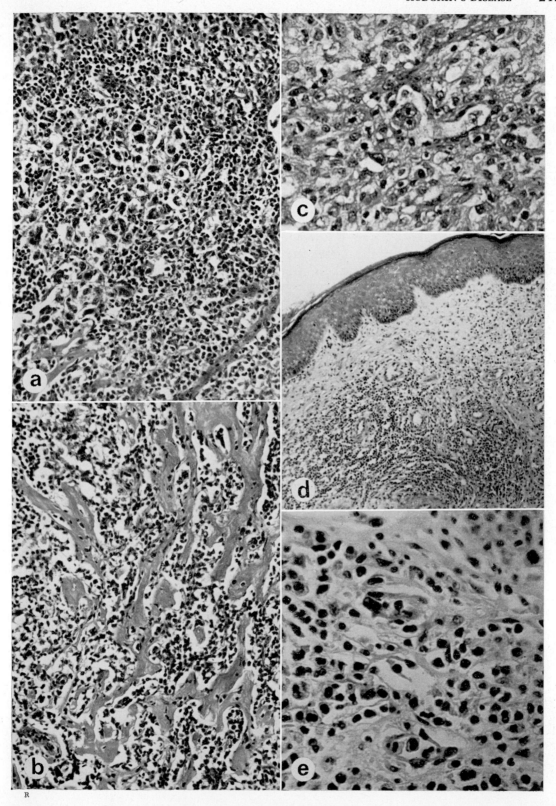

R

MYCOSIS FUNGOIDES

This condition is a type of lymphoma affecting the skin. It may be a manifestation of Hodgkin's disease but its true nature is not really known at present. The lesions commence like those of eczema but in time they become infiltrated by cells and tumour-like, and in most cases the lymph nodes, spleen, liver and other internal organs are also ultimately affected. The lesions are microscopically like those of Hodgkin's disease, reticulum cell sarcoma or lymphosarcoma (Fig. 85).

A case of mycosis fungoides with lesions in the skin and the oral mucosa has been reported by Calhoun and Johnson (1966).

LEUKAEMIA

The primitive precursors of the mature leukocytes may undergo neoplastic change, with the consequent appearance of large numbers of immature white cells in the blood and in tissues throughout the body. Acute leukaemia results when the neoplastic process has affected the most primitive of the white cell precursors, the chronic forms when the less primitive types are involved. Oral lesions occur in about 55 per cent of cases of acute leukaemia and 15 per cent of cases of chronic disease (Sinrod, 1957).

Acute Leukaemia

Although this variety of the disease can occur at any age, it is often seen in younger persons and quite frequently in the first few years of life. The three types of acute leukaemia are distinguished haematologically by the predominance of myeloid, lymphatic or monocytic cells in the blood, but clinically they are identical. There is often a sudden onset with pyrexia and enlargement of lymph nodes and spleen, and swelling of the gingivae is frequently an early symptom, often with ulceration and necrosis. At the same time other areas of the buccal mucosa, for example the cheek, may be ulcerated, and the tonsil is often involved. Excessive bleeding following dental extraction may be an early, or the first, symptom and spontaneous bleeding also occurs. Petechiae and ecchymoses are frequently seen. There is often also marked pallor of the oral mucosa.

The gingival enlargement, which may be so extensive as to envelop the teeth almost completely, is due to infiltration by leukaemic cells and to small haemorrhages (Fig. 86) An unusual case of a localised epulis-like enlargement of the gingiva has been reported by Oldham and John (1966). Toothache, probably due to leukaemic infiltration of the dental pulp, also occurs. The teeth may become loose at an early stage, due to necrosis of the periodontal ligament (Burket, 1944). Many of these changes are determined by trauma, as Duffy and Driscoll (1958) suggest. In their series of 38 cases, gingival lesions were absent in very young patients and in the edentulous. White (1970) has also found that children may not always show florid gingival disease. Enlarged cervical nodes are a much commoner finding.

Fig. 86   **a,** chronic gingivitis. The inflammatory infiltration extends throughout the corium up to the epithelium. × 80. **b,** gingival lesion in myeloid leukaemia. The infiltration stops short of the epithelium, leaving a relatively clear zone of connective tissue. × 80. **c,** gingival lesion in monocytic leukaemia. The general disposition of the infiltrate is similar to that seen in **b. d,** higher magnification, showing the monocytic infiltration. × 500. **e,** higher magnification from **b.** Polymorphs and myelocytes and other immature cells of the granular series are present. × 500.

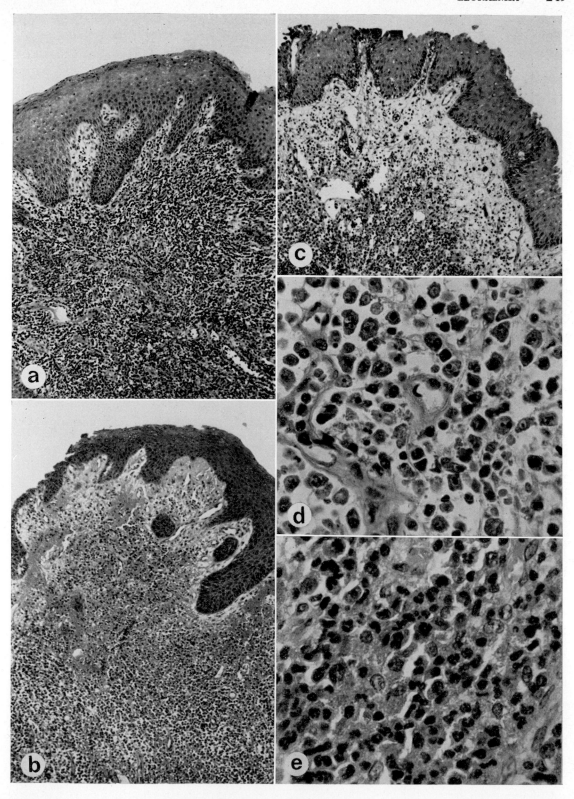

These changes may occur in any type of acute leukaemia, but they are likely to be most severe in the monocytic type (Lynch and Ship, 1967).

Biopsy is usually avoided in leukaemia because of the likelihood of haemorrhage. When the clinician suspects the possibility of leukaemia he will normally confirm the diagnosis by haematological examination. However, biopsy may sometimes have to be done, for example in aleukaemic cases. Microscopic examination shows infiltration by leukaemic cells (Fig. 86). As in lymphosarcoma the infiltration, which is dense, generally leaves a relatively cell-free zone immediately subjacent to the epithelium. The remarks on differential diagnosis made in connection with lymphosarcoma apply equally to the leukaemias.

Chronic Leukaemia

Chronic leukaemia occurs in myeloid and lymphatic forms. The former appears in adults up to middle age, the latter generally in the middle-aged or elderly. The course of both types is much more prolonged than in acute leukaemia where, in the absence of treament, death occurs in 6 months or less. In chronic myeloid leukaemia the patient may live for up to 10 to 15 years, although in most cases 3 to 5 years is a more likely duration. In chronic lymphatic leukaemia the course is more prolonged, for 10 or more years.

Oral lesions are less frequent in chronic leukaemia than in the acute disease, and they are commoner in chronic myeloid than in chronic lymphatic leukaemia. Non-specific acute and chronic gingivitis, however, are frequently present and spontaneous haemorrhages may occur.

Microscopic examination of oral lesions shows infiltration of the tissues by leukaemic cells, similar to leukaemic lesions elsewhere.

REFERENCES

Adatia, A. K. (1968) Dental tissues and Burkitt's tumor. *Oral Surg.*, **25**, 221.

Appel, P. W. (1968) Reticulum-cell sarcoma in the jaws. *Oral Surg.*, **26**, 92.

Barclay, J. K. (1971) Reticulum cell sarcoma: report of case. *J. oral Surg.*, **29**, 734.

Binnie, W. H., Day, R. C. B., and Lynn, A. H. (1971) Lymphosarcoma presenting with oral symptoms. *Brit. dent. J.*, **130**, 235.

Browne, W. G. (1972) Primary reticulum-cell sarcoma of the alveolar mucosa. *Oral Surg.*, **34**, 422.

Burford, W. N. (1947) Lymphosarcoma of the soft palate. *Amer. J. Orthodont. (Oral Surg. Sect.)*, **33**, 24.

Burford, W. N., Ackerman, L. V., and Robinson, H. B. G. (1944) Lymphosarcoma in a child. *Amer. J. Orthodont. (Oral Surg. Sect.)*, **30**, 353.

Burket, L. W. (1944) A histopathologic explanation for the oral lesions in the acute leucemias. *Amer. J. Orthodont. (Oral Surg. Sect.)*, **30**, 516.

Burkitt, D. (1958) A sarcoma involving the jaws in African children. *Brit. J. Surg.*, **46**, 218.

Burkitt, D. (1962) A children's cancer dependent on climatic factors. *Nature*, **194**, 232.

Burkitt, D. (1962) Determining the climatic limitations of a children's cancer common in Africa. *Brit. med. J.*, **2**, 1019.

Burkitt, D., and O'Conor, G. T. (1961) Malignant lymphoma in African children. I. A clinical syndrome. *Cancer*, **14**, 259.

Burstone, M. S., and Baetz, F. O. (1952) A case of primary oral lymphosarcoma. *Oral Surg.*, **5**, 830.

Calderwood, R. G. (1967) Primary reticulum-cell sarcoma of gingiva. *Oral Surg.*, **24**, 71.

Calhoun, N. R., and Johnson, C. C. (1966) Oral manifestation of mycosis fungoides. Report of a case. *Oral Surg.*, **22**, 261.

Campbell, R. L., Kelly, D. E., and Burkes, E. J. (1975) Primary reticulum-cell sarcoma of the mandible. Review of the literature and report of a case. *Oral Surg.*, **39**, 918.

Christiansen, G. W. (1938) Lymphosarcoma of the jaws and palate. *J. amer. dent. Ass.*, **25**, 728.

Coles, W. C., and Schulz, M. D. (1948) Bone involvement in malignant lymphoma. *Radiology*, **50**, 458.

Cook, H. P. (1961) Oral lymphomas. *Oral Surg.*, **14,** 690.

Darlington, C. G., and Lefkowitz, L. L. (1936) A pathological study of "so-called" dental tumors. *Amer. J. clin. Path.*, **6,** 330.

Duffy, J. H., and Driscoll, E. J. (1958) Oral manifestations of leukemia. *Oral Surg.*, **11,** 484.

Eisenbud, L., and Kotch, R. (1954) Hodgkin's "sarcoma" of the cheek. Report of a case. *Oral Surg.*, **7,** 213.

Fanale, S. J., and McCauley, H. B. (1945) Lymphosarcoma of dental interest; report of a case. *J. oral Surg.*, **3,** 186.

Forman, G. H., and Wesson, C. M. (1970) Hodgkin's disease of the mandible. *Brit. J. oral Surg.*, **7,** 146.

Freedman, L. J. (1940) Primary lymphosarcoma of the hard palate. *Amer. J. Roentgenol.*, **43,** 702.

Frisch, J., and Bhaskar, S. N. (1966) Reticulum-cell sarcoma of the gingiva. *Oral Surg.*, **21,** 236.

Gerry, R. G., and Williams, S. F. (1955) Primary reticulum-cell sarcoma of the mandible. *Oral Surg.*, **8,** 568.

Greer, R. O., and Richardson, J. F. (1974) Refractory ulcerative stomatitis: report of a case in a patient with Hodgkin's disease. *J. oral Med.*, **29,** 45.

Harvey, W., and Thomson, A. D. (1965) A case of reticulum cell sarcoma of gums and skin. *Brit. J. oral Surg.*, **3,** 153.

Hatziotis, J., and Asprides, C. (1964) Primary lymphosarcoma of the submaxillary salivary gland. Report of a case. *Oral Surg.*, **17,** 503.

Hellwig, C. A. (1947) Malignant lymphoma. The value of radical surgery in selected cases. *Surg. Gynec. Obstet.*, **84,** 950.

Ivins, J. C., and Dahlin, D. C. (1953) Reticulum-cell sarcoma of bone. *J. Bone Jt. Surg.*, **35A,** 835.

Jackson, H., and Parker, F. (1944) Hodgkin's disease. II. Pathology. *New Engl. J. Med.*, **231,** 35.

Jackson, H., and Parker, F. (1945) Hodgkin's disease. IV. Involvement of certain organs. *New Engl. J. Med.*, **232,** 547.

Jaffe, H. L. (1958) *Tumors and Tumorous Conditions of the Bones and Joints.* London. Henry Kimpton.

Johnson, A. E., Stenstrom, K. W., and Waldron, C. W. (1946) Multiple lymphosarcoma (lymphoblastoma) of the oral and cervical regions. *J. oral Surg.*, **4,** 159.

Khanolkar, V. R. (1948) Reticulum-cell sarcoma of bone. *Arch. Path.*, **46,** 467.

Lynch, M. A., and Ship, I. I. (1967) Initial oral manifestations of leukemia. *J. amer. dent. Ass.*, **75,** 932.

Lynch, M. A., and Ship, I. I. (1967) Oral manifestations of leukemia: a postdiagnostic study. *J. amer. dent. Ass.*, **75,** 1139.

Meyer, G., Roswit, B., and Unger, S. M. (1959) Hodgkin's disease of the oral cavity. *Amer. J. Roentgenol.*, **81,** 430.

O'Conor, G. T. (1961) Malignant lymphoma in African children. II. A pathological entity. *Cancer*, **14,** 270.

Oldham, L., and John, T. J. (1966) An unusual oral manifestation in a case of acute myeloid leukaemia. *Brit. J. oral Surg.*, **4,** 116.

Orsós, S. (1958) Primary lymphosarcoma of the gingivae. *Oral Surg.*, **11,** 426.

Parker, F., and Jackson, H. (1939) Primary reticulum cell sarcoma of bone. *Surg. Gynec. Obstet.*, **68,** 45.

Salman, I., and Darlington, C. G. (1944) Rare (unusual) malignant tumors of the jaws. *Amer. J. Orthodont. (Oral Surg. Sect.)*, **30,** 725.

Sarnat, B. G., and Weinmann, J. P. (1955) Misdiagnosis of oral lymphosarcomatosis. *Arch. Otolaryngol.*, **61,** 654.

Seldin, H. M., Seldin, S. D., and Rakower, W. (1954) Oral lymphosarcoma. *J. oral Surg.*, **12,** 3.

Silverman, L. M. (1955) Lymphosarcoma of gingivae. *Oral Surg.*, **8,** 1108.

Sinrod, H. S. (1957) Leukemia as a dental problem. *J. amer. dent. Ass.*, **55,** 809.

Steg, R. F., Dahlin, D. C., and Gores, R. J. (1959) Malignant lymphoma of the mandible and maxillary region. *Oral Surg.*, **12,** 128.

Steiner, P. E. (1943) Hodgkin's disease. The incidence, distribution, nature and possible significance of the lymphogranulomatous lesions in the bone marrow. A review with original data. *Arch. Path.*, **36,** 627.

Sugarbaker, E. D., and Craver, L. F. (1940) Lymphosarcoma. A study of 196 cases with biopsy. *J. amer. med. Ass.*, **115,** 17.

Szutu, C., and Hsieh, C. K. (1942) Primary reticulum cell sarcoma of bone. Report of two cases with bone regeneration following roentgenotherapy. *Ann. Surg.*, **115,** 280.

Tillman, H. H. (1965) Malignant lymphomas involving the oral cavity and surrounding structures. Report of twelve cases. *Oral Surg.*, **19,** 60.

Tomich, C. E., and Shafer, W. G. (1975) Lymphoproliferative disease of the hard palate. A clinico-pathologic entity. A study of twenty-one cases. *Oral Surg.*, **39**, 754.

White, G. E. (1970) Oral manifestations of leukemia in children. *Oral Surg.*, **29**, 420.

Ziegler, J. L., Wright, D. H., and Kyalwazi, S. K. (1971) Differential diagnosis of Burkitt's lymphoma of the face and jaws. *Cancer*, **27**, 503.

24. Myeloma

Tumours composed of plasma cells generally occur as multiple lesions (myelomatosis) and usually arise in the marrow, particularly in the skull, vertebrae, ribs, sternum and pelvic bones, although any bone may be affected. Cade (1947) has estimated that myelomatous lesions account for 3 per cent of all bone tumours. In some cases solitary tumours occur, in one bone only, but multiple lesions frequently appear subsequently. Soft tissue lesions (plasmacytoma) may also occur, in such tissues as lymph nodes, liver, spleen and other internal organs.

Both the multiple and the solitary lesions occur in the jaws and the soft tissue plasmacytoma may also occur in the oral tissues.

Multiple Myeloma

Radiographic surveys show that the most frequently affected bones are those of the skull, in which there are lesions in over 70 per cent of cases. But as Willis (1967) points out, estimates of involvement of various bones are likely to be on the low side since diffuse myelomatous lesions can readily escape naked-eye detection at autopsy or radiography.

Lesions in the jaws are generally considered as occurring in about 30 per cent of cases, though Cataldo and Meyer (1966) report a much higher incidence when jaw radiography is systematically carried out. The mandible is much more often affected than the maxilla. The lesions are usually multiple and may occur anywhere in the mandible, though the molar and premolar areas and the angle are the regions most commonly affected. The reason for this predilection is thought to be that active red marrow is normally present at these sites.

Clinical Features

Myelomatosis occurs in middle-aged and elderly persons; it is rare under the age of 30. Males are affected about four times as frequently as females. In most cases the patient with jaw lesions has multiple involvement of bones when he is first seen and the oral lesions are merely incidental to the general picture. Occasionally, however, the oral lesions are the first of which complaint is made and examination then leads to the discovery of multiple lesions in other parts of the body. Cases of this type have been reported by Wolff and Nolan (1944), Meloy, Gunter and Sampson (1945), Calman (1952), Silverman and Shklar (1962), Lewin and Cataldo (1967), Wood (1975) and others. Bruce and Royer (1953) report on a series of 17 cases. Pain is a common early symptom and it may be very severe. Numbness of the lip or chin may be present, and loosening of the teeth. Pathological fractures may be the first sign (Henderson and Rowe, 1969). There may be severe haemorrhage after extractions. At the outset the lesion is entirely intraosseous, but in due course it causes swelling of the jaw with destruction of bone. On palpation, the swelling is tender and eggshell crackling may be elicited. Eventually the cortex is perforated and the tumour appears as a fleshy mass that may grow widely, enveloping teeth and ulcerating. Sometimes, however, it remains as a quite small, firm lump in the gum. Occasionally, the lesion breaks through the bone in more than one place and if there has been little expansion of the jaw, the "epulides" as they have sometimes been termed, may constitute the main intraoral finding. Such lesions can also occur in the gum in the absence of an intraosseous lesion (Burford and Ackerman, 1945; Moss, 1958).

Amyloidosis may occur in myelomatosis and the tongue may be affected. Brunsting and Macdonald (1947) and Cahn (1957) describe cases of this type, in which the tongue was rubbery and enlarged to about twice its normal size, causing impairment of speech, mastication and deglutition. Dockerty and colleagues (1968) point out that the induration produced by amyloidosis may be suggestive of carcinoma. They have also found that macroglossia due to amyloidosis may be an early manifestation of myelomatosis. It may even precede the bone lesions (Buchanan and colleagues, 1969).

Radiological examination of the skull and other bones may show the characteristic punched-out areas of rarefaction, devoid of osteoblastic activity, together with some degree of generalised osteoporosis. In some cases, however, there is a more diffuse rarefaction without localised osteolytic areas. The changes in the jaws may be similarly variable, and though sometimes the characteristic appearances are seen, in other cases the radiograph may be more suggestive of ameloblastoma or a giant cell lesion, or of metastatic carcinoma (Fig. 87).

Where the oral lesion is simply the presenting manifestation of widespread disease the diagnosis does not present much difficulty, as in addition to the clinical and radiological features of the disseminated lesions one or more of the other features of the condition are likely to be present. These include the characteristic changes in the serum protein distribution, Bence Jones proteinuria, elevated serum calcium level, excess of plasma cells in marrow puncture films and anaemia. The hyperproteinaemia is due to an increase in the globulins, generally the gamma globulins. The abnormal nature of the excessive globulin is indicated by the fact that patients with myelomatosis are particularly susceptible to intercurrent infections. The protein abnormality is also the cause of the amyloidosis that occurs in some 10 per cent of patients.

Pathology. Myelomatous lesions destroy the bone, replacing it with soft fleshy purplish red tissue. Microscopically, the lesion consists of a dense mass of cells which in most cases resemble the familiar plasma cells of chronic inflammatory lesions. However, the tumour cells are rather larger than inflammatory plasma cells and binucleate forms are more often seen. Mitoses are present, though they are not usually numerous, and the occasional giant cell may be seen. The stroma is very scanty.

In other cases the resemblance to plasma cells is much less obvious, the tumour cells being round or oval with a spherical nucleus and basophilic cytoplasm. It is in lesions of this type that confusion may arise, for example with reticulum cell sarcoma, or with Ewing's tumour or neuroblastoma. Jaffe (1958) therefore recommends that a diagnosis made initially on a biopsy specimen should be confirmed by sternal marrow puncture or by direct smears from the specimen, stained with Wright stain.

Behaviour. Myelomatosis is a fatal condition and in most cases the duration is not longer than 3 or 4 years. However, there do occur instances in which the course is prolonged, especially since the introduction of cytostatics, though the ultimate outcome cannot be in doubt.

Solitary Myeloma

In a small number of cases there occurs a lesion in the jaws that conforms to the solitary type of growth described by Lichtenstein and Jaffe (1947), Ritz and Meyer (1952), Naylor and Chester-Williams (1954) and others, but even after many years further growths are very likely to appear. It is highly probable that if most cases of solitary growths be followed over a sufficiently long period, obvious disseminated disease will ultimately be found. Nevertheless, there are well documented cases where after many years there have been no recurrences or new foci after resection or radiotherapy of a solitary lesion, or even where a solitary lesion has existed for years in the absence of further lesions. Cases of this type have been reported by Willis (1941), Raven and Willis (1949), Lumb (1952), Pankovich and Griem (1972) and others.

A small number of jaw lesions come into this category also (Stewart and Taylor, 1932; Spitzer and Price, 1948; Christopherson and Miller, 1950; Lane, 1952; Davis and Havens, 1954;

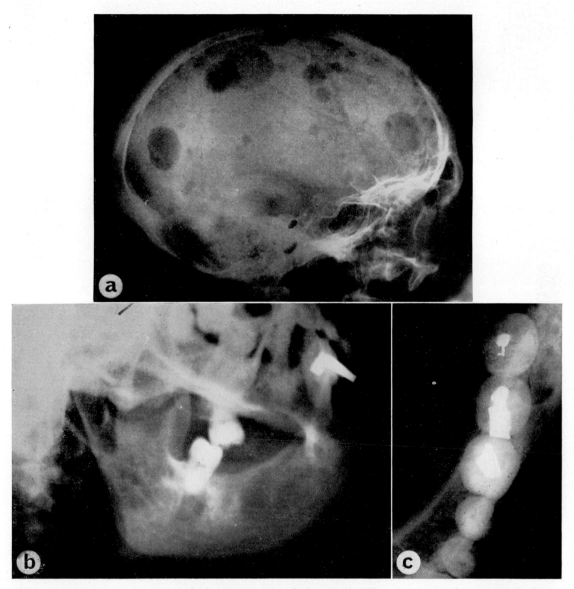

Fig. 87 Myelomatosis. **a,** typical appearance of the skull. The clear-cut, almost punched-out radiolucencies are characteristic. **b, c,** similar appearances are often seen in jaw lesions, but sometimes, as here, the radiolucent areas may be rather less well defined.

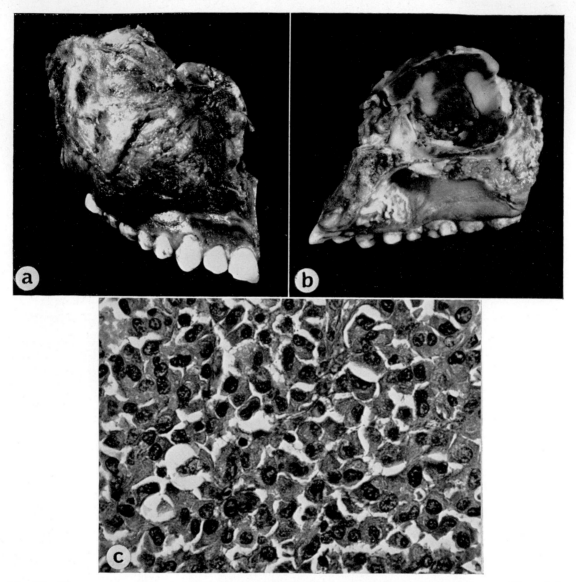

Fig. 88.   Plasmacytoma of the maxillary region. This African male of 22 years had a diffuse swelling of the right maxillary region of 2 months duration. There was a small projection of growth in the upper buccal sulcus and a polypoidal mass was seen in the right nostril. No other lesions were detected on radiographic skeletal survey. Bone marrow biopsy was normal. The plasma proteins, calcium, phosphate and phosphatase were normal. There was no proteinuria. **a, b,** the maxilla was excised. It was largely destroyed and replaced by a fleshy tumour with several well defined lobulated areas, and there were polypoidal extensions of growth towards the right ethmoid cells. It was thought probable that the lesion had arisen in the naso-pharynx and had then invaded bone. Natural size. **c,** section of the tumour, showing a uniform mass of plasma cells. $\times$ 500.

Hinds, Pleasants and Bell, 1956; Whitlock and Hughes, 1960; Webb and colleagues, 1966). Notable among these cases is Christopherson and Miller's patient with a mandibular lesion; this patient was free from recurrence or further lesions 16 years after its excision. Whitlock and Hughes's patient also had a mandibular lesion. This had been present for 16 years, and 5 years after its removal by curettage the patient was well and free from any further lesions.

In most cases of solitary myeloma there is absence of the haematological and biochemical changes that characterise many cases of multiple myelomatosis. Exceptionally, however, such changes may be found, as for example, in Lumb's (1948) patient with a large sacral lesion. In this case there was Bence Jones proteinuria and blockage of the renal tubules by proteinaceous deposits. Slight Bence Jones proteinuria was noted in Whitlock and Hughes's patient and electrophoresis showed a raised gamma globulin with some increase in the beta globulin. Similarly, in Lane's (1952) case, a slightly abnormal electrophoretic pattern was noted, but in both these cases the serum protein pattern returned to normal some time after operation.

Plasmacytoma

Lesions in the soft tissues occur chiefly in the upper respiratory and alimentary tract, including the nares, sinuses, tonsils, palate, tongue, gingivae, and the floor of the mouth. They have also been found in the pleura, mediastinum, thyroid, spermatic cord, ovary, intestines, kidney and skin. The published cases have been reviewed by Hellwig (1943) and Poole and Marchetta (1968). Reports of oral lesions are cited by Stiff and Ferraro (1972).

The lesions are often polypoid or pedunculated but may be sessile or present as diffuse swellings beneath the mucosa. Multiple lesions are rare. Ewing and Foote (1952) note that the main symptom is obstruction rather than bleeding or discharge, unless the adjacent bone is involved, when bleeding and ulceration are more likely. Pain is not a prominent feature, again unless bone is invaded.

Microscopically, the lesions consist of solid masses of plasma cells. Sometimes multinucleated cells are present and some mitoses may be noted (Fig. 88). As Stout and Kenney (1949) and others have pointed out, these lesions have to be differentiated from chronic inflammatory foci, particularly in the mouth where such lesions are common. Inflammatory lesions, however, are more vascular than the plasmacytoma and even though they may consist largely of plasma cells other inflammatory cells are always present, at least to some extent. Poswillo (1968) has reported cases of diffuse plasma cell infiltration of the gingivae, which he considers to differ both from plasmacytoma and inflammatory accumulations of plasma cells. Similarly, Bhaskar, Levin and Frisch (1968) describe what they call plasma cell granuloma of the periodontal tissues, but there seems no good reason for considering these lesions to be distinct entities and other than examples of chronic inflammation with pronounced plasma cell infiltration. It should in fact be noted that a dense plasma cell infiltration is such a common feature of inflammatory lesions in the oral soft tissues, and especially the gingivae, that in these areas the diagnosis of plasmacytoma should be made with great caution.

The behaviour of the plasmacytoma is unpredictable and cannot be related to variations in the cellular picture, such as numbers of mitoses. Some lesions appear to be benign and do not recur after complete removal. Others show evidence of local malignancy, with invasion and destruction of adjacent tissue. The regional lymph nodes may be involved. Lesions in bone may also be present and the picture may then be indistinguishable from multiple myelomatosis (Stewart and Taylor, 1932; Blacklock and Macartney, 1932; Lumb, 1952).

REFERENCES

Bhaskar, S. N., Levin, M. P., and Frisch, J. (1968) Plasma cell granuloma of periodontal tissues. Report of 45 cases. *Periodontics*, **6**, 272.

Blacklock, J. W. S., and Macartney, C. (1932) Plasmacytoma of the naso-pharynx. *J. Path. Bact.*, **35**, 69.

Bruce, K. W., and Royer, R. Q. (1953) Multiple myeloma occurring in the jaws. A study of 17 cases. *Oral Surg.*, **6**, 729.

Brunsting, L. A., and Macdonald, I. D. (1947) Primary systematized amyloidosis with macroglossia: a syndrome related to Bence Jones proteinuria and myeloma. *Proc. Mayo Clin.*, **22**, 67.

Buchanan, J., Gibson, I. I. J. M., Gibson, T., and Russell, A. R. (1969) Macroglossia in myelomatosis. *Brit. J. plastic Surg.*, **22**, 157.

Burford, W. N., and Ackerman, L. V. (1945) Plasma-cell myeloma with involvement of the gum of the mandible. *Amer. J. Orthodont. (Oral Surg. Sect.)*, **31**, 541.

Cade, S. (1947) Primary malignant tumours of bone. *Brit. J. Radiol.*, **20**, 10.

Cahn, L. (1957) Oral amyloid as a complication of myclomatosis. *Oral Surg.*, **10**, 735.

Calman, H. I. (1952) Multiple myeloma. Report of a case first observed in the maxilla. *Oral Surg.*, **5**, 1302.

Cataldo, E., and Meyer, I. (1966) Solitary and multiple plasma-cell tumors of the jaws and oral cavity *Oral Surg.*, **22**, 628.

Christopherson, W. M., and Miller, A. J. (1950) A re-evaluation of solitary plasma-cell myeloma of bone. *Cancer*, **3**, 240.

Davis, G. D., and Havens, F. Z. (1954) Plasma cell myeloma of the mandible. *Proc. Mayo Clin.*, **29**, 569.

Dockerty, M. B., Parkhill, E. M., Dahlin, D. C., Woolner, L. B., Soule, E. H., and Harrison, E. G. (1968) *Tumors of the Oral Cavity and Pharynx.* Atlas of Tumor Pathology. Section 4. Fascicle 10b. Washington, D.C. Armed Forces Institute of Pathology.

Ewing, M. R., and Foote, F. W. (1952) Plasma-cell tumors of the mouth and upper air passages. *Cancer*, **5**, 499.

Hellwig, C. A. (1943) Extramedullary plasma cell tumors as observed in various locations. *Arch. Path.*, **36**, 95.

Henderson, D., and Rowe, N. L. (1969) Myelomatosis affecting the jaws. *Brit. J. oral Surg.*, **6**, 161.

Hinds, E. C., Pleasants, J. E., and Bell, W. E. (1956) Solitary plasma-cell myeloma of the mandible. *Oral Surg.*, **9**, 193.

Jaffe, H. L. (1958) *Tumors and Tumorous Conditions of the Bones and Joints.* London. Henry Kimpton.

Lane, S. L. (1952) Plasmacytoma of the mandible. *Oral Surg.*, **5**, 434.

Lewin, R. W., and Cataldo, E. (1967) Multiple myeloma discovered from oral manifestations: report of case. *J. oral Surg.*, **25**, 68.

Lichtenstein, L., and Jaffe, H. L. (1947) Multiple myeloma. A survey based on thirty-five cases, eighteen of which came to autopsy. *Arch. Path.*, **44**, 207.

Lumb, G. (1948) Solitary plasmocytoma of bone with renal changes. *Brit. J. Surg.*, **36**, 16.

Lumb, G. (1952) The pathology of the myelomata (plasma cell tumours). *Ann. roy. Coll. Surg. Engl.*, **10**, 241.

Meloy, T. M., Gunter, J. H., and Sampson, D. A. (1945) Mandibular lesion as first evidence of multiple myeloma. *Amer. J. Orthodont. (Oral Surg. Sect.)*, **31**, 685.

Moss, R. L. (1958) Multiple myeloma with maxillary myelomatous epulis and malignant pheochromocytoma. Report of a case. *Oral Surg.*, **11**, 951.

Naylor, A., and Chester-Williams, F. E. (1954) Myelomata of bone. A review of 25 cases. *Brit. med. J.*, **1**, 120.

Pankovich, A., and Griem, M. (1972) Plasma cell myeloma. *Radiology*, **104**, 521.

Poole, A. G., and Marchetta, F. C. (1968) Extramedullary plasmacytoma of the head and neck. *Cancer*, **22**, 14.

Poswillo, D. (1968) Plasmacytosis of the gingiva. *Brit. J. oral Surg.*, **5**, 194.

Raven, R. W., and Willis, R. A. (1949) Solitary plasmocytoma of bone. *J. Bone Jt. Surg.*, **31B**, 369.

Ritz, N. D., and Meyer, L. M. (1952) Solitary plasmacytoma of bone with subsequent multiple myeloma. *Acta haemat.*, **8**, 224.

Silverman, L. M., and Shklar, G. (1962) Multiple myeloma. Report of a case. *Oral Surg.*, **15**, 301.

Spitzer, R., and Price, L. W. (1948) Solitary myeloma of the mandible. *Brit. med. J.*, **1**, 1027.

Stewart, M. J., and Taylor, A. L. (1932) Observations on solitary plasmocytoma. *J. Path. Bact.*, **35**, 541.

Stiff, R. H., and Ferraro, E. F. (1972) The extramedullary plasmacytoma, benign or malignant? *J. oral Med.*, **27**, 22.

Stout, A. P., and Kenney, F. R. (1949) Primary plasma-cell tumors of the upper air passages and oral cavity. *Cancer*, **2**, 261.

Webb, H. E., Devine, K. N., and Harrison, E. G. (1966) Solitary myeloma of the mandible. *Oral Surg.*, **22**, 1.

Whitlock, R. I. H., and Hughes, N. C. (1960) Solitary myeloma of mandible. Report of a case. *Oral Surg.*, **13**, 23.

Willis, R. A. (1941) Solitary plasmocytoma of bone. *J. Path. Bact.*, **53**, 77.

Willis, R. A. (1967) *Pathology of Tumours*. 4th Edition. London. Butterworth & Co. (Publishers) Ltd.

Wolff, E., and Nolan, L. E. (1944) Multiple myeloma first discovered in the mandible. *Radiology*, **42**, 76.

Wood, G. D. (1975) Myelomatosis. A case report. *Brit. dent. J.*, **139**, 472.

25. Ewing's Tumour

Most pathologists concede to Ewing's tumour an independent existence though some, including Willis (1967), are uncertain that there is such an entity. The tumour was first characterised as a definitive condition by Ewing in 1921 and though the histological criteria for its diagnosis have undergone some changes since the original description, the lesion as now conceived is generally agreed as constituting a specific primary malignant tumour of bone. It occurs in childhood and adolescence, twice as often in males as in females, and mostly in the long bones, tibia, humerus, femur or fibula. Less often, the ribs, pelvis, vertebrae or cranial bones are affected, and very occasionally the jaws. Pain is the chief complaint, together with the presence of a swelling that has often been increasing in size fairly rapidly. The swelling may be tender and sometimes there is hyperaemia of the overlying tissues, suggesting an inflammatory condition. There may also be constitutional symptoms such as moderate pyrexia, leucocytosis, anaemia and increased sedimentation rate. In jaw tumours paraesthesia of the lips and chin may be present. Metastases occur both by the lymphatics and the blood stream, to almost any tissue, but a peculiarity of the tumour is its proclivity to metastasise to other bones. The condition is usually fatal within 2 years, though some cases are more prolonged.

The incidence of jaw lesions is low. The tumour may occur in either the mandible, particularly the horizontal ramus, or the maxilla, but much more frequently in the former. In the early stages, while the tumour is still intraosseous, the swelling is firm. When the tumour breaks through the cortex, however, it spreads extensively in the soft tissues and forms a soft mass that may ulcerate. In maxillary tumours the sinus may be filled by growth while in mandibular tumours a very large intra-oral mass may ultimately result. Radiologically, osteolytic destruction is the principal feature. In early cases this may not be very marked, and if there is some surrounding sclerosis the appearances may closely resemble those of chronic osteomyelitis. However, the bone destruction is progressive and often rapid, so that soon a large defect develops, with widening or destruction of the cortex. New bone formation may be seen, either in the form of concentric "onion peel" layers deposited parallel to the periosteum or as perpendicular striae of the sunray type that may suggest a diagnosis of osteosarcoma.

Pathologically, the findings in jaw tumours correspond to those in other bones. The tumour forms a greyish-white mass in which there may occur areas of haemorrhage or degeneration and subsequently cyst formation. Microscopically, the tumour consists of solid masses of small round cells of uniform size, with little cytoplasm and rather indistinct margins. Mitoses are present, though not in large numbers. There is very little stroma between the tumour cells (Fig. 89). It is this cellular uniformity which has caused much of the difficulty in the diagnosis of Ewing's tumour, since other tumours may have a very similar appearance. Amongst the important differential diagnoses are metastatic carcinoma, neuroblastoma and reticulum cell sarcoma. The question of carcinoma arises particularly in older patients and every care has to be taken to exclude the possibility of an occult or clinically silent primary tumour elsewhere. Similarly, a metastatic lesion may be the first evidence of neuroblastoma in children. The estimation of urinary catecholamines may be helpful, as these are increased in many cases of neuroblastoma. In reticulum cell sarcoma reticulin fibres are often disposed regularly around the cells, whereas these fibres are not thus seen in Ewing's tumour. Glycogen may be demonstrated within the cells in Ewing's tumour, but not in reticulum cell sarcoma or neuroblastoma. Lichtenstein and

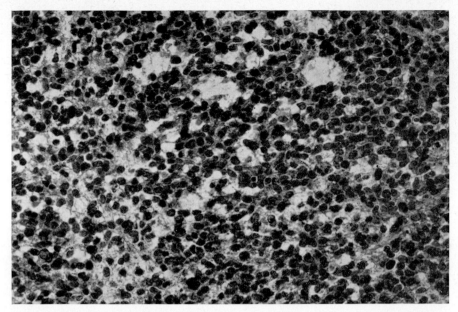

Fig. 89   Ewing's tumour. The tumour presented as a rapidly enlarging swelling of 6 weeks duration in the middle of the mandible in a girl of 3 years of age. It consists of sheets of quite uniform small round cells with little cytoplasm and indistinct outlines. × 300.

Jaffe (1947), Jaffe (1958), Evans (1966) and Lichtenstein (1972) deal with these points in detail

The outlook in Ewing's tumour is poor. Although the tumour as a rule responds to local irradiation, this is only temporary. There is, however, evidence that better results might be obtained with combined chemotherapy and radiotherapy (Freeman and colleagues, 1972; Fernandez and colleagues, 1974).

For case reports of Ewing's tumour in the jaws, see Geschickter (1935), Salman and Darlington (1944), Mann, Ash and Bernier (1944), Oehlers (1950), and Thoma and Goldman (1960). The literature is summarised by Crowe and Harper (1965) and by Roca and colleagues (1968), with further reports from Hunsuck (1968), Brownson and Cook (1969) and Potdar (1970). The last named author describes a series of nine cases. A metastatic lesion in the mandible from a primary rib tumour has been recorded by Carl and colleagues (1971).

REFERENCES

Brownson, R. J., and Cook, R. P. (1969) Ewing's sarcoma of the maxilla. *Ann. Otol. Rhinol. Laryngol.*, **78**, 1299.

Carl, W., Schaaf, N. G., Gaeta, J., and Sinks, L. F. (1971) Ewing's sarcoma. *Oral Surg.*, **31**, 472.

Crowe, W. W., and Harper, J. C. (1965) Ewing's sarcoma with primary lesion in mandible: report of case. *J. oral Surg.*, **23**, 156.

Evans, R. W. (1966) *Histological Appearances of Tumours*. 2nd Edition. Edinburgh. E. & S. Livingstone Ltd.

Ewing, J. (1921) Diffuse endothelioma of bone. *Proc. N.Y. Path. Soc.*, **21**, 17.

Fernandez, C. H., Lindberg, R. D., Sutow, W. W., and Samuels, M. L. (1974) Localized Ewing's sarcoma—treatment and results. *Cancer*, **34**, 143.

Freeman, A. I., Sachatello, C., Gaeta, J., Shah, N. K., Wang, J. J., and Sinks, L. F. (1972) An analysis of Ewing's tumor in children at Roswell Park Memorial Institute. *Cancer*, **29**, 1563.

Geschickter, C. F. (1935) Tumors of the jaws. *Amer. J. Cancer*, **26**, 90.

Hunsuck, E. E. (1968) Ewing's sarcoma of the maxilla. Report of a case. *Oral Surg.*, **25**, 923.

Jaffe, H. L. (1958) *Tumors and Tumorous Conditions of the Bones and Joints*. London. Henry Kimpton.

Lichtenstein, L. (1972) *Bone Tumours*. 4th Edition. St. Louis. The C.V. Mosby Company.

Lichtenstein, L., and Jaffe, H. L. (1947) Ewing's sarcoma of bone. *Amer. J. Path.*, **23**, 43.

Mann, J. B., Ash, J. E., and Bernier, J. L. (1944) *Atlas of Dental and Oral Pathology*. 3rd Edition. Chicago. American Dental Association.

Oehlers, F. A. C. (1950) A case of Ewing's tumour with primary lesion in the mandible. *Brit. dent. J.*, **88**, 146.

Potdar, G. G. (1970) Ewing's tumors of the jaws. *Oral Surg.*, **29**, 505.

Roca, A. N., Smith, J. L., MacComb, W. S., and Jing, B.-S. (1968) Ewing's sarcoma of the maxilla and mandible. Study of six cases. *Oral Surg.*, **25**, 194.

Salman, I., and Darlington, C. G. (1944) Rare (unusual) malignant tumors of the jaws. *Amer. J. Orthodont. (Oral Surg. Sect.)*, **30**, 725.

Thoma, K. H., and Goldman, H. M. (1960) *Oral Pathology*. 5th Edition. St. Louis. The C. V. Mosby Company.

Willis, R. A. (1967) *Pathology of Tumours*. 4th Edition. London. Butterworth & Co. (Publishers) Ltd.

26. Giant Cell Lesions

Giant cell lesions in the oral tissues occur as intraosseous growths within the jaws and as extrabony lesions in the soft tissues. The intrabony lesions comprise the giant cell tumour of bone, the giant cell granuloma and the focal giant cell lesion or "brown tumour" of hyperparathyroidism. The soft tissue giant cell lesion is the giant cell epulis or peripheral giant cell granuloma.

GIANT CELL TUMOUR OF BONE

The work of Jaffe and his colleagues particularly, and of others, has done a great deal to increase our understanding of giant cell lesions of bone (Jaffe, 1953; Jaffe, Lichtenstein and Portis, 1940; Coley, 1960; Lichtenstein, 1950, 1951, 1953). These workers have defined the true giant cell neoplasm and have shown that in the past many other lesions, both neoplastic and non-neoplastic, have frequently been diagnosed as giant cell tumours of bone simply because of the presence of giant cells. These lesions included fibromas, bone cysts, fibrous dysplasia, the bone lesions of hyperparathyroidism and other conditions. The definitive recognition of such conditions has been of great importance, because of marked differences in their behaviour and prognosis. Following on this work, the diagnosis of giant cell tumour of bone has been made much less frequently in recent years than was formerly the case, owing to a clearer appreciation by pathologists of the heterogeneous nature of the group of lesions that have only the presence of some giant cells in common. This is particularly so in the case of the jaws, for in these bones it now appears that true giant cell tumours are very rare, whereas once they were diagnosed with some frequency.

The commonest sites for giant cell tumour are the lower end of the femur, the upper end of the tibia and the lower end of the radius. Other long bones may occasionally be affected. The incidence of the tumour in the jaws is difficult to determine, because of the diagnostic confusion that has prevailed in the past. Bernick's (1948) review of 816 cases of giant cell tumour reported in the literature since 1900 showed that 11·3 per cent of these tumours occurred in the jaws, but it is certain that many of the lesions reported prior to 1948 as true giant cell tumours of the jaws would not now be so diagnosed. In fact, in recent years very few giant cell lesions of the jaws have been reported as true tumours, for the majority of authors have agreed with Jaffe as to the rarity of this lesion. Waldron (1953), for example, reviewed his own material, comprising 28 jaw lesions originally diagnosed as giant cell tumours, and concluded that in only 5 of the cases could the lesions be considered as identical with the bona fide giant cell tumour of long bones. Austin, Dahlin and Royer (1959) in a series of 968 benign jaw tumours found 34 intraosseous and 30 soft tissue giant cell granulomas, but only two true giant cell tumours. Jaffe himself considered that only one of the giant cell lesions of the jaw that he had seen was a true tumour.

There has been some reaction to these views. For example, Morton (1956), Bernier (1958), Shklar and Meyer (1961) and others suggest that true giant cell tumours do occur more frequently in the jaws than has recently been supposed. Waldron and Shafer (1966) take the view that the giant cell lesion in the jaws is probably identical with the "benign giant cell tumour" of other bones. Nevertheless, though some giant cell lesions in the jaws have certainly behaved rather aggressively, it is undoubted that unequivocal metastasising lesions are excessively rare.

Clinical Features

Giant cell tumours occur principally between the ages of 20 and 40 years. Jaffe (1953) and Lichtenstein (1972) stress that they are very rare in children under the age of 10 and are uncommon below the age of 15 to 20.

The principal symptom is swelling of the bone, accompanied in some cases by pain. The swelling may be tender, and eggshell crackling may be elicited in large tumours. Radiologically, there is an area of translucency with thinning and expansion of the cortex, but little or no periosteal new bone formation. The radiolucent area may show a soap bubble or honeycomb appearance, but this is inconstant. The appearances are thus not specific, and in the jaws could be caused by a number of other lesions such as ameloblastoma, myxoma and some cysts.

Pathology

The tumour forms a maroon or reddish-brown fleshy mass that replaces the spongiosa of the bone. Expansion and thinning of the cortex occur, with ultimate perforation and the protrusion of a soft subperiosteal mass. The periosteum generally remains intact. Necrosis, haemorrhage, fibrosis and cyst formation can all occur, usually in larger growths of some duration.

Microscopically, the tumour consists of numerous giant cells lying in a cellular matrix composed of spindle-shaped cells and scanty collagen. The giant cells measure about 100μ in diameter and contain numerous vesicular nuclei, up to 40 or 50 or more, which are situated towards the centre of the cell, leaving a clear area of cytoplasm around the periphery. Occasionally, the nuclei in a cell are pyknotic. The cytoplasm is granular and vacuoles are often present. An important feature of the histological architecture is the even distribution of the giant cells throughout the tumour. A considerable number of the cells are nearly always to be seen in every microscopic field. The matrix cells are mainly spindle-shaped with large elongated nuclei, though cells with rounded or ovoid nuclei are also present. The nuclei are very similar to those of the giant cells. There is a scanty collagenous matrix between the tumour cells and numerous thin-walled blood vessels are also present (Fig. 90). Bone or osteoid tissue, other than that formed reactively, is usually absent.

Histogenesis

Speculations on the nature of the giant cell tumour are of some antiquity. The lesion was first described early in the nineteenth century as a benign neoplasm, but later opinion changed to regard it as a malignant tumour. Hence the names "myeloid sarcoma" and "giant cell sarcoma," which persisted well into the present century. The concept of the lesion as a neoplasm, however, was challenged by Barrie (1920), Konjetzny (1922) and others, who regarded the condition as an inflammatory or reparative reaction, or perhaps as an expression of an abnormal healing process following on intramedullary haemorrhage (Codman, 1925). Nevertheless, many investigators still regarded the lesion as a neoplasm, though once again as a benign one. Bloodgood (1910, 1919) introduced the term "giant cell tumour" and claimed that it could be treated conservatively with success. However, experience showed that liability to recurrence was in fact a feature of these

Fig. 90   Giant cell tumour of bone. **a,** tumour of lower end of femur. The giant cells are quite evenly distributed throughout a spindle cell matrix. × 80. **b,** higher magnification, showing the multinucleated giant cells and the round, ovoid and spindle cells of the intervening tissue. These cells, in this specimen, are quite regular in size, shape and staining propensities. Mitoses are very infrequent. As this was a large tumour, perforating the cortex over an extensive area, amputation was performed. This patient was alive and well 6 years later. × 200, **c,** giant cell tumour of the humerus. This tumour, which metastasised, shows histological evidence of its malignancy. The spindle cells show anisocytosis and hyperchromatism, and mitoses are seen. × 200. **d,** detail from c. × 500.

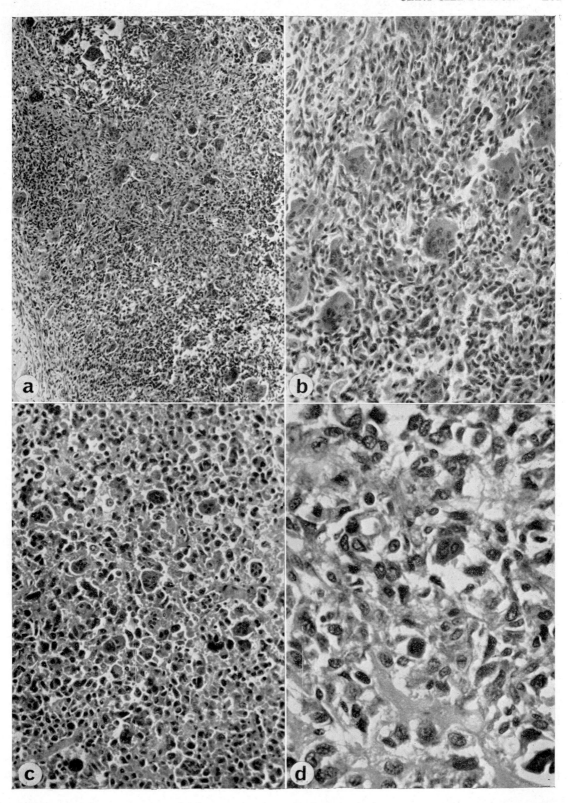

were under 30 years of age, the extremes being 7 and 67 years. As has been noted, true giant cell tumour very rarely occurs below the age of 15. The granuloma occurs more often in females than in males (68 per cent females in Waldron and Shafer's series) and more often in the mandible than in the maxilla. It occurs only in the tooth-bearing area of the jaws and the vast majority of lesions are anterior to the first permanent molar region.

As in giant cell tumour the main symptom is swelling, sometimes accompanied by pain, and some tenderness on palpation. Growth may sometimes be rapid. Although there does not appear to be any particular connection between the lesion and pregnancy, should a lesion be present it may grow more rapidly during pregnancy (Henry, 1964; McGowan, 1969). The teeth may become loose and exfoliate. The cortical plate of bone is not usually perforated, though this does sometimes occur. Marble and colleagues (1969) report a case in which the cortex was eroded and a large soft tissue mass protruded from the palate. Similarly, the lesion may occasionally present as an epulis.

Radiologically, the appearances are similar to those noted for giant cell tumour of bone, a radiolucent defect being present (Fig. 91). Though this has often been described as character-istically multilocular, Austin, Dahlin and Royer (1959) found such an appearance in only one of their 34 cases. In most of the cases the radiolucency was sharply delineated. However, the multilocular appearance was more frequent in Waldron and Shafer's cases. The outline may also present a notched or lobulated appearance.

Pathology

The gross appearance of giant cell granuloma is similar to that of giant cell tumour of bone, but though the cortex is thinned and expanded perforation is much less frequent.

Microscopically, although some granulomas of the jaws and some giant cell tumours of other bones show very close resemblances, there are often differences. In the giant cell granuloma, the giant cells are usually less in number and are more irregularly distributed than in the giant cell tumour (Fig. 92). The giant cells themselves are often smaller than the giant cells of the neoplasm and are unevenly distributed throughout the lesion, so that in a given microscopic field none might be seen while in another perhaps half a dozen might be present. In the neoplasm, on the other hand, numerous evenly distributed giant cells are present in practically every field. The irregular distribution of the giant cells seems to be related to the presence of haemorrhage, for they are aggregated around areas where this has occurred and they may contain ingested red cells and vacuoles of fat. In some cases, however, giant cells may be as abundantly present as in the true tumour.

The giant cells are distributed in a collagenous tissue that contains many small spindle-shaped cells with oval or fusiform nuclei. These have a distinct nuclear membrane and small nucleolus. Whereas in the giant cell tumour the spindle cells may show irregularity in size and shape, nuclear hyperchromatism and mitoses, such features are noted much less frequently in the spindle cells of the granuloma. Appreciable quantities of collagen are present, with small areas of haemorrhage, oedema and sometimes microcyst formation. Trabeculae of osteoid or bone are

Fig. 92.   Giant cell granuloma. **a,** the lesion is similar to giant cell tumour of bone, in that it consists of giant cells in a matrix of spindle and ovoid cells, but the giant cells are relatively fewer in number and form focal accumulations, as shown here, whereas in the tumour they tend to be distributed more evenly. × 80. **b,** in some cases, however, the giant cells are as numerous as in the true tumour, and as diffusely distributed. × 80. **c,** a focus of giant cells around a small area of haemorrhage. The matrix contains an appreciable amount of collagen. The spindle and ovoid cells are regular in size and shape. No mitoses are seen. × 200. **d,** detail from **c.** × 500.

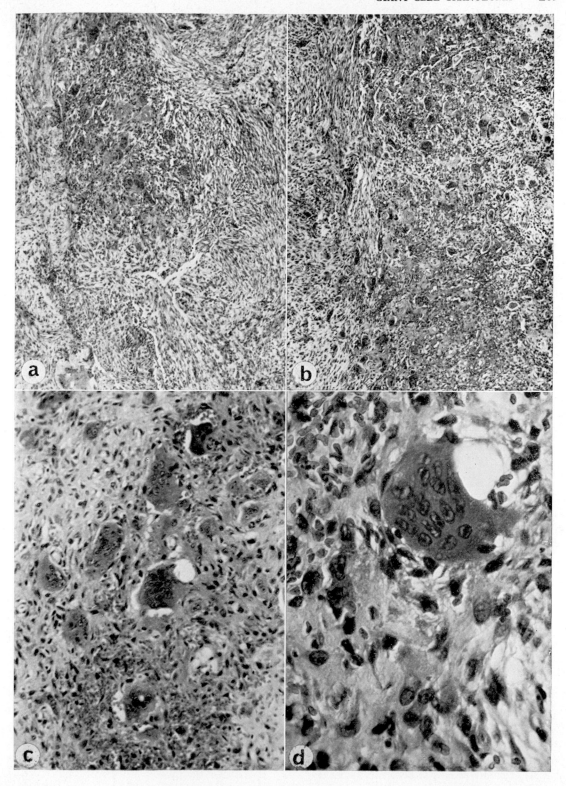

frequently seen. In the giant cell tumour there is little or no ground substance, though occasionally at the periphery bony trabeculae may be present.

Nature and Behaviour

Many authors have followed Jaffe in considering the giant cell granuloma to be a local repara-tive reaction, possibly to intramedullary haemorrhage or trauma, the giant cells being thought not to represent an essential part of a neoplastic condition, as in the giant cell tumour, but rather to be related to the occurrence of haemorrhage in the interior of the bone. However, this view is unlikely to be correct, since the lesion is essentially destructive rather than reparative. Moreover, although the giant cells may contain fragments of erythrocytes, phagocytosis does not seem to be their principal activity (Adkins and colleagues, 1969).

Some authorities believe that the benign giant cell tumour of bone and the giant cell granu-loma of the jaws are of similar, if not identical, nature, both lesions being granulomatous and not neoplastic (Waldron and Shafer, 1966; Shafer, Hine and Levy, 1974). Those long bone lesions with evidence of malignancy they consider to be osteosarcomas or other neoplasms containing numerous giant cells. However, there is abundant evidence that giant cell tumours of bone that appear perfectly benign histologically can metastasise. There is, on the contrary, no evidence of unequivocal metastasis in the case of a jaw lesion. Furthermore, a proportion of long bone tumours that appear initially to be benign giant cell tumours later develop histological evidence of malignancy, whereas such changes in histology have not been reported definitely in jaw lesions. Undoubtedly, there are many similarities between the jaw lesion and giant cell tumours in other bones; they can show close resemblances histologically, and ultrastructure and histochemical studies show that the giant cells of both lesions are very similar to each other and to osteoclasts (Matsumura and colleagues, 1971; Soskolne, 1972), but the differences in behaviour, both histological and clinical, indicate that the lesions are not identical. It is also of interest to note that lesions that are considered to be identical with, or very similar to, the jaw lesions have been described in other bones and are thought to be granulomas rather than neoplasms. Hirschl and Katz (1974) review the literature on these granulomas and report a lesion in the temporal bone.

With regard to behaviour, giant cell granuloma is, as already indicated, an essentially benign condition. It can be treated satisfactorily by enucleation or curettage, after which the cavity readily heals. The recurrence rate may be in the region of 13 per cent (Andersen, Fejerskov and Philipsen, 1973), but the recurrences can again be treated by similar measures; wide and mutilat-ing excisions would not seem to be called for. Radiotherapy can also effect a cure, but the possi-bility of postradiation sarcoma, though small, does exist.

"BROWN TUMOUR" OF HYPERPARATHYROIDISM

In addition to the generalised osteoporosis of hyperparathyroidism, focal lesions similar in histological structure to the giant cell granuloma occur in various bones, including the jaws. When the focal lesions are solitary, as not infrequently happens, a jawbone is very often the site of such a lesion and it may in fact constitute the presenting symptom. This was so in 7 out of 22 patients in Black and Ackerman's (1950) series of cases of parathyroid adenoma, and Bridge (1968) and others have reported similar cases. It has been suggested that this particular liability of the jaws to develop lesions is due to the fact that the turnover of bone is considerable, even in the edentulous state, probably due to masticatory stresses (Weinmann, 1945; Cohen, 1959) or other trauma (Bramley and Dwyer, 1970).

Radiologically, the focal lesion in the jaws appears as a radiolucent area that may be either sharply defined or less well demarcated (Fig. 93). It may be diagnosed tentatively as a cyst of dental origin or as an ameloblastoma or other neoplasm, if the generalised osteoporosis that is also present escapes notice. The porosity produces a more uniform opacity in place of the normal trabecular pattern. Another important radiological feature in hyperparathyroidism is the absence of the lamina dura around the teeth, though this is not an early sign, and in advanced cases there is an apparent increase in the density of the teeth. In some cases resorption of the roots may be noted and this may be so extensive as to lead to exfoliation of the teeth.

Macroscopically, the "brown tumour" forms a mass that expands the bone and may perforate the cortex. Histologically, the appearances are often identical with those of giant cell granuloma and Jaffe considered the brown tumour to be, in effect, a giant cell reparative granuloma itself, representing a reparative scarring reaction in an area damaged by the local effects of hyperparathyroidism (Fig. 93).

OTHER JAW LESIONS IN WHICH GIANT CELLS MAY BE PRESENT

Generally speaking, the diagnosis of giant cell lesions in the jaws is a less difficult task than in other bones, for the reason that the possibilities are less numerous. Thus, benign chondroblastoma and osteoblastoma apparently occur only very rarely in the jaws. These are lesions which have from time to time been confused with giant cell tumour in the long bones. Aneurysmal bone cyst, fibrous dysplasia, cherubism and other fibro-osseous lesions do occur in the jaws and may contain giant cells, but again as in the giant cell granuloma these cells are generally present only focally, and in relatively small numbers, compared with giant cell tumour. However, in some cases the giant cells in aneurysmal bone cyst or cherubism may be so uniformly distributed that the histological distinction from giant cell tumour may present considerable difficulty. In these cases it is particularly important to consider fully the clinical and radiological features. Finally, it will be remembered that, as Thomson and Turner-Warwick (1955) pointed out, areas of osteoclastic resorption are frequently present at the periphery of any bone lesion.

However this may be, the macroscopic and microscopic features of the "brown tumour" may be identical with those of giant cell granuloma and of giant cell tumour of bone. The possibility of hyperparathyroidism should therefore be kept in mind in all cases where a lesion of the jaws turns out to be of the giant cell type. Although the giant cell epulis or peripheral giant cell granuloma is not related to hyperparathyroidism, it should be noted that a "brown tumour" that has perforated the cortex may present apparently as a soft tissue lesion that may be described clinically as an epulis. If multiple epulides are present, or if there is recurrence after excision, again the possibility of hyperparathyroidism should be considered. Recurrence is not necessarily prompt; in the patient whose lesions are illustrated in Fig. 93, this took some time in the case of the first lesion. Buckerfield (1971) reports a case in which parathyroidectomy could not be done, but the local lesions in the jaws were excised. There was no recurrence after one year. It is also of importance to note that more than one estimation of the serum calcium level may be necessary to detect hypercalcaemia, even though the existence of bone lesions indicates that the hyperparathyroid state has been in existence for some time.

GIANT CELL EPULIS

The giant cell epulis is a not uncommon lesion of the oral tissues. It is also known as osteoclastoma, peripheral giant cell tumour or peripheral giant cell granuloma, and was formerly known as myeloid epulis or myeloid sarcoma but these terms have now been discarded.

Clinical Features

The average age of patients with giant cell epulis is between 30 and 40 years. The age distribution is quite wide, for the lesion occurs not infrequently in children and adolescents. Females are affected more often than males, according to the analyses of Baxter (1930), Bernick (1948), Cooke (1952), Brown, Darlington and Kupfer (1956) and Andersen and colleagues (1973). Cooke found the sex incidence to be more or less equal between the ages of 6 and 15 years, but in the older age groups there was a marked preponderance of women in the child-bearing period. The sex ratio taken over all cases showed that females were affected two to three times more often than males.

In an analysis of 720 cases from the literature, Giansanti and Waldron (1969) found that the lesion may occur anywhere in the gingival or alveolar mucosa, although more lesions occur anteriorly than posteriorly. The lower jaw is more often affected than the upper. Early lesions may appear as discoloration and slight swelling of the buccal aspect of the gingiva, while later the lesion increases in size and becomes rounded and very often pedunculated. Sometimes it grows in an hour-glass manner, with the waist of the lesion between two teeth and the globular extremities presenting buccally and lingually.

Pathology

In most cases it is possible to remove the lesion completely while preserving the teeth (Fig. 94), but sometimes, and particularly in recurrent cases, it is necessary to extract the adjoining teeth. In such cases the specimen consists of a tooth or teeth with the growth *in situ*, and it is probable that the lesion has originated in the peridontal ligament or the muco-periosteum. The lesion is characteristically of deep red or maroon appearance and is soft in consistency. Occasional lesions contain a fair proportion of fibrous tissue and tend to be paler and firmer. Ulceration of the surface is not uncommon. The cut surface is reddish-brown and homogeneous in appearance, or it may exhibit a peripheral brownish zone broken by paler radiating streaks.

Microscopically, the lesion consists of large numbers of giant cells in a stroma of collagen fibres and spindle cells (Fig. 95). To this extent the picture resembles the giant cell tumour of bone, but the giant cells are often even more numerous than in the tumour and may be rather larger. The arrangement of the nuclei, filling the cell except for a narrow zone of cytoplasm around the periphery, is similar, but the cytoplasm tends to stain rather less densely and the cell

Fig. 93., Giant cell lesions in a woman of 46 years, with hyperparathyroidism. The first manifestation was a soft red nonfluctuant gingival swelling in the left maxillary second premolar-second molar area. The tumour, which extended into the antrum, was excised. At this time no other lesions were present and radiographic skeletal survey and the blood chemistry were normal. Healing was satisfactory but 9 months later a similar swelling appeared, on this occasion in the right maxillary premolar region. This lesion extended into the antrum, the floor of the orbit and the wall of the nose. Radiographic survey showed in addition a large cyst in the body of the right side of the mandible and a smaller cyst more posteriorly, a large cyst in the left maxilla and several smaller cysts in the region of the right maxillary antrum. The skull bones showed evidence of decalcification. The cervical trachea was deviated by a mass in the left side of the neck. Serum calcium 15·4 mg. A left parathyroid adenoma was removed and the patient made a good recovery. **a,** radiograph of the intitial lesion, showing obliteration of the left maxillary antrum by a radiopaque mass. **b,** nine months later, the right maxillary antrum is obliterated by a similar mass. This is also seen in **c,** where the normal bone pattern is obscured, with destruction of the horizontal plate of the palate. There is also progressive loss of the lamina dura around the teeth. **d,** showing deviation of the oesophagus. **e,** microscopic appearance of the initial lesion. It consists of large multinucleated giant cells in an ovoid and spindle cell stroma. × 80. **f,** detail from **e.** × 500.

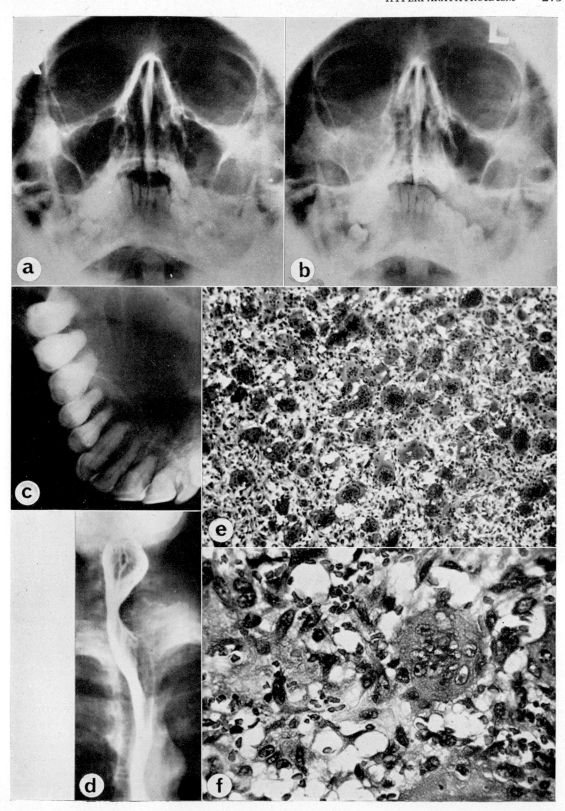

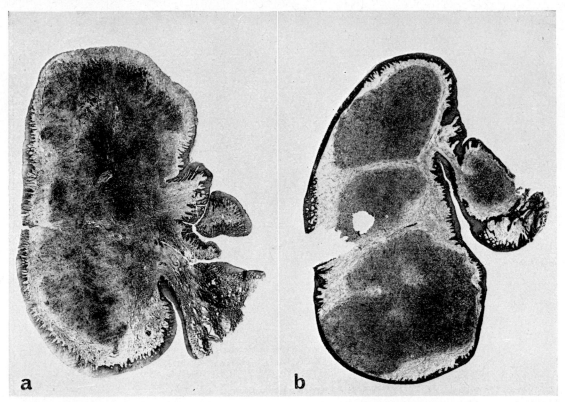

Fig. 94.   Giant cell epulis. **a,** tumour from a man of 58 years, which presented as a firm, non-tender, pedunculated swelling of the gingiva, slightly redder than the normal mucosa. This low power photomicrograph shows the tumour tissue forming a circumscribed mass, separated from the epithelium by a narrow zone of fibrous tissue. × 6. **b,** tumour from a woman of 48 years. The lesional tissue forms several discrete masses. × 85.

outline is sometimes less clear cut. Although Pepler (1958) has shown that these cells contain a non-specific esterase that is not present in the bone lesion, Wertheimer (1967) has demonstrated this enzyme activity in both intraosseous and soft tissue lesions. In many cases the giant cells appear to be almost confluent, with a minimum of matrix.

The matrix consists of spindle-shaped cells with oval nuclei similar to those of the giant cells, and a variable amount of collagen fibre. The lesion is generally very vascular, numerous capillary vessels being present. Small areas of haemorrhage are frequently seen and haemosiderin is often present, sometimes within the giant cells, more often in the connective tissue at the margins of the lesions. In some areas the matrix is more markedly collagenous and there the giant cells are

Fig. 95.   **a,** microscopically, giant cell epulides vary considerably with regard to numbers of giant cells and general cellularity. The lesion shown here has large numbers of giant cells, in almost syncytial masses in places, with intervening spindle and ovoid cells. × 200. **b,** a much more collagenous lesion, with fewer giant cells and an abundant fibro-cellular matrix. × 80. **c,** detail from **a,** showing the giant cells and spindle cells. × 500. **d,** another area from the lesion shown in **a.** There is active formation of osteoid and bone. × 200.

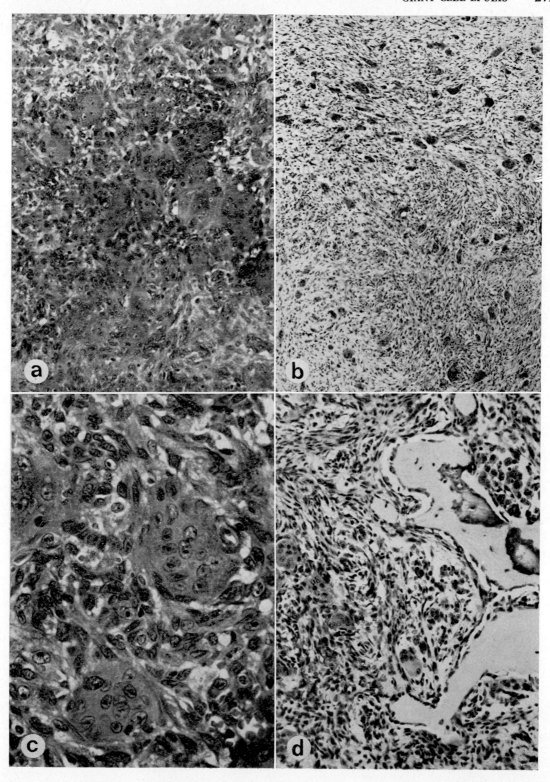

more widely separated and vessels are less numerous. Osteoid tissue and bone are often formed in the collagenous areas. Inflammatory infiltration is frequently present, due to surface ulceration.

The entire lesion is situated in the subepithelial connective tissue of the gingiva, separated from the overlying epithelium by a narrow zone of fibrous tissue. There is no capsule.

Histogenesis

The general behaviour and appearance of the giant cell epulis account for the formerly widely held view that the lesion is a neoplasm. Although many now believe that it is granulomatous and reactive in nature and not neoplastic, its true nature is still unknown.

The quite frequent occurrence of the lesion in young persons and its usual location in those areas where the deciduous teeth are situated, that is, anterior to the molar region, have suggested that it represents an abnormality of the processes concerned in the resorption of these teeth. Geschickter and Copeland (1949) considered that this is a hyperplasia of the osteoclasts that normally act in the shedding of the deciduous teeth. However, it is clear that the lesion does also occur in the molar region, so that this theory is probably incorrect.

Jaffe, Lichtenstein and Portis (1940) and Willis (1967) believe the lesion to represent a variety of granulation tissue and Cooke (1952) also considers it to be of this nature. Cooke thinks that the excessive and aberrant osteogenic granulation tissue arises from the alveolar mucoperiosteum, the cause of the excessive overgrowth possibly being trauma from extraction of a tooth, the shedding of a deciduous tooth, or irritation from calculus or an ill-fitting denture. When the exciting stimulus has subsided, or has been removed, healing by fibrosis takes place. Bernier and Cahn (1954) agree that trauma appears to be the exciting cause of the condition, and Bhaskar and colleagues' (1971) review of 50 cases also implicated trauma as a not infrequent feature. Weinmann and Sicher (1955) also looked on the lesion as a granulomatous condition, but they postulated a state of latent hyperparathyroidism that resulted in minor injuries leading to the production of this special type of granulation tissue because of increased parathyroid activity. This view has not been generally accepted.

Behaviour

The lesion is benign and though unencapsulated it does not infiltrate surrounding tissues, tending to grow outwards. It does not recur if completely removed, but lesions that have originated rather deeply are not uncommonly incompletely removed, with subsequent recurrence, mainly because the surgeon has hoped to avoid removing teeth.

REFERENCES

Adkins, K. F., Martinez, M. G., and Hartley, M. W. (1969) Ultrastructure of giant-cell lesions. A peripheral giant-cell reparative granuloma. *Oral Surg.*, **28**, 713.

Adkins, K. F., Martinez, M. G., and Robinson, L. H. (1969) Cellular morphology and relationships in giant-cell lesions of the jaws. *Oral Surg.*, **28**, 216.

Andersen, L., Fejerskov, O., and Philipsen, H. P. (1973) Oral giant cell granulomas. A clinical and histological study of 129 new cases. *Acta path. microbiol. scand.*, Sect. A. **81**, 606.

Austin, L. T., Dahlin, D. C., and Royer, R. Q. (1959) Giant-cell reparative granuloma and related conditions affecting the jawbones. *Oral Surg.*, **12**, 1285.

Barrie, G. (1920) Multiple hemorrhagic foci of bone. Chronic hemorrhagic osteomyelitis. *Ann. Surg.*, **71**, 581.

Baxter, G. R. (1930) A study of myeloid epulis and its relationship to myeloid sarcoma of the long bones. *Brit. dent. J.*, **51**, 49.

Bernick, S. (1948) Growths of the gingiva and palate. II. Connective tissue tumors. *Oral Surg.*, **1**, 1098.

Bernick, S. (1948) Central giant cell tumors of the jaws. *J. oral Surg.*, **6**, 324.

Bernier, J. L. (1958) *The Management of Oral Disease*. 2nd Edition. New York. The C.V. Mosby Co.

Bernier, J. L., and Cahn, L. R. (1954) The peripheral giant cell reparative granuloma. *J. amer. dent. Ass.*, **49**, 141.

Bhaskar, S. N., Cutright, D. E., Beasley, J. D., and Perez, B. (1971) Giant cell reparative granuloma (peripheral): report of 50 cases. *J. oral Surg.*, **29**, 110.

Black, B. K., and Ackerman, L. V. (1950) Tumors of the parathyroid. A review of twenty-three cases. *Cancer*, **3**, 415.

Bloodgood, J. C. (1910) Benign bone cysts, ostitis fibrosa, giant cell sarcoma and bone aneurysm of the long pipe bones. *Ann. Surg.*, **52**, 145.

Bloodgood, J. C. (1919) Bone tumors. Central (medullary) giant-cell tumor (sarcoma) of lower end of ulna, with evidence that complete destruction of the bony shell or perforation of the bony shell is not a sign of increased malignancy. *Ann. Surg.*, **69**, 345.

Bramley, P., and Dwyer, D. (1970) Primary hyperparathyroidism. Its effect on a mother and her children. *Oral Surg.*, **30**, 464.

Bridge, A. J. (1968) Primary hyperparathyroidism presenting as a dental problem. *Brit. dent. J.*, **124**, 172.

Brown, G. N., Darlington, C. G., and Kupfer, S. R. (1956) A clinicopathologic study of alveolar border epulis with special emphasis on benign giant-cell tumor. *Oral Surg.*, **9**, 765, 888.

Buckerfield, J. P. (1971) Primary hyperparathyroidism causing bony swelling in the edentulous jaw. A case report. *Brit. dent. J.*, **131**, 497.

Codman, E. A. (1925) The nomenclature used by the Registry of Bone Sarcoma. *Amer. J. Roentgenol.*, **13**, 105.

Cohen, B. (1959) A study of bone lesions in a case of hyperparathyroidism. *Oral Surg.*, **12**, 1347.

Coley, B. L. (1960) *Neoplasms of Bone and Related Conditions*. 2nd Edition. New York. Paul B. Hoeber, Inc.

Coley, B. L., Higinbotham, N. L., and Kogure, T. (1958) Giant cell tumor of bone. *Amer. J. Surg.*, **96**, 479.

Cooke, B. E. D. (1952) The giant-cell epulis: histogenesis and natural history. *Brit. dent. J.*, **93**, 13.

Dahlin, D. C., Cupps, R. E., and Johnson, E. W. (1970) Giant-cell tumor: a study of 195 cases. *Cancer*, **25**, 1061.

Geschickter, C. F., and Copeland, M. M. (1949) *Tumors of Bone*. 3rd Edition. Philadelphia. J. B. Lippincott Company.

Giansanti, J. S., and Waldron, C. A. (1969) Peripheral giant cell granuloma: review of 720 cases. *J. oral Surg.*, **27**, 787.

Hanaoka, H., Friedman, B., and Mack, R. P. (1970) Ultrastructure and histogenesis of giant-cell tumor of bone. *Cancer*, **25**, 1408.

Henry, T. C. (1964) A giant cell reparative granuloma? *Brit. J. oral Surg.*, **2**, 94.

Hirschl, S., and Katz, A. (1974) Giant cell reparative granuloma outside the jaw bone. Diagnostic criteria and review of the literature with the first case described in the temporal bone. *Human Path.*, **5**, 171.

Hutter, R. V. P., Worcester, J. N., Francis, K. C., Foote, F. W., and Stewart, F. W. (1962) Benign and malignant giant cell tumors of bone. A clinicopathological analysis of the natural history of the disease. *Cancer*, **15**, 653.

Jaffe, H. L. (1953) Giant-cell tumour (osteoclastoma) of bone: its pathologic delimitation and the inherent clinical implications. *Ann. roy. Coll. Surg. Engl.*, **13**, 343.

Jaffe, H. L. (1953) Giant-cell reparative granuloma, traumatic bone cyst, and fibrous (fibro-osseous) dysplasia of the jawbones. *Oral Surg.*, **6**, 159.

Jaffe, H. L., Lichtenstein, L., and Portis, R. B. (1940) Giant cell tumor of bone. Its pathologic appearance, grading, supposed variants and treatment. *Arch. Path.*, **30**, 993.

Konjetzny, G. E. (1922) Die sogenannte "lokalisierte Ostitis fibrosa" (Ein Beitrag zur Kenntnis der Solitären Knochenzysten und der sogenannten "schaligen myelogenen Riesenzellensarkome"). *Arch. klin. Chir.*, **121**, 567.

Lichtenstein, L. (1950) Aneurysmal bone cyst. A pathological entity commonly mistaken for giant-cell tumor and occasionally for hemangioma and osteogenic sarcoma. *Cancer*, **3**, 279.

Lichtenstein, L. (1951) Giant-cell tumor of bone. Current status of problems in diagnosis and treatment. *J. Bone Jt. Surg.*, **33A**, 143.

Lichtenstein, L. (1953) Aneurysmal bone cyst. Further observations. *Cancer*, **6**, 1228.

Lichtenstein, L. (1972) *Bone Tumors*. 4th Edition. St. Louis. The C. V. Mosby Company.

McGowan, D. A. (1969) Central giant cell tumour of the mandible occurring in pregnancy. *Brit. J. oral Surg.*, **7**, 131.

Marble, H. B., Baker, R. D., Scofield, H. H., and Luther, N. K. (1969) Central giant-cell reparative granuloma with extraosseous manifestations: report of case. *J. oral Surg.*, **27**, 215.

Matsumura, T., Sugahara, T., Wada, T., and Kawakatsu, K. (1971) Recurrent giant-cell reparative granuloma: report of a case and histochemical patterns. *J. oral Surg.*, **29**, 212.

Morton, J. J. (1956) Giant cell tumor of bone. *Cancer*, **9**, 1012.

Pepler, W. J. (1958) The histochemistry of giant-cell tumours (osteoclastoma and giant-cell epulis). *J. Path. Bact.*, **76**, 505.

Schajowicz, F. (1961) Giant-cell tumors of bone (osteoclastoma). A pathological and histochemical study. *J. Bone Jt. Surg.*, **43A**, 1.

Shafer, W. G., Hine, M. K., and Levy, B. M. (1974) *A Textbook of Oral Pathology*. 3rd Edition. Philadelphia. W. B. Saunders Company.

Shklar, G., and Meyer, I. (1961) Giant-cell tumors of the mandible and maxilla. *Oral Surg.*, **14**, 809.

Soskolne, W. A. (1972) Some observations on the pathogenesis and morphology of giant cell granulomas. *Proc. roy. Soc. Med.*, **65**, 1130.

Soskolne, W. A. (1972) Peripheral giant cell granulomas: an ultrastructural study of three lesions. *J. oral Path.*, **1**, 133.

Spjut, H. J., Dorfman, H. D., Fechner, R. E., and Ackerman, L. V. (1971) *Tumors of Bone and Cartilage*. Atlas of Tumor Pathology. Second Series. Fascicle 5. Washington, D.C. Armed Forces Institute of Pathology.

Stewart, M. J. (1922) The histogenesis of myeloid sarcoma. *Lancet*, **2**, 1106.

Thomson, A. D., and Turner-Warwick, R. T. (1955) Skeletal sarcomata and giant-cell tumour. *J. Bone Jt. Surg.*, **37B**, 266.

Waldron, C. A. (1953) Giant cell tumors of the jawbones. *Oral Surg.*, **6**, 1055.

Waldron, C. A., and Shafer, W. G. (1966) The central giant cell reparative granuloma of the jaws. An analysis of 38 cases. *Amer. J. clin. Path.*, **45**, 437.

Weinmann, J. P. (1945) Bone changes in the jaw caused by renal hyperparathyroidism. *J. Periodont.*, **16**, 94.

Weinmann, J. P., and Sicher, H. (1955) *Bone and Bones*. 2nd Edition. London. Henry Kimpton.

Wertheimer, F. W. (1967) Enzyme histochemistry of giant-cell reparative granulomas. *Oral Surg.*, **23**, 464.

Willis, R. A. (1967) *Pathology of Tumours*. 4th Edition. London. Butterworth & Co. (Publishers) Ltd.

27. Melanoma

The pigment-producing cells of the skin, the melanocytes, originate in the neural crest and migrate during embryonic life to their final position in the epidermis. There they are interspersed among the cells of the basal layer, and similar cells have also been shown to occur in the oral mucosa (Laidlaw and Cahn, 1932; Cattoni, 1953). In addition, cells that carry melanin, though they do not produce it, are present in the dermis. These are the melanophages. The melanocytes have fine dendritic processes, and the melanin they produce is transferred along these processes to the adjacent cells of the epidermis, so that in routine sections pigment can be seen in the epidermal cells whereas the melanocytes themselves appear as clear cells interspersed here and there among the basal cells. Pigment similarly derived from melanocytes is sometimes present in the cells of such tumours as papilloma, basal cell carcinoma and squamous cell carcinoma, but in the naevus and the malignant melanoma the pigment is produced by the lesional cells themselves.

PIGMENTED NAEVUS
(Benign melanoma; mole)

Naevi or birth marks are not true neoplasms but are disturbances of development. The name is often applied also to vascular and other blemishes of the skin, but we are here concerned only with pigmented naevi, which are so common that the vast majority of individuals have at least one or two tiny pigmented spots and many people have appreciable numbers. Larger lesions are less common, but are frequent enough.

Pigmented naevi fall into three groups: dermal, junctional and compound. The basic feature of the *dermal naevus* is the naevus cell. This is a rounded, ovoid or polyhedral cell with a hyperchromatic nucleus, and occasionally binucleated or multinucleated types are seen. Melanin is present, but often in small amounts. In fact, there may be more pigment in macrophages in the adjacent tissues than in the naevus cells themselves. The naevus cells are arranged in characteristic groups or clusters situated in the dermis, just below the epithelium but with a clear area of fibrous tissue between the basal layer and the groups of naevus cells. The epithelium itself appears quite normal (Fig. 96).

The origin of naevus cells is not yet known. Possibly they are derived from melanocytes which have migrated from the epidermis into the connective tissue. It is also possible that they may be derived from the Schwann cells of the dermal nerves, or even from both sources.

Dermal naevi occur anywhere in the skin and vary very considerably in size from small flat or raised spots to large lesions that may involve an extensive area of skin. They very rarely become malignant.

The *junctional naevus* is characterised by the presence of proliferating melanocytes, these cells forming clusters in the region of the junction of dermis and epidermis. In the *compound naevus* the melanocytes "drop" down from the junctional area into the dermis, so that groups of these cells are present both in the basal area of the epithelium and in the dermis.

Both junctional and compound naevi are common in children and young adults, although they are also seen in older people. The importance of the various types of naevus is their differing propensities for malignant change. As already noted, dermal naevi very rarely become malignant;

T

when such change does occur in a pre-existing benign naevus there has been junctional activity. However, it must be noted that, even so, the number of naevi showing junctional activity that do become malignant is small, and particularly in children where such activity is common, malignant change is rare. In fact, the *juvenile melanoma* of children, which is a compound naevus showing pronounced junctional activity and at one time not infrequently diagnosed as malignant, has been recognised as an entity; it is quite benign. The naevi that may become malignant, then, are those that show junctional activity and that occur in adults. Lesions on the soles and skin of the leg generally are more prone to malignant change, but this may occur in lesions in any area. Chronic irritation may be a predisposing factor: for example, continued friction by the clothing.

Pigmented naevi occur in the oral mucosa as well as in the skin, but are not very common. They present as small brown raised areas in the lip (Field and Ackerman, 1943), palate (Couch and Kaufman, 1956), gingiva (Allen and Bruce, 1954) and buccal mucosa (Greene and colleagues, 1953; Akamine, 1962). Recent reviews are given by Weathers and Waldron (1965), who point out the important fact that oral naevi, like those of the skin, are not always pigmented. King and colleagues (1967), Nagel (1972) and Gossman and Miller (1975), also review recent cases. A juvenile melanoma of the tongue in a 7-year-old girl has been reported by Jernstrom and Aponte (1956).

BLUE NAEVUS

On their way to the epidermis from the neural crest, some migrating melanocytes may remain in the subepidermal connective tissue and it is probably from such cells that blue naevi arise. As the name implies, these naevi are deeply pigmented, appearing blue or even almost black, due to the fact that they are situated deeply in the dermis. The lesion has been found at all ages though it has probably been present since birth, and may appear anywhere in the skin as a small smooth rounded swelling less than 1 cm in diameter. Microscopically, the lesion consists of melanin-containing elongated or fusiform cells with dendritic processes. The cells are often arranged in fascicles rather like smooth muscle or nerve, and around these melanocytes are variable numbers of melanophages.

The blue naevus is a benign lesion though, very rarely, malignant transformation has occurred.

The occurrence of a blue naevus in the oral tissues was first described by Scofield (1959) and just over twenty examples have subsequently been recorded. Teles and colleagues (1974) have summarised the reported cases. In most cases the lesion has been in the hard palate. The soft palate and lip have also been affected.

MALIGNANT MELANOMA

Malignant melanomas are rare tumours. Some undoubtedly arise in pre-existing pigmented naevi, but there is considerable variation in the figures quoted. Some authorities suggest that as many as 50 per cent of malignant melanomas have originated in this way, others put the figure as low as 5 per cent, but even if the higher figure should eventually prove to be the better estimate, this would not alter the fact that the proportion of benign naevi that become malignant is very low.

Malignant melanoma is well known as one of the most aggressive of all tumours, many cases running a very rapid course with a fatal outcome. However, there do occur tumours that are considerably less aggressive and this, with modern methods of treatment, makes the outlook rather less gloomy. In the skin, tumours of the head and neck tend to have a better prognosis than those of the trunk, females tend to do better than males and patients with smaller tumours have a

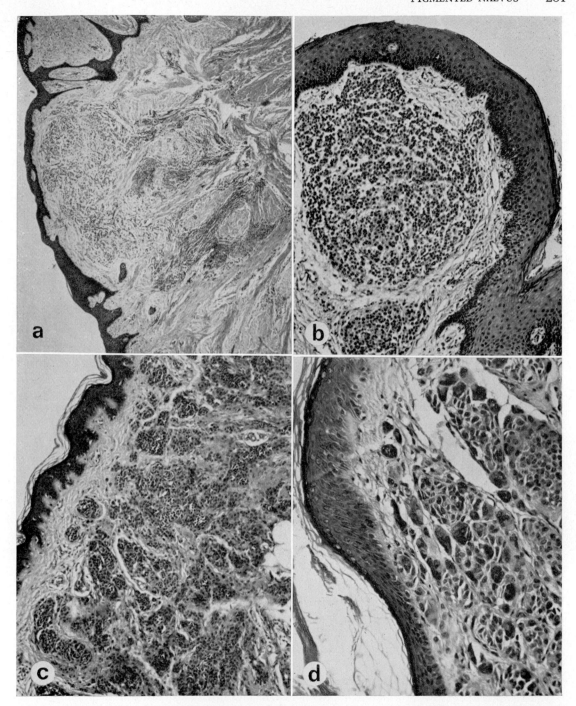

Fig. 96. Pigmented naevus. **a, b,** naevi of the gingiva, showing the collections of naevus cells in the corium. × 30 and × 80. **c,** naevus of lip. The naevus cells are larger and more pleomorphic than those in **a** and **b.** × 50. **d.** detail from **c.** × 200.

better survival rate than those with larger ones (Lehman, Cross and Richey, 1966; Cochran, 1969). The sole of the foot is a well known area of ominous significance, for melanomas here are nearly always malignant, and the same is true of subungual growths of the hands and feet. When the tumour occurs as the result of malignant change in an existing naevus, this is signified by the naevus beginning to grow rapidly, becoming darker and tending to ulcerate or bleed. Invasion of the lymphatics occurs very early and the regional nodes are usually enlarged. Blood-borne metastases also occur, often being widespread.

In the oral tissues, malignant melanoma accounts for 1 to 2 per cent of all malignant tumours. A review and analysis of 105 published cases by Chaudhry, Hampel and Gorlin (1958) gives a comprehensive picture of the condition. Duckworth (1962), Borello and colleagues (1966), Soman and Sirsat (1974), Jackson and Simpson (1975) and Liversedge (1975) review the subsequent literature and Eneroth (1975) reports a series of 23 patients, one of the largest so far published. In Japan, oral malignant melanoma is relatively common, while at the same time malignant melanoma of the skin appears to be less frequent than in Caucasians (Takagi, Ishikawa and Mori, 1974).

Chauhdry and colleagues' review showed that oral melanoma was twice as common in males as in females, and Eneroth's series gives a similar ratio. The sex incidence in most series of cutaneous tumours is equal, or there may be a preponderance of males. However, the number of oral tumours is relatively small. The peak age incidence of oral tumours is the sixth decade, the range being between the years of 20 and 90. The tumours in infants reported by Krompecher (1918) and Soderberg and Padgett (1941) appear to be examples of the benign pigmented tumour of infants (p. 110) rather than melanomas.

The upper jaw is affected in about 80 per cent of cases, the hard palate being the commonest site. Less frequently the alveolar ridge, the soft palate and other areas of the upper jaw are involved. The lower jaw, cheeks, tongue and floor of mouth account for the remaining 20 per cent of cases. The reason for the much higher incidence of the tumour in the upper jaw than in the lower is unknown. Chaudhry, Burke and Gorlin (1960) suggest that it may be due to the presence of an increased number of active melanoblasts in this area. Primary malignant melanoma of the parotid gland (p. 336) has been reported by Greene and Bernier (1961).

The lesion takes the form of a dark brown or bluish-black area that may be only slightly raised or may form a larger mass with a nodular or papillary surface. Occasionally multiple lesions may be present (Baldridge and Waldron, 1954; Moore and Martin, 1955) and rare lesions may be devoid of pigment. The growth is painless, with the result that often the patient's attention is drawn to its existence only when ulceration and bleeding occur. An important feature is the pre-existence of pigmentation of the oral mucosa. Gotshalk, Tessmer and Smith (1940) have reported a case in which pigmented spots in the mucosa of the palate had been present since birth and malignant melanoma appeared at the age of 25. A number of observers have noted that in nearly 30 per cent of all cases the appearance of the tumour has been preceded for a few months or years by mucosal pigmentation (Baxter, 1941; Hobaek, 1949; Sirsat, 1953; Moore and Martin, 1955; Trodahl and Sprague, 1970; Takagi, Ishikawa and Mori, 1974). However, intraoral pigmentation, which has long been recognised as common in dark skinned races, is also found normally in a proportion of white persons (Masson, 1948).

With continued growth, which is rapid, invasion and extensive destruction of bone occurs, accompanied by loosening and exfoliation of the teeth. Metastases in both the regional lymph nodes and in distant sites occur, the usual sites being lung, liver, brain and bone. Baxter (1941) found that about half the patients had enlarged cervical nodes when first examined, and about three-quarters of all patients developed regional lymph node metastases at some time in the course of the disease.

Very occasionally melanoma appears as a much less aggressive growth than is usual. Tumours of this type generally arise on the basis of a pre-existing Hutchinson's malignant lentigo. This is a condition which appears as a pigmented spot, usually on the face, but any skin area may be affected and lesions have been reported in the oral mucosa (Robinson and Hukill, 1970). The malignant lentigo appears after puberty and often remains unchanged for many years. It may in fact regress, but sometimes it develops into an invasive tumour. However, the tumours that develop in this way are of very much slower growth than the usual type of melanoma and often do not metastasise. Grinspan and colleagues (1969) report a case of this nature and feel that a number of oral melanomas have developed on the basis of malignant lentigo.

The histological picture in malignant melanoma can be very varied (Fig. 97). Masses of cells are present in the dermis and epidermis; the cells are round, polyhedral or fusiform with hyperchromatic nuclei, and quite often there is a good deal of pleomorphism with the presence of oddly-shaped cells and mononucleated and multinucleated giant cells. Mitotic figures are often numerous. Melanin is nearly always present in the tumour cells, often plentifully but sometimes in very small amounts and thus difficult to detect. Rarely, it may be entirely absent. The arrangement of the tumour cells varies. They may form solid masses or take up a fascicular arrangement reminiscent of fibrosarcoma or they may be in an alveolar arrangement.

In those areas of the lesion where the epidermodermal junction remains relatively unobscured there is practically always marked junctional activity. That is to say, there are proliferating melanocytes in and around the basal layer of the epidermis and these cells may also infiltrate all layers of the epidermis. It has already been noted that those naevi that may become malignant are the ones showing junctional changes, but that the actual proportion of such lesions that do in fact transform in this way is very small. Many workers believe that all malignant melanomas begin with junctional changes, whether in a pre-existing junctional naevus or arising *de novo*. Considerable histological experience of these lesions is necessary to assess the significance of any junctional activity, and the established malignant melanoma, particularly poorly pigmented growths, may simulate a variety of neoplasms. Thus the spindle cell type of growth may suggest fibrosarcoma or undifferentiated lesions may suggest anaplastic carcinoma. Another danger in the histological diagnosis of melanoma is "overdiagnosis." It has already been noted how until comparatively recently many juvenile melanomas were diagnosed as malignant melanomas (Spitz, 1948). A similar lesion is now known to occur in adults (Allen and Spitz, 1953) and here again these "spindle cell naevi," as they are termed in adults, have sometimes been diagnosed as malignant melanoma. They occur anywhere, and Echevarria and Ackerman (1967) report a series of 26 cases, including 4 lesions of the cheek and 1 of the upper lip.

Secondary melanoma in the oral tissues has occasionally been noted. De Cholnoky (1941) has reported a malignant melanoma of the toe that metastasised to the mandible. In Bluestone's (1953) patient the primary tumour occurred in the skin of the lumbar region and one of the many metastases was in the mandible. Heslop (1964) has reported a secondary oral lesion from a primary growth in the calf.

The prognosis of malignant melanoma in the oral tissues, as for melanoma of other mucous membranes, is very poor (Allen and Spitz, 1953). Chaudhry, Hampel and Gorlin found that the average duration of life from the time of diagnosis was 18·3 months in 24 patients. Only 3 patients were alive after 5 years. This contrasts with, for example, the results in a series of skin tumours such as that of Lane, Lattes and Malm (1958). The five-year cure rate was 10 per cent for patients with clinically evident lymph node metastases, but a good deal better than this for other patients. Those authors quote the five-year survival rates from a number of published series; the average is about 29 per cent.

INTESTINAL POLYPOSIS WITH MELANIN PIGMENTATION
(PEUTZ-JEGHERS SYNDROME)

It is convenient here to describe briefly this familial condition. Transmitted as a mendelian dominant, it is characterised by the presence of melanin spots in the skin and oral mucosa and adenomatous polyps in the intestine (Jeghers, 1944; Jeghers, McKusick and Katz, 1949).

The pigmented spots are similar to freckles and, like them, are often present at birth. However, while freckles occur particularly on the convexities of the face, the pigmentation in this syndrome occurs especially around the mouth, nostrils and eyes and may also involve the hands, feet and abdomen. Pigmentation of the oral mucosa is practically always present, occurring particularly on the lips and cheeks. The gingivae and hard palate may also be affected, but rarely the tongue. The intraoral pigmentation remains throughout life, though the pigmentation of the skin, like ordinary freckles, tends to fade away at puberty. Histologically, the pigmented spots appear to be very similar to labial lentigo (Shapiro and Zegarelli, 1971).

The intestinal polyps may occur anywhere in the gastrointestinal tract from the stomach to the anus, but the small intestine is the favourite site. Macroscopically the polyps show the usual characteristics of the ordinary adenoma but they are frequently present in large numbers and may even be confluent, when the appearances may closely resemble polyposis coli. Microscopically, the polyps appear to be hamartomatous rather than neoplastic, as Bartholomew, Dahlin and Waugh (1957) and Morson (1959) have pointed out. However, Dormandy (1957) has shown that even where the small intestine appears normal to the naked eye, microscopic examination may show extensive disorganisation of the mucosa with apparent invasion of muscle, and similar appearances may be seen in some of the polyps. Because of this, mistaken histological diagnoses of malignancy have been made, but the small intestine polyps, unlike those in polyposis coli and despite their microscopic appearances, very rarely become malignant. The few cases in which malignant change has occurred are discussed by Reid (1965). Polyps occurring in the colon, on the other hand, do become malignant rather more frequently.

The condition may be symptomless, but often there are recurrent attacks of abdominal pain. Intussusception frequently occurs.

Oral pigmentation in general is the subject of useful reviews by Dummett and Barens (1967, 1971).

REFERENCES

Akamine, R. N. (1962) Compound nevus of the buccal mucosa. Report of a case. *Oral Surg.*, **15**, 27.
Allen, R. R., and Bruce, K. W. (1954) Nevus of the gingiva: report of a case. *J. oral Surg.*, **12**, 257.

Fig. 97.   **a,** junctional activity in a melanoma. × 200. **b,** detail from another field of the same tumour. × 300. **c,** melanoma of gingiva in a man of 30 years. The patient was referred to hospital for extraction of a lower third molar tooth, because of pericoronitis. On examination, there was a slightly raised and ulcerated brown patch on the mucosa lingual to this tooth, which was loose. The tooth and affected area of mucosa were removed. Microscopic examination showed melanoma, with superficial ulceration. × 30. **d,** higher magnification of a field from **c.** × 200. The mandible was now resected from the ascending ramus to the canine region and a block dissection of the cervical glands carried out. A few months later there was a recurrence in the mucosa covering the stump of the mandible in the canine area. A further resection, across the midline, was performed and cytotoxic agents given by arterial perfusion. Somewhat later, the glands on both sides of the neck enlarged and fungated and a fungating mass appeared on the stump of the remaining portion of mandible. The patient died 18 months after the first appearance of the tumour.

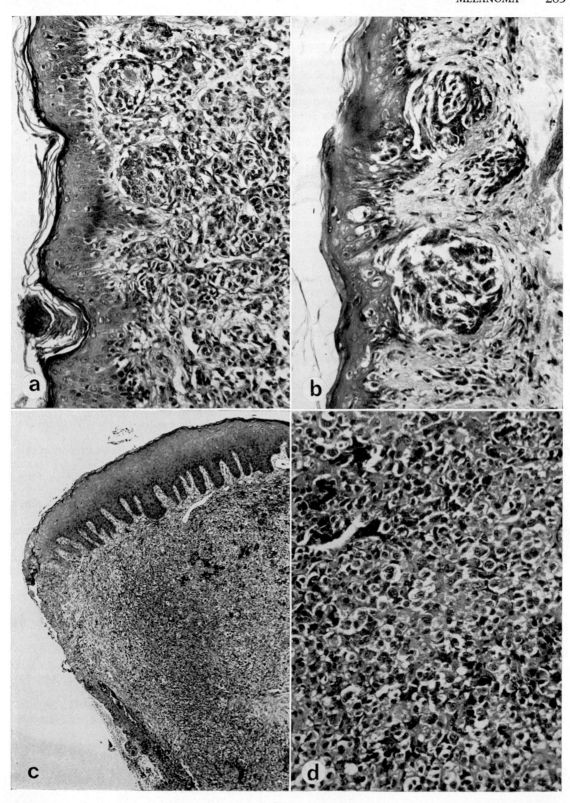

28. Teratoma

EPIGNATHUS

Teratomatous lesions occurring in the mouth in the newborn are generally known as epignathi, though strictly speaking this term implies a growth on the jaws. In fact, as Erich (1945) points out, the majority of these rare growths arise from the sphenoid bone, some arise from the hard or the soft palate or the pharynx and only a few originate in the jaws. From the site of origin the tumour grows into the mouth or nasal cavity or into the cranial cavity. Some tumours grow in both directions, filling the oral cavity and also extending intracranially.

The tumours vary in structural complexity. The simpler types of growth are compatible with life if they can be promptly removed. These growths are usually evident at birth or soon after, as polypoid masses filling the mouth or protruding from it. Smaller growths may lie farther back in the oral cavity and may not be immediately evident. Growths of this type consist mainly of adipose tissue, often with a central area of cartilage or bone, and are covered by stratified squamous epithelium with pilosebaceous follicles. In some growths nervous tissue is present. Cases of this type have been reported by Hankins and Harding (1932), Stokoe (1937), Foster (1944), Dohlman and Sjövall (1953), Kesson (1954) and others. Rarely, the growth may consist almost entirely of nervous tissue. Bratton and Robinson (1946) reported two cases of this type, the growths consisting of neuroglial tissue. In one infant the lesion was in the soft palate, in the other the lesion was situated in the skin of the side of the nose. Similar growths in the tongue have been reported by Peterer (1922) and Bras, Butts and Hoyte (1969). A growth of the tongue, composed of bone, cartilage, skin, glandular tissue, adipose and connective tissue has been reported by Miller and Owens (1966).

Tumours of any greater degree of complexity than those just mentioned are practically always fatal and are seen therefore in the fetus or stillborn infant. Various tissue combinations occur. In Wynn and colleagues' (1956) case, the grapefruit-size tumour protruding from the mouth arose from the palate and bore a well-formed finger with a finger nail on its upper surface. Microscopically, it consisted of connective tissue, smooth muscle, skin and dermal appendages, and cysts lined by columnar epithelium. The finger had fairly well-formed joints. A tumour containing bones and teeth is described by Ochsner and Ayers (1951) but these tissues were identified radiologically and not, apparently, histologically. A more complex growth is described by Erich (1945). This tumour arose from the sphenoid and filled the pharynx, mouth and nose. It was covered by skin with sebaceous glands and hair follicles and consisted of connective tissue, fat, bone, nerves, liver, brain tissue and structures similar to choroid plexus. A partially formed eye was present and also mucous glands and cysts lined by squamous epithelium. Willis (1962) mentions other cases and gives references to the earlier literature.

OTHER TERATOMAS

Teratomas in various parts of the body may contain teeth. Ovarian dermoid cysts are the commonest teratomas in which dental structures may develop; probably about 15 per cent of these cysts contain teeth. Detailed accounts of the dental tissues in ovarian dermoids have been given by Kronfeld (1940), Babbush and August (1963), Main (1970) and others. The teeth vary

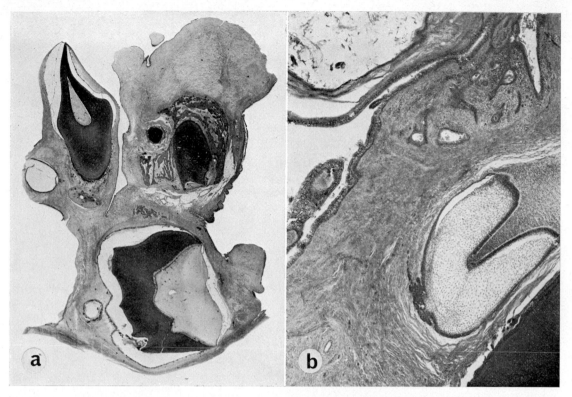

Fig. 98. Teeth in an ovarian dermoid cyst. **a,** an incisor and a molar type tooth are present, and another tooth is situated in a bony crypt. × 4. **b,** higher magnification to show a tooth germ adjacent to the dentine of another tooth, at lower right. There is a keratin-filled cyst at upper left. × 30.

considerably in number; there may be one or two, or larger numbers, up to about twenty (Pullon and Child, 1972). They develop in the cyst wall, and are distributed randomly and without any apparent orientation. Much less commonly the teeth are arranged in a bony structure resembling maxilla or mandible (Pullon and Child, 1972; Whitehouse and Schofield, 1974). They are generally smaller than normal teeth and although there may be some divergences from the normal pattern, structurally they are well formed (Fig. 98).

The occurrence of teeth in other teratomas is much less frequent. They have been found in the pituitary and pineal regions, third ventricle, sacrococcygeal area, anterior mediastinum, stomach, face and external auditory meatus. The literature is surveyed by Gorlin and Wolfson (1966).

REFERENCES

Babbush, C. A., and August, R. V. (1963) Ectopic teeth. A case of bilateral benign cystic teratomas containing dental and periodontal structures. *Oral Surg.*, **16,** 586.

Bras, G., Butts, D., and Hoyte, D. A. (1969) Gliomatous teratoma of the tongue. Report of a case. *Cancer*, **24,** 1045.

Bratton, A. B., and Robinson, S. H. G. (1946) Gliomata of the nose and oral cavity: a report of 2 cases. *J. Path. Bact.*, **58,** 643.

Dohlman, G., and Sjövall, A. (1953) Large epignathus-teratoma successfully operated upon immediately after birth. *Glasgow med. J.*, **34,** 122.

Erich, W. E. (1945) Teratoid parasites of the mouth (episphenoids, epipalati (epurani), epignathi). *Amer. J. Orthodont. (Oral Surg. Sect.)*, **31,** 650.

Foster, J. H. (1944) Congenital dermoid tumor of the nasopharynx. *Ann. Otol.*, **53,** 578.

Gorlin, R. J., and Wolfson, J. J. (1966) Teeth in extraovarian teratomas. *Amer. J. Roentgenol.*, **97,** 248.

Hankins, F. D., and Harding, W. G. (1932) Teratoid tumor of the pharynx. Report of a case in a fetus of six months. *Arch. Otolaryngol.*, **16,** 46.

Kesson, C. W. (1954) Asphyxia neonatorum due to a nasopharyngeal teratoma. *Arch. Dis. Child.*, **29,** 254.

Kronfeld, R. (1940) Ovarian dermoid containing teeth. *J. dent. Res.*, **145,** 1953.

Main, D. M. G. (1970) Tooth identity in ovarian teratomas. *Brit. dent. J.*, **129,** 328.

Miller, A. P., and Owens, J. B. (1966) Teratoma of the tongue. *Cancer*, **19,** 1583.

Ochsner, A., and Ayers, W. B. (1951) Case of epignathus. Survival of the host after its excision. *Surgery*, **30,** 560.

Peterer, F. (1922) Ueber glioma linguae. *Zeit. Path.*, **26,** 214.

Pullon, P. A., and Child, P. L. (1972) An unusual dental variant of ovarian teratoma. Report of a case. *Oral Surg.*, **34,** 800.

Stokoe, J. (1937) Nasopharyngeal teratoma. *Brit. med. J.*, **2,** 909.

Whitehouse, W. L., and Schofield, J. J. (1974) Teeth of a teratoma—a case report. *Brit. J. oral Surg.*, **11,** 256.

Willis, R. A. (1962) *The Pathology of the Tumours of Children.* Edinburgh and London. Oliver and Boyd.

Wynn, S. K., Waxman, S., Ritchie, G., and Askotzky, M. (1956) Epignathus. Survey. *Amer. J. Dis. Child.*, **91,** 495.

VI
METASTATIC TUMOURS IN THE ORAL TISSUES

29. Metastatic Tumours in the Oral Tissues

Secondary tumours may occur in the soft tissues of the oral region or in the jaws. They account for about 1 per cent of malignant tumours of the oral cavity (Frank, Brini and Nicolas, 1961). They are usually solitary deposits, but more than one may occur, rarely. The literature of multiple metastases in the oral tissues is summarised by McMillan and Edwards (1975).

Soft tissue deposits are rare. Hatziotis and colleagues (1973) have reviewed the literature and found reports of forty-eight cases between the years 1945 and 1970. The primary tumours occurred in a wide variety of sites, the commonest being lung, followed by kidney, stomach and liver. The metastatic deposits occurred most frequently in the gingiva, the tongue was next most often involved, then the lip. Other reports of metastatic neoplasms in the oral soft tissues include cases of carcinoma of thyroid (Al-Ani, 1973), malignant melanoma (Mosby, Sugg and Hiatt, 1973), lymphangiosarcoma (Wertheimer and Crayle, 1973), carcinoma of breast (Perlmutter, Buchner and Smukler, 1974) and carcinoma of the head of the pancreas (Schofield, 1974). Zegarelli and colleagues (1973) report on twelve cases of secondary deposits in the tongue. These were in patients with known primary tumours and most of them had widespread metastases. The lingual metastases in eight patients were discovered only at autopsy, while in each of the remaining four cases the tongue lesion was suspected at some stage to be a primary tumour. Thus it may very well be that metastases in the soft tissues of the mouth occur more often than might be thought, remaining clinically silent in an appreciable proportion of cases.

Metastatic tumours occur in the jaws more frequently than in the soft tissues and there are reports in the literature recording secondary deposits from a wide variety of primary sites. Although jaw metastases are not common, it is probable that, like the soft tissue deposits, they occur more frequently than has been thought. Moorman and Shafer (1954), for example, examined the jaws radiologically in 10 patients with advanced carcinomas of various organs and found evidence of mandibular deposits in 3 of the cases, though oral symptoms had been absent. On the other hand, secondary deposits in the jaws may give rise to symptoms while the primary growth still remains silent. It is necessary, therefore, to bear this possibility in mind when examining biopsy specimens from supposed primary tumours of the jaw. Secondary deposits occur much more often in the mandible than in the maxilla, and particularly in the molar region. Clausen and Poulsen (1963) found 77 cases affecting the mandible and 17 the maxilla in their review of the literature. Although pain is the commonest symptom, it is not an invariable feature (Cash, Royer and Dahlin, 1961). Alteration of sensation of the lip, when it occurs, is always a suspicious symptom, as is loosening of the teeth. Pathological fracture occasionally occurs.

Willis (1941) has shown, in 500 consecutive necropsies on cases of malignant disease, that the three most frequent sites for blood-borne metastases are the liver (40 per cent), lungs (32 per cent) and bone (15 per cent). Jaffe (1958) puts the overall figure for bone metastases very much higher, at 70 per cent, and if only the most common carcinomas metastasising to bone be considered, the figure is nearer 85 per cent. The bones most often affected are those with a high content of red marrow. It may be that the low marrow content of the jaws and their lesser degree of vascularity as compared with some other bones is the reason why they are comparatively seldom the site of metastases.

The commonest sites for primary growths that metastasise to bone are breast, bronchus, prostate and thyroid, though the figures given in recent series of cases tend to vary as to order of frequency (Abrams, Spiro and Goldstein, 1950; Sharp, Bullock and Hazlet, 1956; Clain, 1965). So far as the jaws are concerned, the commonest primary site for carcinoma appears to be the breast. Appenzeller, Weitzner and Long (1971) and Batsakis (1974) have tabulated carcinomas that metastasised to the jaws and found that breast was the primary site in 15 to 30 per cent of cases. Lung and kidney were the next most frequent sites. In small numbers of cases the primary tumour arose in stomach, colon, rectum, thyroid, testis and skin (melanoma). Liver, pancreas, bladder, ovary and uterus have figured as primary sites in solitary instances, or two or three cases only have been recorded. Following are some of the reports that have appeared in the literature.

Breast: Adair and Herrmann (1946); Cook (1949); Salman and Langel (1954); Blackwood (1956); Cohen (1958); Cawson (1959); Blake and Blake (1960); Heslop (1965); Epker, Merrill and Henny (1969); van der Kwast and van der Waal (1974). Bronchus: MacGregor and Lewis (1972) review the literature. Thyroid: Stern and Shepard (1941); Byars and Sarnat (1946); McDaniel, Luna and Stimson (1971); Hanratty (1971). Adrenal: Delaire and colleagues (1960). Kidney: Salman and Darlington (1944); Stewart and Bruce (1953); Mallett (1961); Milobsky and colleagues (1975). Bladder: Seldin and Rakower, (1953). Prostate: Thoma and Goldman (1960); Sorbera and Taylor (1966); Snyder, Merkow and White (1971). Stomach: Salman and Darlington (1944); Catone and Henny (1969). Pancreas: Hayes, Pinson and Leffall (1966). Colon: Bruce and McDonald (1954); Hägglund (1959); Sage and Hoggins (1961). Rectum: Salman and Darlington (1944); Meyer and Shklar (1958). Liver: Appenzeller, Weitzner and Long (1971) review the literature. Gall bladder: Rominger, Lockwood and Canino (1961). Testis: Cameron and Stetzer (1947); Cawson (1959); Bernstein, Montgomery and Balogh (1966); Lainson and colleagues (1975). Cervix uteri: Holland (1953); Salman and Langel (1954). Choriocarcinoma: Catania (1953); Ramanathan, Eravelly and Ken (1968).

Carcinomas of adjacent structures such as lip, gingiva and salivary gland often involve the jaws by direct extension, but carcinoma of the lower lip may also metastasise to the mandible by way of the lymphatics through the mental foramen (Geschickter and Copeland, 1949). Carcinoma of the parotid may give rise to haematogenous deposits in the mandible as well as involving it by direct extension (Burford, Ackerman and Robinson, 1944). Carcinomas of the nasal mucosa and the tonsil have metastasised to the jaws (Bernard, 1931; Geschickter and Copeland, 1949).

Tumours other than carcinomas do not of course metastasise so frequently to the skeleton and correspondingly secondary deposits in the jaws form a small proportion of all such metastases in bone. Metastases in the jaws have been described from the following tumours: fibrosarcoma, primary in breast (Thoma and Goldman, 1960); chondrosarcoma, primary in tibia (Goldstein and Goldstein, 1943; Kemper and Bloom, 1944; Robinson, 1947); osteosarcoma (Cataldo, Savage and Shklar, 1965; Snyder and Marks, 1968; Ohba and colleagues, 1975); Ewing's tumour (Burford and Ackerman, 1945); neuroblastoma (Angelopoulos, Tilson and Stewart (1972) review the literature); medulloblastoma (Eversole and colleagues, 1972); ganglioneuroma (Young, 1967; Mitcherling and colleagues, 1974).

The histological appearances in jaw metastases follow the general pattern of all secondary growths in bone. Thus both osteoplastic and osteolytic lesions are to be observed, especially the latter (Cohen, 1958). Osteoplastic metastases are particularly associated with carcinoma of the prostate. Breast tumours, especially scirrhous growths, and carcinomas of the urinary tract also tend to produce osteoplastic metastases. As Cohen points out, the bone in osteoplastic secondary deposits is always well formed and regular, thus differing markedly from the irregular malignant bone of osteosarcoma. Cawson (1959) draws attention to the fact that in osteoplastic metastases the histological features of Paget's disease may be closely simulated. Not only may the bone show such changes, but hypercementosis of the teeth may also occur.

Visceral metastases from carcinoma in the oral cavity are uncommon. Traditionally, it has been taught that cancer of the mouth does not metastasise below the clavicle, but this generalisation is not true. However, it is the case that visceral metastases practically never occur at an early stage of the disease. Castigliano and Rominger (1954) have analysed a series of 752 cases of carcinoma in the oral cavity and have found that of the 321 patients known to have died of cancer visceral metastases were present in 17, an incidence of 5·3 per cent. The organs chiefly involved were the lungs and bones. The incidence of visceral metastases, they consider, is probably increasing owing to improved treatment of the local lesion and its cervical metastases leading to a longer life span for these patients.

The incidence of metastases in Topazian's (1961) series was higher, being 24 per cent of 83 cases. Carcinoma of the tonsil, floor of mouth, palate and tongue were the tumours that metastasised to distant sites with the greatest frequency.

REFERENCES

Abrams, H. L., Spiro, R., and Goldstein, N. (1950) Metastases in carcinoma. Analysis of 1000 autopsied cases. *Cancer*, **3**, 74.

Adair, F. E., and Herrmann, J. B. (1946) Unusual metastatic manifestations of breast carcinoma. I. Metastasis to the mandible with a report of five cases. *Surg. Gynec. Obstet.*, **83**, 289.

Al-Ani, S. (1973) Metastatic tumors to the mouth: report of two cases. *J. oral Surg.*, **31**, 120.

Angelopoulos, A. P., Tilson, H. B., and Stewart, F. W. (1972) Metastatic neuroblastoma of the mandible: review of literature and report of case. *J. oral Surg.*, **30**, 93.

Appenzeller, J., Weitzner, S., and Long, G. W. (1971) Hepatocellular carcinoma metastatic to the mandible: report of case and review of literature. *J. oral Surg.*, **29**, 668.

Batsakis, J. G. (1974) *Tumors of the Head and Neck*. Baltimore. The Williams & Wilkins Company.

Bernard, R. (1931) La résection économique dans l'exérèse des cancers de l'amygdale ayant envahi la branche montante du maxillaire. *Presse Méd.*, **39**, 1013.

Bernstein, J. M., Montgomery, W. W., and Balogh, K. (1966) Metastatic tumors to the maxilla, nose and paranasal sinuses. *Laryngoscope*, **76**, 621.

Blackwood, H. J. J. (1956) Metastatic carcinoma of the mandibular condyle. *Oral Surg.*, **9**, 1318.

Blake, H., and Blake, F. S. (1960) Breast carcinoma metastatic to maxilla. Report of a case. *Oral Surg.*, **13**, 1099.

Bruce, K. W., and McDonald, J. R. (1954) Metastatic adenocarcinoma of the mandible from the sigmoid colon. *Oral Surg.*, **7**, 772.

Burford, W. N., and Ackerman, L. V. (1945) Ewing's tumor of the mandible. *Amer. J. Orthodont.* (*Oral Surg. Sect.*), **31**, 544.

Burford, W. N., Ackerman, L. V., and Robinson, H. B. G. (1944) Mixed tumors of the submaxillary gland and oral cavity. *Amer. J. Orthodont.* (*Oral Surg. Sect.*), **30**, 377.

Byars, L. T., and Sarnat, B. G. (1946) Mandibular tumors. A clinical, roentgenographic, and histopathologic study. *Surg. Gynec. Obstet.*, **83**, 355.

Cameron, J. R., and Stetzer, J. J. (1947) Metastatic carcinoma of mandible. *J. oral Surg.*, **5**, 227.

Cash, C. D., Royer, R. Q., and Dahlin, D. C. (1961) Metastatic tumors of the jaws. *Oral Surg.*, **14**, 897.

Castigliano, S. G., and Rominger, C. J. (1954) Distant metastasis from carcinoma of the oral cavity. *Amer. J. Roentgenol.*, **71**, 997.

Cataldo, E., Savage, M., and Shklar, G. (1965) Osteogenic sarcoma of femur metastatic to mandible. Report of a case. *Oral Surg.*, **19**, 86.

Catania, A. F. (1953) Three nonvital teeth associated with chorio-epithelioma. *J. oral Surg.*, **11**, 324.

Catone, G. A., and Henny, F. A. (1969) Metastatic gastric adenocarcinoma of the mandible: report of a case. *J. oral Surg.*, **27**, 36.

Cawson, R. A. (1959) Secondary carcinoma of the mandible. *Dent. Practit.*, **9**, 240.

Clain, A. (1965) Secondary malignant disease of bone. *Brit. J. Cancer*, **19**, 15.

Clausen, F., and Poulsen, H. (1963) Metastatic carcinoma to the jaws. *Arch. path. microbiol. scand.*, **57**, 361.

Cohen, B. (1958) Secondary tumours of the mandible. *Ann. roy. Coll. Surg. Engl.*, **23**, 118.

Cook, T. J. (1949) Adenocarcinoma with metastasis to the mandible. *Oral Surg.*, **2,** 780.

Delaire, J., Gaillard, A., Renaud, Y., and Billet, J. (1960) Métastase au maxillaire supérieur d'un sympathome embryonnaire. *Rev. Stomat.*, **61,** 32.

Epker, B. N., Merrill, R. G., and Henny, F. A. (1969) Breast adenocarcinoma metastatic to the mandible. Report of seven cases. *Oral Surg.*, **28,** 471.

Eversole, L. R., Sabes, W. R., Brandebura, J., and Massey, G. B. (1972) Medulloblastoma: extradural metastasis to the jaw. Report of a case. *Oral Surg.*, **34,** 634.

Frank, R. H., Brini, A., and Nicolas, P. (1961) Métastase à la mugueuse buccale du maxillaire inférieur d'un gliome de la rétine. *Rev. Stomat.*, **62,** 21.

Geschickter, C. F., and Copeland, M. M. (1949) *Tumors of Bone*. 3rd Edition. Philadelphia. J. B. Lippincott Company.

Goldstein, I. H., and Goldstein, M. C. (1943) Jaw metastases in chondroblastic osteogenic sarcoma. *Amer. J. Orthodont. (Oral Surg. Sect.)*, **29, 57**.

Hägglund, G. (1959) Adenocarcinoma of the mandible, a metastasis from a primary tumor in the sigmoid colon. *Oral Surg.*, **10,** 1228.

Hanratty, W. J. (1971) Oral manifestations of giant cell carcinoma of the thyroid gland. *Brit. J. oral Surg.*, **8,** 281.

Hatziotis, J. C., Constantinidou, H., and Papanayotou, P. H. (1973) Metastatic tumors of the oral soft tissues. Review of the literature and report of a case. *Oral Surg.*, **36,** 544.

Hayes, R. L., Pinson, T. J., and Leffall, L. D. (1966) Adenocarcinoma of the pancreas metastatic to the mandible. *Oral Surg.*, **21,** 61.

Heslop, I. H. (1965) Secondary neoplasia of the jaws. *Brit. J. oral Surg.*, **2,** 47.

Holland, D. J. (1953) Metastatic carcinoma to the mandible. *Oral Surg.*, **6,** 567.

Jaffe, H. L. (1958) *Tumors and Tumorous Conditions of the Bones and Joints*. London. Henry Kimpton.

Kemper, J. W., and Bloom, H. J. (1944) Metastatic osteochondroma of maxilla from primary tumor of tibia. Report of case. *Amer. J. Orthodont. (Oral Surg. Sect.)*, **30,** 704.

Lainson, P. A., Khowassah, M.A., and Tewfik, H. H. (1975) Seminoma metastatic to the jaws. Report of a case. *Oral Surg.*, **40,** 404.

McDaniel, R. K., Luna, M. A., and Stimson, P. G. (1971) Metastatic tumors in the jaws. *Oral Surg.*, **31,** 380.

MacGregor, A. J., and Lewis, D. A. (1972) Metastasis of carcinoma of the lung by implantation in tooth sockets. *Brit. J. oral Surg.*, **9,** 195.

McMillan, M. D., and Edwards, J. L. (1975) Bilateral mandibular metastases. *Oral Surg.*, **39,** 959.

Mallett, S. P. (1961) A renal-cell metastatic carcinoma involving the mandible and submaxillary gland. *Oral Surg.*, **14,** 4.

Meyer, I., and Shklar, G. (1958) Involvement of the mandible and oral mucosa in a case of rectal adenocarcinoma with generalized metastases. *Oral Surg.*, **11,** 69.

Milobsky, S. A., Milobsky, L., and Epstein, L. I. (1975) Metastatic renal adenocarcinoma presenting as periapical pathosis in the maxilla. *Oral Surg.*, **39,** 30.

Mitcherling, J. J., Greenwold, W. E., Keen, R. R., and Jordan, J. E. (1974) Metastatic ganglioneuroblastoma: report of case and review of the literature. *J. oral Surg.*, **32,** 578.

Moorman, W. C., and Shafer, W. G. (1954) Metastatic carcinoma of the mandible. *J. oral Surg.*, **12,** 205.

Mosby, E. L., Sugg, W. E., and Hiatt, W. R. (1973) Gingival and pharyngeal metastasis from a malignant melanoma. Report of a case. *Oral Surg.*, **36,** 6.

Ohba, T., Katayama. H., Nakagawa, E., and Takeda, N. (1975) Mandibular metastasis of osteogenic sarcoma. Report of a case. *Oral Surg.*, **39,** 821.

Perlmutter, S., Buchner, A., and Smukler, H. (1974) Metastasis to the gingiva. Report of a case of metastasis from the breast and review of the literature. *Oral Surg.*, **38,** 749.

Ramanathan, K., Eravelly, J., and Ken, T. P. (1968) Metastatic choriocarcinoma involving the maxilla. Report of a case. *Oral Surg.*, **26,** 688.

Robinson, H. B. G. (1947) Metastasis of chondromyxosarcoma to the jaw and tooth. *Amer. J. Orthodont. (Oral Surg. Sect.)*, **33,** 558.

Rominger, C. J., Lockwood, D. W., and Canino, C. W. (1961) Carcinoma of the gallbladder with mandibular metastasis: report of case. *J. oral Surg.*, **19,** 425.

Sage, R. H., and Hoggins, G. S. (1961) Metastatic carcinoma of the mandible. *Oral Surg.*, **14,** 589.

Salman, I., and Darlington, C. G. (1944) Rare (unusual) malignant tumors of the jaws. *Amer. J. Orthodont. (Oral Surg. Sect.)*, **30,** 725.

U

Salman, I., and Langel, I. (1954) Metastatic tumors of the oral cavity. *Oral Surg.*, **7**, 1141.

Schofield, J. J. (1974) Oral metastatic deposit from carcinoma of the head of the pancreas. *Brit. dent. J.*, **137**, 355.

Seldin, H. M., and Rakower, W. (1953) Metastatic carcinoma of the mandible. *J. oral Surg.*, **11**, 336.

Sharp, G. S., Bullock, W. K., and Hazlet, J. W. (1956) *Oral Cancer and Tumors of the Jaw*. New York. McGraw-Hill.

Snyder, S. L., and Marks, I. (1968) Osteogenic sarcoma metastatic to the mandible. *Oral Surg.*, **25**, 216.

Snyder, S. R., Merkow, L. P., and White, N. S. (1971) Prostatic carcinoma metastatic to the mandible: report of case. *J. oral Surg.*, **29**, 205.

Sorbera, R. J., and Taylor, R. G. (1966) Carcinoma of the prostate metastatic to the oro-facial region and mandible. *Brit. J. oral Surg.*, **4**, 121.

Stern, L., and Shepard, A. (1941) Metastatic carcinoma of the mandible. *J. amer. dent. Ass.*, **28**, 707.

Stewart, E. E., and Bruce, K. W. (1953) Mandibular tumor metastasized from a hypernephroma. *J. oral Surg.*, **11**, 252.

Thoma, K. H., and Goldman, H. M. (1960) *Oral Pathology*. 5th Edition. London. Henry Kimpton.

Topazian, D. S. (1961) Distant metastasis of oral carcinoma. *Oral Surg.*, **14**, 705.

Van der Kwast, W. A. M., and van der Waal, I. (1974) Jaw metastases. *Oral Surg.*, **37**, 850.

Wertheimer, F. W., and Crayle, L. J. (1973) Lymphangiosarcoma of the gingiva. *Int. J. oral Surg.*, **2**, 159.

Willis, R. A. (1941) A review of 500 consecutive cancer necropsies. *Med. J. Aust.*, **2**, 258.

Young, W. G. (1967) Histopathologic study of ganglioneuroma in the mandible. *J. oral Surg.*, **25**, 325.

Zegarelli, D. J., Tsukada, V., Pickren, J. W., and Greene, G. W. (1973) Metastatic tumor to the tongue. Report of twelve cases. *Oral Surg.*, **35**, 202.

VII
SALIVARY GLAND TUMOURS

30. Salivary Gland Tumours

CLASSIFICATION AND NOMENCLATURE

The nomenclature of the tumours of salivary tissue has been, in the past, a matter of excessive complexity, stemming largely from the great variety of histological patterns that these tumours display and from the many views that have been held concerning their histogenesis. It would serve no useful purpose to go into the matter in detail here, though mention must be made of some of the commoner synonyms that are in use. A few remarks on nomenclature are therefore included in the descriptions of the various types of tumours. The terminology used here is based on the nomenclature recommended by the World Health Organization (Thackray and Sobin, 1972).

Epithelial Tumours
Adenoma
    Pleomorphic adenoma
    Monomorphic adenoma
      Adenolymphoma
      Oxyphilic adenoma
      Other types of adenoma
Mucoepidermoid tumour
Acinic cell tumour
Carcinoma
    Adenoid cystic carcinoma
    Adenocarcinoma
    Epidermoid carcinoma
    Undifferentiated carcinoma
    Carcinoma in pleomorphic adenoma.

Connective Tissue and Other Primary Tumours
    Fibroma; Fibrosarcoma; Lipoma; Neurilemmoma; Haemangioma; Melanoma; Lymphoma.

Although not a neoplastic condition, lymphoepithelial lesion is also considered in this chapter, as it is characterised by salivary gland enlargement and comes into the differential diagnosis of salivary gland tumours.

INCIDENCE

According to Frazell (1954) tumours of the major salivary glands account for 5 per cent of all benign and malignant tumours, excluding those of the skin. Malignant tumours of the major salivary glands comprise about 10 per cent of cancers of intraoral and neighbouring structures. Other observers cited by Frazell have found the incidence of salivary gland tumours to be between 0·1 and 2 per cent of all neoplasms. In those countries in which incidence figures have been determined, they occur in less than 3 per 100,000 of the population (Eneroth, 1964). In general, tumours of the minor salivary glands are much less common than those of the major glands, accounting for some 15 to 20 per cent of all salivary tumours, though some recent reports suggest that the relative frequency of tumours of the minor glands may be greater in some areas such as South Africa (Schulenberg, 1954), Uganda (Davies, Dodge and Burkitt, 1964), Egypt (Aboul-Nasr, 1961), West Indies (Gore, Annamunthodo and Harland, 1964) and India (Potdar and Paymaster, 1969).

Of the three major salivary glands, the parotid is much more often the site of tumours than the others; between 85 and 90 per cent of all tumours occur in it (see the large series of Harvey, Dawson and Innes, 1938; Foote and Frazell, 1954; Eneroth, 1971; Thackray and Lucas, 1974). Most of the remaining tumours occur in the submandibular gland, while tumours of the sublingual gland are rare.

The glands of the palate are more frequently the site of tumours than any of the other intraoral glands. About 55 per cent of intraoral salivary tumours occur in the palate and about 15 per cent in the lip, which is the next commonest site. The upper lip is much more frequently affected than the lower, the latter being the most infrequent site of all for salivary tumours (Krolls and Hicks, 1973). In Eggers' (1938) survey of the literature, only 4 out of 64 tumours were found to occur in the lower lip. In Bernier's (1946) series of 38 tumours 3 were in the lower lip. The remaining tumours are distributed about equally among the other glands in the floor of the mouth, the retromolar region, the cheek, tongue and peritonsillar area (Rawson, Howard, Royster and Horn, 1950; Ranger, Thackray and Lucas, 1956; Chaudhry, Vickers and Gorlin, 1961; Stuteville and Corley, 1967; Luna, Stimson and Bardwil, 1968; Potdar and Paymaster, 1969; Frable and Elzay, 1970; Spiro and colleagues, 1973). Uncommonly, tumours may occur in the mandible, apparently as intraosseous growths. Such tumours possibly arise from salivary tissue derived from the sublingual or submandibular glands that may occupy a recess or defect in the bone (Jacobs, 1955; Richard and Ziskind, 1957; Seward, 1960; Simpson, 1965; and others). Or it is possible, as suggested by Hayes (1961) and Bhaskar (1963), that oral epithelium may be included in the developing mandible or that odontogenic cysts may undergo neoplastic change.

The different types of tumour vary in distribution. Pleomorphic adenomas account for 60 to 70 per cent of all tumours of the major glands, but for a smaller proportion (about 55 per cent) of the tumours of the minor glands. Mucoepidermoid tumours, on the other hand, constitute up to about 5 per cent of tumours of the major glands but occur more frequently in the minor glands, accounting for as much as 25 to 30 per cent of all tumours in some recent series, but this figure is almost certainly unduly high. Adenoid cystic carcinoma also shows a notable difference in incidence. Up to 5 per cent of major gland tumours are adenoid cystic carcinomas but in the minor glands the figure is between 15 and 25 per cent. Carcinomas of various types are commoner in the major glands, accounting for up to 15 per cent of tumours, whereas in the minor glands they account for no more than 5 per cent. Adenomas of various types are uncommon in the minor glands. Chaudhry, Vickers and Gorlin (1961) give a comprehensive statistical review of the incidence of tumours in the minor salivary glands. Evans and Cruickshank (1970) give a general review of incidence in all sites.

EPITHELIAL TUMOURS

Pleomorphic Adenoma

The term pleomorphic adenoma or mixed tumour is used to describe those tumours of salivary tissue in which epithelial elements occur in a matrix of mucoid, myxoid or chondroid tissue and in which a variety of histological appearances may be observed. Although many would feel that these tumours are of purely epithelial origin, the matter cannot be regarded as finally settled; in any event the term "mixed" is used rather as an appropriate description of the varied cellular picture than with any histogenetic implications. The many synonyms that are met with, particularly in the less recent literature, spring from the varied theories that have been held, from time to time, about the nature and origin of mixed tumours. Thus one encounters titles such as chondroma, endothelioma, myxoma, fibromyxoepithelioma, myxochondrocarcinoma, branchioma, enclavoma and the like, indicating beliefs in mesodermal, diploblastic or embryonic rests origins for the tumours. On the other hand, adenoma, complex adenoma or pleomorphic adenoma indicate the purely epithelial origin of the tumour while at the same time emphasising the variable histological picture.

Clinical Features

Pleomorphic adenomas occur at all ages, even occasionally in the new-born (Howard and colleagues, 1950; Karlan and Snyder, 1968). In Frazell's (1954) series the youngest patient was 7 and the oldest 82 years of age. The age groups most frequently affected are the fifth and sixth decades. Most published series of cases show a distinct preponderance of women (60 per cent).

Most pleomorphic adenomas of the major glands occur in the parotid, particularly in the tail of the gland. In the minor glands the palate is the site of election. Multiple tumours are rare; Frazell mentions a patient with two typical tumours in one parotid gland and a third tumour in the other gland, and another patient with a tumour of the parotid and also a tumour of the submandibular gland. In one of Gardner, Siegler and Spire's (1964) patients a tumour was present in each parotid gland. Bilateral tumours of the palate have been reported by Praytor (1966). Multiple tumours of different histological type are very rare. Lumerman and colleagues (1975) cite the published cases.

Pleomorphic adenomas generally grow slowly and painlessly and often they have been present for years before the patient seeks advice. In some cases, however, there is a history of more recent rapid growth after a long period of quiescence, or on the other hand, a phase of active growth may be followed by a prolonged period during which there is little change. Tumours vary in size from a centimetre or less in diameter in the case of some growths of the minor glands up to the large masses that are still occasionally to be seen in the parotid gland. The intraoral location of the tumours of the minor glands generally ensures that they are not permitted to attain the size that some parotid tumours reach, though occasionally palatal tumours may reach surprising dimensions, almost filling the mouth. Ulceration of the overlying skin or mucosa is uncommon.

Pathology

Macroscopic appearance. Pleomorphic adenomas are generally irregularly rounded or ovoid structures with a smooth, lobulated or nodular surface. The connective tissue capsule does not always envelop the tumour completely, for there may occur areas in which it is deficient and where the tumour is contiguous with normal salivary tissue (Fig. 99). Furthermore, some of the nodules noted on the surface of the tumour may appear to be separate from the remainder of the growth and enveloped completely in their own subpartitions of capsule.

Fig. 99. Examples of pleomorphic adenoma, showing the variable arrangement of the capsule. **a,** a tumour of the palate. In the area shown here the capsule is indistinct and tumour tissue is in close apposition to normal gland elements. × 80. **b,** a tumour of the palate, showing how a plane of cleavage can occur below the surface of the growth, leaving tumour tissue adherent to the capsule. × 80. **c,** a parotid tumour with a small nodule of growth lying beyond the capsule. × 80. **d** and **e,** sections from a parotid tumour, showing that what appear to be separate tumour masses at one level are connected at a deeper level. × 2·5.

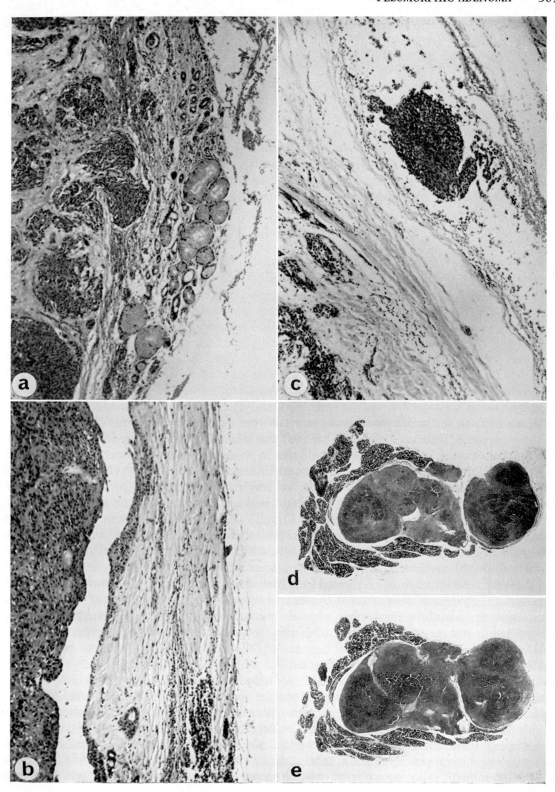

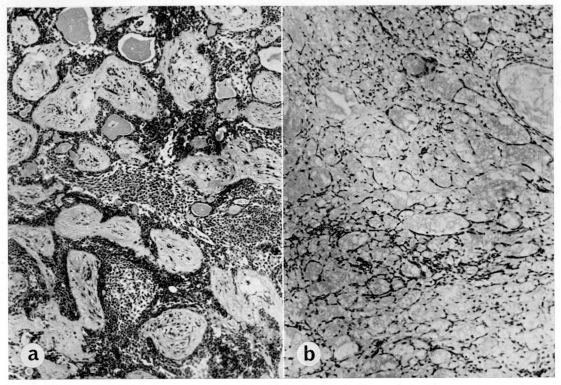

Fig. 101 **a,** a palatal tumour, consisting of strands and sheets of epithelial cells in a collagenous matrix, The cells in the larger sheets are of the myoepithelial type. Some irregular duct-like spaces are present. containing homogenous eosinophilic material. × 80. **b,** a parotid tumour, consisting of numerous fine interlacing strands of cells in a mucoid matrix. × 80.

columnar cells with eosinophilic and finely granular cytoplasm, similar to those seen in adenolymphoma. Very often these duct-like or tubular structures contain eosinophilic material that gives a positive PAS reaction (Fig. 102a, b).

Squamous areas are not uncommon and vary in extent from the presence of small foci of epidermoid cells to fully developed epithelial pearls. Adipose tissue is occasionally present (Fig. 102c).

In about 1 per cent of cases, according to Foote and Frazell, the tumour is almost entirely made up of spindle cells growing in anastomosing bands and bundles, sometimes with the nuclei in palisade arrangement, the appearance then being very similar to that of benign smooth muscle tumours (Fig. 102d).

Sebaceous glands normally occur in the parotid gland (Hamperl, 1931; Hartz, 1946; Lee, 1949). Meza-Chávez (1949) found them in over a quarter of the glands examined, arising from

Fig. 102 **a,** a parotid tumour showing well formed ducts, each with an inner layer of cells like those in normal ducts and an outer layer of cells resembling myoepithelial cells. × 200. **b,** palatal tumour with numerous duct-like structures. These are more irregular and less like normal ducts than in **a.** × 80. **c,** a palatal tumour showing squamous metaplasia and keratinisation. Fat is also present. × 80. **d,** a parotid tumour, consisting largely of spindle cells. × 200.

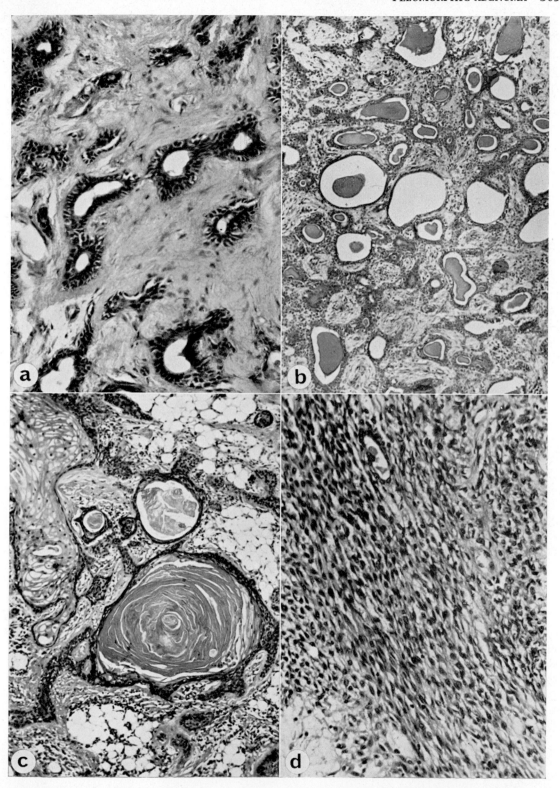

intercalated and striated ducts that ended blindly. They were often to be found in parotid glands that were the seat of pleomorphic adenomas. Patey and Thackray found sebaceous glands in all their cases of parotid tumours, varying in number from a few glands up to as many as three or four thousand. Sebaceous glands also occur, but less frequently, in the submandibular and sublingual glands (Linhartova, 1974).

Intercellular material is generally prominent in pleomorphic adenoma, except in those cases where extensive epithelial proliferation constitutes the bulk of the growth. In such cases there is only a small quantity of delicate connective tissue between the cell groups. Where more abundant intercellular material is present it may consist almost entirely of fibrous tissue of normal appearance but very often a variety of changes can be noted. Hyalinisation often seems to have occurred, but the apparently structureless eosinophilic material can be seen, by diffracted light, to contain foci of fibrillar appearance. The fibrils are arranged in sheaves or radiating stellate formations, and they can be strikingly demonstrated by Van Gieson's stain (Thackray and Lucas, 1974). The hyaline areas also frequently contain elastic tissue, sometimes in large amounts, as demonstrated by Azzopardi and Zayid (1972). Other changes include cartilaginous metaplasia or ossification. Perhaps the most characteristic appearance is the presence of large areas of mucoid or myxochondroid material, often constituting the greater part of the tumour, with the epithelial cells scattered singly or in strands or sheets in the mucoid background. The cells frequently have stellate processes which appear to run into and blend with the intercellular material, giving the impression that the cells melt, as it were, into the background. Since the cells themselves often contain mucin droplets within their cytoplasm this impression is heightened. Many cells, however, persist, and are engulfed in the matrix which may thus, with its cell inclusions, come to resemble hyaline cartilage.

Histochemical studies on pleomorphic adenoma have been reported by a number of workers. Hemplemann and Womack (1942) found that the mucoids in duct-like structures or otherwise closely associated with the epithelial cells could be distinguished by titration of metachromasia from the mucoid forming the intercellular or stromal material of the tumour. For this reason they believed that mixed tumours were in fact of diploblastic origin. Grishman (1952) also found that the intercellular mucin could be distinguished from that associated with the epithelial cells. The former type of mucin she considered to be a secretion of myoepithelial cells. On the other hand, Lennox, Pearse and Richards (1952) in a study of the comparable "mixed" tumours of the skin, considered the mucin to be an entirely epithelial product but of highly labile nature. Contact with the stroma might modify it in such a way that it could come to show many of the physical and chemical attributes of a so-called connective tissue mucin. In this way an epithelial mucin might pass through a series of physical changes, ultimately to produce cartilage. The same type of change could probably also occur in salivary gland tumours. Another view is that of Yates and Paget (1952), who believe that the chondroid material in salivary tumours develops from the connective tissue stroma under the organiser influence of the epithelial elements of the tumour. Azzopardi and Smith (1959) support the view that the intercellular mucinous material of the myxochondroid areas is a product of the myoepithelial cell, being probably chondroitin sulphate A or B. Erichsen (1955) and Cotchin (1958) also concluded from a study of mixed tumours of the mammary gland in dogs that myoepithelium is responsible for the connective tissue type of mucin seen in these tumours.

Histogenesis

Although most workers now believe these salivary tumours to be of purely epithelial origin this is by no means an entirely modern concept, for it represents some of the earliest scientific thinking on the histogenesis of these neoplasms. It is, moreover, a view that has always continued to have its adherents, even during the periods when counter-theories were enjoying much support and popularity.

The epithelial theory of origin was first put forward because of the similarities between normal salivary tissue and salivary tumours, and its early expression can be found in some of the first papers on the subject. At the same time, however, the extremely complex histological appearance of many salivary tumours had stimulated theories of origin that ascribed an important role to mesenchyme or postulated a mixed origin, from both mesenchyme and epithelium. Thus Billroth (1859) and Virchow (1863) ascribed the origin of salivary tumours to the connective tissue in the salivary glands and they were followed by many others, with very diverse views being put forward. From this period date the concepts of vascular endothelial origin and branchial arch origin, with nomenclature to suit—angiosarcoma, endothelioma and the like. The purely mesenchymal theory is now defunct but the notion that salivary tumours really are "mixed," in the sense that they derive from both epithelium and mesenchyme, has persisted. Amongst those who have adhered to such views may be mentioned McFarland (1926, 1942) and Ewing (1940), and as new methods and techniques have come into use there have not failed to appear those who have found in them support for these views. Fully documented surveys of the historical aspects of the subject are given by Ahlbom (1935) and Mylius (1960).

Although the epithelial theory has now gained many adherents there is still much discussion with regard to the particular cells which give rise to tumours and the nature of the mucoid and cartilaginoid changes so often observed in the tumours. With regard to the cells of origin, the idea that the tumours arise from adult glandular epithelium was put forward by the early workers and has since been held by a succession of pathologists. This view is supported by the general resemblance of the tumour cells to the cells of normal salivary tissue and the frequent presence in tumours of ductular and acinar structures very similar to those of normal salivary glands. Moreover, Zymbal (1933), Willis (1967) and others have pointed out that direct transitions between tumour and normal salivary tissue can be seen, and Willis in particular believes that an entire field of salivary tissue, ducts and lobules of acini alike, may simultaneously undergo neoplastic transformation.

On the other hand, some authors have suggested that the tumours might arise from particular cells. Thus Sheldon (1943), Bauer and Fox (1945), Bauer and Bauer (1953) and others have suggested on morphological grounds that the myoepithelial cells may give rise to pleomorphic adenomas. The possible role played by these cells has also been discussed by Grishman (1952) and Azzopardi and Smith (1959). However, Murata and Miyaji (1966) have shown that while in normal salivary gland alkaline phosphatase is present in the myoepithelial cells, this enzyme is absent from the epithelium of pleomorphic adenomas. The concept of genesis of tumours from the cells of a primitive replacement epithelium that is presumably always present in normal glandular tissue for repair purposes was suggested by Harvey, Dawson and Innes (1938). Embryonic epithelial cells have also been suggested in the various enclavement theories as the cells of origin of mixed tumours. These theories postulate remnants of the branchial arches or portions of primitive salivary gland lying dormant in the tissues.

The presence and nature of the mucoid and chondroid material in pleomorphic adenomas has received much notice from the supporters of the epithelial theory and has generally been attributed to the secretory activity of the tumour cells, or even to metaplasia. Most of the more recent authors do not consider the cartilage-like material to be real cartilage, but merely to have some resemblance to it. Thus Willis (1967) shares the view of Fry (1928), Patey (1931), Zymbal (1933), Stein and Geschickter (1934) and others that the cartilage-like tissue represents only further change of the type that produced the mucinous matrix. The epithelial cells thus become widely separated and bear a superficial resemblance to cartilage cells.

Recent ultrastructure studies have not been able to resolve the problem. Welsh and Meyer (1968) made an electron microscope study of the myxochondroid areas and found a mixture of epithelial and myoepithelial cells, together with true cartilage cells. Since no intermediate forms were found they concluded that the chondrocytes were not derived from the epithelial or myo-epithelial cells, and that the tumours were thus truly mixed. Similar findings are recorded by Fukushima (1968). On the other hand, Doyle and colleagues (1968) could find no chondrocytes, but they did identify neoplastic myoepithelial cells in a cartilage-like matrix. They concluded that the myoepithelial cells had undergone partial metaplasia to produce typical chondroid matrix. In another ultrastructure investigation, Deppisch and Toker (1969) could find no evidence to support a myoepithelial histogenesis for the cells in the myxoid stroma. Likewise, Kondo, Muragishi and Imaizuma (1971) and Chisholm and colleagues (1974) could not support the myoepithelial theory. Thus, this branch of microscopic anatomy leaves us still with conflicting and contradictory answers to some important questions. In any event, none of these studies excludes the possibility that cartilage cells might be formed by metaplasia of the connective tissue stroma.

Behaviour

A number of attempts have been made to correlate the microscopic appearances of pleo-morphic adenoma with clinical behaviour, depending on such features as the proportion of mucoid or chondroid material to cells, the appearance of the cells themselves, the presence of differentiated structures of duct-like or acinar type and so on. However, these attempts have not been generally successful, and little guidance can be obtained with regard to the probable behaviour of a given tumour from the histological appearances alone. The course of these lesions appears rather to depend on the type of treatment given and figures quoted for recurrence rates vary considerably. For parotid tumours, the rate for most of the series reported in the literature is between 25 and 50 per cent, though in Foote and Frazell's (1953) cases the rate was 5 per cent. However, much depends on the length of follow-up; a recurrence rate of 1 per cent per year up to 25 years seems to be a fairly constant figure.

The recurrence rate for tumours of the minor glands has also been high, particularly in the earlier reports, and many of the records are incomplete. However, more recent reports such as those of Harrison (1956), Brown, Bishop and Girardeau (1959) and Fine, Marshall and Horn (1960) have shown very much better results. In Morgan and Mackenzie's (1968) series, for example, 9 out of 11 patients were free from disease 10 years after local excision of parotid tumours, and 32 out of 35 were similarly free following local excision plus radiotherapy. In the minor salivary gland tumours, there were no recurrences 5 years after treatment of the 17 patients with these tumours. The earlier high figures for recurrence in all probability reflect the outcome of the operation of simple enucleation, which was formerly the standard operative procedure for these growths. The likelihood of procedures of this type leaving tumour fragments or cells behind in the tumour bed appears to be considerable, as has already been pointed out, and it seems reason-able to expect that recurrence rates in future will be lower than those mentioned, owing to the growing recognition that extracapsular dissection or occasionally more radical procedures must be employed. At the same time, in the evaluation of published series the need for adequate follow-up periods has to be kept in mind. Recurrence after operation of any type of salivary tumour may be long delayed. In one of McFarland's (1943) cases, for example, the period between operation and recurrence was 47 years and though this may be an extreme example, it is certainly true to say that a follow-up period of less than 5 years is of little value. Ten years is a preferable period and even then recurrences may be still to come.

Another cause of recurrence, and probably a not infrequent one, is rupture or fragmentation during removal of tumours with an appreciable myxoid component. The soft or diffluent material then spills into the wound and the seeded tumour cells lead to multiple tumour nodules appearing later in the operation area.

Recurrent tumours, like primary growths, grow slowly and sometimes intermittently. They are much more difficult to deal with than primary tumours, since the multiple nodules extend over a relatively wide field and therefore require more extensive excision which, both in the major and the minor glands, soon takes the operation into areas where it becomes very difficult to avoid mutilation while at the same time achieving complete extirpation of tumour.

Although pleomorphic adenoma is essentially a benign tumour, very rarely there may occur bloodborne metastasis. Thackray (1957) noted a metastasis from a parotid tumour to the iliac bone, Foote and Frazell reported lung metastasis and Youngs and Scheuer (1973) a liver metastasis. All three of the patients had had parotid tumours, removed many years previously. These metastases, which were identical histologically with the respective primary tumours, are to be regarded as exceptional curiosities. The rare instances of benign tumours producing metastases in this way differ from the usual type of metastasis in malignant tumours, in that they are not associated with the progressive course to death that characterises malignancy.

Carcinoma arising in Pleomorphic Adenoma

There is some variation in opinion about the incidence of malignancy in pleomorphic adenoma. Probably some of the earlier reports of such tumours included neoplasms that are now generally considered to be distinct from pleomorphic adenoma. Thus Mulligan (1943) reviewed the literature and collected 21 cases of pleomorphic adenoma in which there had been metastasis. He considered at least 12 of these tumours to have been adenoid cystic carcinomas. On the other hand, Ahlbom (1935) had never seen a histologically benign tumour become malignant. None of the 100 pleomorphic adenomas in the series reported by Rawson, Howard, Royster and Horn (1950) metastasised. However, in Foote and Frazell's large series, 57 tumours were diagnosed as malignant mixed, out of the total of 877 tumours of all types. In Luna, Stimson and Bardwil's (1968) series of 68 tumours of the intraoral glands, malignant mixed tumours accounted for 11 per cent of the total number. Foote and Frazell point out that since only very small areas of such malignant tumours may show the usual appearances of pleomorphic adenoma, many growths are diagnosed simply as salivary gland carcinoma. This may account for the relatively small number of malignant pleomorphic tumours recorded as such in the literature. On the other hand, it is rare for tumours showing only typical pleomorphic structure to give rise to metastases, although such cases do occur, as already noted. Other instances of pleomorphic adenomas giving rise to metastases are reported by Fine and Marshall (1961), who record a parotid tumour of typical pleomorphic appearance that produced multiple skeletal metastases and Gerughty and colleagues (1969) have seen metastatic deposits of typical pleomorphic structure. Vertebral metastases seem to be a feature of these cases (Thomas and Coppola, 1965). However, it is not certain that carcinomatous change had not occurred in the primary tumours in these patients. In Moberger and Eneroth's (1968) series, malignant tumours constituted some 2 per cent of 1,633 pleomorphic tumours. Of the 9 cases studied fully, the primary tumour was of typical pleomorphic type, with occasional small areas showing cytological evidence of malignancy. However, in every one of these cases the secondary deposits showed carcinoma alone and never any pleomorphic structure. In three of the cases the metastases appeared as adenoid cystic carcinoma, in two as mucoepidermoid tumour and in four as poorly differentiated or anaplastic carcinoma.

Thackray and Lucas (1974) found that carcinoma arose in pleomorphic adenoma in 5·4 per cent of cases, but point out that the published figures vary widely, as just noted. Such figures cannot be taken as a precise indication of the likelihood of malignant change in pleomorphic adenoma; a

component that is so often a notable feature of that tumour. These have been termed monomorphic adenomas, as being the obvious antonym to pleomorphic adenoma.

In pleomorphic adenoma the cellular pattern is characteristically very varied; in the same tumour there may be seen ducts, cells arranged in sheets, strands or islands, areas of keratinisation, foci of adipose tissue and other features, as well as cartilaginous, myxoid or mucoid areas, all irregularly mixed together. In the monomorphic adenomas, the variability of the cellular pattern of the pleomorphic adenoma is absent; instead of the juxtaposition of ducts, sheets or strands of cells and the like the pattern is uniform. If the adenoma is composed of tubules for example, then these structures are distributed regularly throughout the whole tumour; it it is a trabecular adenoma, the trabeculae form a very regular and uniform pattern throughout the whole, or almost the whole, growth. In this way, a number of recognisable patterns are formed.

The recognisable, and indeed characteristic nature, of the overall patterns of the monomorphic adenomas is supplemented by another point of distinction between these tumours and pleomorphic adenoma. This is the absence of myxochondroid tissue. Of course, not all pleomorphic adenomas contain this tissue, or it may be present in such small quantities that it can be found only after prolonged search. However, the epithelium in these tumours shows the same varied pattern as in pleomorphic adenomas in which the typical myxochondroid tissue is also present, that is to say, it consists of ducts, keratin-filled cysts, sheets and strands of myoepithelial cells and other arrangements typically associated with pleomorphic adenoma, so that there is no difficulty in making that diagnosis, despite the absence from the section examined of myxochondroid tissue. Thus, the diagnosis of monomorphic adenoma does not depend simply on the absence of myxochondroid; it is necessary that the epithelium should be arranged throughout the tumour in one or other of the various patterns considered characteristic for these adenomas.

Monomorphic adenomas may be composed of oxyphilic, sebaceous, mucous, myoepithelial or basal-type cells, and may be named accordingly; or alternatively, they may be designated according to cellular pattern rather than cell type, for example, as trabecular, tubular or canalicular adenomas. Both types of nomenclature have been used in the literature, and sometimes they have been combined. What for one author is a basal cell adenoma is for another a trabecular adenoma of basal cell type, and perhaps for a third, a canalicular adenoma. Thus there is at present little uniformity in terminology, but this is understandable in a group of tumours that are not very common and are only currently becoming generally recognised. In the WHO classification (Thackray and Sobin, 1972) the group of monomorphic adenomas is subdivided into three categories. Adenolymphoma is considered as a member of the group since the neoplastic element —as opposed to the reactive lymphocytic component—is the epithelium, and this is uniform and regular. Oxyphilic adenoma likewise consists of a single, regularly arranged, cell type. The remaining members of the group comprise the "other types."

Adenolymphoma

This tumour was first described by Albrecht and Arzt in 1910 as a papillary cystadenoma, though it is often known after Warthin (1929) who described further cases under the name of papillary cystadenoma lymphomatosum. Many other synonyms have been used.

Clinical Features

Most patients are aged between 50 and 70 years. There is a striking sex difference; 85 to 90 per cent of patients are males.

Practically all the tumours occur in connection with the parotid gland, being situated very often in the lower pole or close to it but just outside the capsule. A few tumours have been reported in association with the submandibular gland, but it is possible that in these cases, as

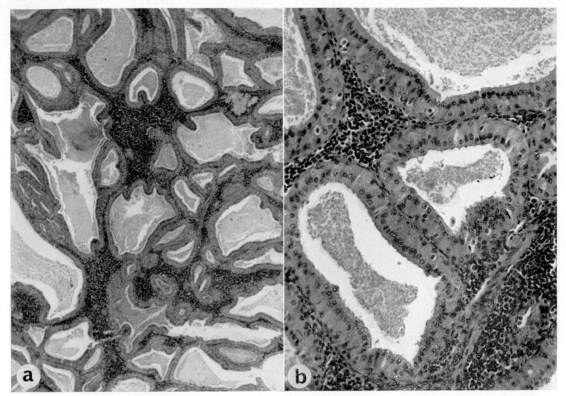

Fig. 104   Adenolymphoma. **a,** the tumour is composed of columnar or cubical epithelial cells forming double-layered columns or processes, with intervening lymphoid tissue. × 30. **b,** detail from **a.** × 200.

Martin and Ehrlich (1944), Thompson and Bryant (1950) and others have pointed out, the tumours have really arisen in that portion of the lower pole of the parotid that is very close to the submandibular gland. The tumour can also occur outside the parotid gland or its immediate neighbourhood. Bernier and Bhaskar (1958) have reported 4 cases in which the tumour occurred in lymph nodes unrelated to any of the salivary glands. In some 5 to 10 per cent of cases bilateral tumours in the parotid glands are found and, uncommonly, there may be multiple discrete tumours (Foote and Frazell, 1954; Patey and Thackray, 1958; Kleinsasser and colleagues, 1966).

There are very few reports of tumours in the minor salivary glands. Hart and Andrews (1968) record a tumour in the oral mucosa opposite the lower right canine, and though very small it appeared to fulfil all the criteria for the diagnosis. The authors consider it to have arisen from minor salivary gland ductal epithelium and accompanying nodes of the buccal chain of lymphatics. A tumour of the lip has been reported by Veronesi and Corbetta (1960).

The lesion appears as a painless circumscribed mass, not attached to the skin or underlying tissues. The facial nerve is not involved. The rate of growth is slow.

Pathology

The tumour presents as a circumscribed oval or rounded mass measuring up to some 5 to 6 cm in length but very rarely more. Large tumours, comparable with some of the examples of pleomorphic adenomas, are not seen. The surface is smooth and even, or it may be slightly lobulated. There is a thin capsule, which may be incomplete. The tumour is soft and compressible and may even be fluctuant when there has been much cyst formation. The patient may report that it varies in size. The cut surface characteristically shows numerous cystic spaces though occasionally there is one large cyst only, or none at all. The cysts often contain papillary ingrowths from the wall and are filled with mucoid or gelatinous fluid, or with thicker caseous-like material of typical brownish colour. The intercystic tissue is greyish-white.

The microscopic picture with its two elements, the epithelial and the lymphoid, is very characteristic (Fig. 104). The epithelial element consists of columnar and cubical or polyhedral cells arranged generally in double-layered columns or processes. These cells have finely granular and pronouncedly eosinophilic cytoplasm and round or oval vesicular nuclei with prominent nucleoli. Electron microscopically, they have been shown to contain large numbers of mitochondria of abnormal type (Schiefer, Hübner and Kleinsasser, 1968). The cell columns are arranged in convoluted patterns which, together with the lymphoid element, form the solid portion of the tumour and protrude in papillary manner into the cystic spaces. The columns consist of a layer of tall columnar cells regularly arranged in a palisade manner and a layer of smaller cubical or polygonal cells. The tall columnar cells clothe those aspects of the cell columns that face the cavities of the cystic spaces and the smaller cells form a basal layer. The nuclei of the tall columnar cells are arranged in an even row towards the free margins of the cells. The cells of the basal layer are fewer in number than those of the columnar layer, they are less regularly arranged and their nuclei do not present the same regimented appearance as do those of the columnar cells. Often there are more than the two rows of cells just described, sometimes quite large cell masses being formed. In some of these squamous metaplasia may be noted. In some areas, owing to distension of the cystic spaces, the lining cells may become cubical or flattened. The cysts themselves contain amorphous material, sometimes showing cholesterol clefts.

The presence of ciliated cells has been reported by Warthin (1929), though this occurrence must be rare as most other investigators have failed to find such cells. Mucus-secreting cells are occasionally seen, occurring here and there between the eosinophilic cells. The occurrence of sebaceous-like cells has been reported by Rawson and Horn (1950).

The lymphoid element of the tumour is separated from the epithelium by a thin basement membrane. It is usually plentiful and consists of a reticulum diffusely infiltrated with lymphocytes and showing numerous germinal centres. That the lymphoid element in some tumours represents organised lymphatic tissue and not merely infiltrations of lymphocytic cells is indicated by the presence of a capsule and subcapsular and medullary lymph sinuses. These features can be demonstrated in specimens that have not yet grown so large as to obliterate them (Thompson and Bryant, 1950; Bernier and Bhaskar, 1958).

Plasma cells and eosinophils may be noted amongst the lymphoid cells and if there has been secondary infection or if radiotherapy has been given, quite often there are areas of fibrosis (Patey and Thackray, 1970). Sometimes the lymphatic element may be very scanty, or even absent. Bernier and Bhaskar report six tumours of this type, four from the parotid area and two from the cheek. Apart from the absence of lymphatic tissue the appearances are indentical with the usual type of adenolymphoma.

Histogenesis

As with other salivary tumours, there has been much controversy about the histogenesis of adenolymphoma. Some of the names that have been used for the tumour, congenital epithelial cyst of the neck, branchioma, orbital inclusion cyst, oncocytoma, for example, give some indication of the range of views that has been held on the subject. However, opinion has come round again to the original view of Albrecht and Arzt, that the tumour arises from salivary tissue and this may be in lymph nodes as well as in the salivary glands themselves. Neisse (1898) had already shown that lymph nodes in the parotid gland in the fetus may contain salivary tubules and that these structures could also be found in the preparotid lymph nodes. Nicholson (1922,

1923) and later Thompson and Bryant (1950) and others confirmed these findings. Lang (1929) and Ewing have also found salivary tissue in cervical nodes. The occurrence of adenolymphoma in those lymph nodes in which salivary tissue is well known to occur thus renders unnecessary some of the more complicated hypotheses just mentioned. The occasional finding of the tumour in nodes further removed from the parotid is also accounted for by the normal occurrence of salivary tissue in those structures.

In the salivary glands, it seems probable that the tumour develops from oncocytic duct epithelium, with accompanying accumulation of lymphoid tissue, quite apart from pre-existing lymph nodes.

Shklar and Chauncey (1965) have investigated the enzyme activity of adenolymphoma, and find that the epithelial component gives similar reactions to the ductal epithelium of the normal parotid gland. They suggest that the lesion is a developmental malformation arising from the ducts of normal parotid gland and including lymphoid tissue from primordial branchial arches or from contiguous lymph nodes. The view has also been put forward that the lymphoid element of adenolymphoma might represent a delayed hypersensitivity reaction (Allegra, 1971; Sikorowa, 1973).

Behaviour

Adenolymphoma is a slowly growing and benign tumour. Excision is curative, but recurrences have been noted in some cases. These may be due to the growth of independent tumour foci elsewhere in the gland. Malignant transformation is very rare; instances in which this appears to have occurred are reported by Ruebner and Bramhall (1960), de la Pava and colleagues (1965) and others. In Ruebner and Bramhall's case a papillary carcinoma appeared. In de la Pava's case there was squamous metaplasia of the columnar epithelium, which developed into squamous cell carcinoma. Gadient and Kalfayan (1975) cite the reported cases.

OXYPHILIC ADENOMA

This tumour consists of large granular eosinophilic cells or oncocytes, of the type found in normal salivary glands in later life.

Clinical Features

Oxyphilic adenomas are quite rare tumours, accounting for one per cent or less of parotid tumours. The great majority occur in the parotid gland, but tumours have been reported in other sites such as palate, submandibular gland, tonsillar region, cheek, nasal mucosa and larynx. Bilateral parotid tumours have been reported (Boley and Robinson, 1954) and they were present in over one-third of the patients in Blanck, Eneroth and Jakobsson's (1970) series.

The tumour occurs in patients who are usually aged 60 years or over; it is very rare below the age of 50. It is slightly commoner in women; this contrasts with the striking male preponderance of adenolymphoma.

The tumour grows very slowly, as a painless smooth swelling, not attached to the skin or deep structures and not tender.

Pathology

The tumour is generally round or ovoid, smooth or nodular, and may measure up to some 5 cm in its longest dimension; exceptionally it may be multinodular (Meza-Chávez, 1949; Schwartz and Feldman, 1969). It is well encapsulated and demarcated from the surrounding tissues. The cut surface is usually a dark reddish-brown shade and without areas of haemorrhage or of the mucoid of the pleomorphic adenoma. It is divided into lobules by fine connective tissue

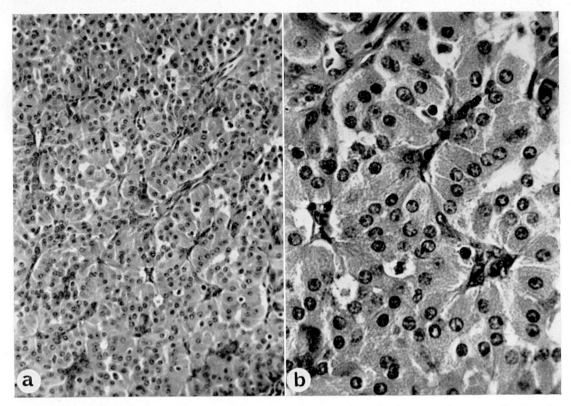

Fig. 105   Oxyphilic adenoma of the parotid. **a,** the tumour consists of columns and groups of cells, often in attempted acinar formation. × 200. **b,** the cells are large, round or polygonal, with finely granular cytoplasm and vesicular nuclei. × 500.

bands. The cells of which the tumour is composed, and which give it its name, are strikingly eosinophilic. They are arranged in columns or small rounded groups somewhat suggestive of an acinar arrangement, but frequently no lumen is seen. A very delicate stroma is present between the columns and groups. The cells themselves are large and round or polygonal, with a finely granular and eosinophilic cytoplasm. The nucleus is vesicular and contains one or more nucleoli. Mitoses are very seldom seen. Among the cells, there are some with dense hyperchromatic nuclei and deeply eosinophilic cytoplasm, appearing as if they had been compressed. These are sometimes referred to as "dark cells," in contrast to the more numerous "light cells" (Fig. 105).

The mucoid and stromal changes of pleomorphic adenoma are not seen in oxyphilic adenoma, though Christopherson (1949) has reported a case in which areas of cartilage were present. Lymphoid cells may be present, in varying amounts. Usually there is no more than a scanty infiltration of lymphocytes and they rarely form follicles, as occurs in adenolymphoma.

Histogenesis

Hamperl (1931, 1936) gave the name "oncocyte" to the epithelial parenchymal cells that, in certain organs, undergo a peculiar change. These cells become enlarged and the cytoplasm is filled with numerous eosinophilic granules. The nucleus is like those of the surrounding cells, or it may stain more deeply or may even be pyknotic. Oncocytes are found in many tissues, including the salivary glands, pancreas, thyroid, parathyroid, anterior and posterior lobes and stalk of the pituitary, testis, fallopian tube, liver and stomach. In the salivary glands, the duct epithelial cells most often undergo this oncocytic change, but the cells of groups of acini may also lose their zymogen granules and become swollen and eosinophilic. Hamperl described an adenoma of the salivary glands composed of cells of this type and also found them in adeno-lymphoma. Because of this Jaffé (1932) introduced the term oncocytoma for the tumour now known as adenolymphoma. Ackerman (1943) deprecated this usage and considered that the designation oncocytoma should be restricted to the tumour here described, although oxyphilic adenoma is now the preferred designation. Moreover, the term oncocytoma may be extended to tumours occurring in other organs, but which are composed entirely of oncocytes (Hamperl, 1962).

The occurrence of oncocytes is related to age. They are seen only occasionally under the age of 50, but thereafter they appear to increase and are practically always present in persons over 70 years of age. This age relationship may explain why the tumour practically always occurs in persons over 60. Further observations on oncocytes in tumours and normal salivary gland and their incidence in relation to age have been made by Meza-Chávez (1949).

The nature of the oncocytic change is not yet clear. Balogh and Roth (1965) have shown that the oncocytes in oxyphilic adenoma (and the granular cells in adenolymphoma) have a high level of mitochondrial enzymic activity. Electron microscopy showed the cytoplasm to be almost completely filled with mitochondria. It would seem, therefore, that the oncocyte is not a cell showing degenerative changes, as has often been supposed because of the increasing numbers with age.

Behaviour

In most cases the tumour is benign though there may be recurrences if excision has been incomplete, but this may be delayed for years (McFarland, 1927; Buxton, Maxwell and French, 1953). Since scattered foci of oncocytes are commonly found in glands that contain an oxyphilic adenoma, it seems quite likely that these apparent recurrences may be due to the development of a new primary lesion rather than to incomplete removal of the original growth, as may some-times occur in adenolymphoma.

Malignant oxyphilic tumours have been described. Hamperl (1962) has recorded two such tumours of the nasal mucosa, Marucci, Fontana and Marcato (1962) and Bazaz-Malik and Gupta (1968) have reported malignant parotid tumours and Briggs and Evans (1967) record a locally malignant palatal tumour. It is questionable, however, whether such tumours really are the malignant counterparts of oxyphilic adenoma. Foci of oncocytes are quite commonly seen in pleomorphic adenomas. Mucoepidermoid tumours and adenocarcinomas may also contain oncocytic areas. Metastases from such tumours may be composed almost entirely of oncocytes and thus could erroneously be considered as malignant oncocytoma.

OTHER TYPES OF ADENOMA

As well as the highly distinctive adenolymphoma and oxyphilic adenoma, there occur other types of monomorphic adenoma; as these tumours are increasingly recognised, it is becoming apparent that some of them are no less distinctive in their own fashion than the two more familiar tumours already described. These other adenomas present clinically in much the same manner as do pleomorphic adenomas and such, in fact, is the usual pre-operative diagnosis. Like pleo-morphic adenoma, they occur rather more often in women than in men, but in an older age group. Most tumours occur in patients aged between 50 and 70 years. They account for rather less than 2 per cent of parotid tumours (Thackray and Lucas, 1974) but are more common than this in the minor salivary glands (Eneroth and colleagues, 1972).

Pathology

Monomorphic adenomas of these other types occur as round or ovoid, smooth-surfaced, encapsulated tumours. On section, the cut surface is whitish or pale pink and of homogeneous appearance. Small cysts are present, and rarely the tumour forms a nodule in the wall of a single large cyst. Microscopically, the striking features are the uniform nature of the cellular arrangement and the clear circumscription and encapsulation of the tumour mass (Fig. 106a). It has already been pointed out that these tumours have been reported in the literature under a confusing variety of designations which indicate either the histological configuration or the supposed cell type. The terminology used here is based on the WHO classification (Thackray and Sobin, 1972) and the AFIP Fascicle on salivary gland tumours (Thackray and Lucas, 1974), with such additions as appear necessary.

Alveolar Adenoma. In some adenomas the cells are arranged in solid masses, in which an alveolar arrangement may be discerned (Fig. 106b).

Tubular Adenoma. Tumours of this type consist of numerous and uniformly distributed small ducts, each of which has a central lumen bordered by an inner lining of ductal epithelium surrounded by one or more rows of smaller cells, usually interpreted as being myoepithelial. There is a scanty fibous stroma. These tumours are variously described in the literature as tubular, ductular or canalicular adenomas.

Trabecular Adenoma. These growths are composed of strands or trabeculae of cells of myoepithelial type. Very occasionally tubules with a lumen, or simply small groups of cells of duct lining type, may be seen. When present, the ducts are formed by a double layer of cells, those of the outer layer being the same as the cells that form the trabeculae (Fig. 106c).

Canalicular Adenoma. This designation has been used by some authors for the adenomas described here as tubular. It has also been used for a type of adenoma that occurs much more frequently in the glands of the upper lip than in any of the other salivary glands. The tumours consist of tubules or ducts lined by cuboidal or columnar cells, often lacking the outer zone of the myoepithelial cells that are seen in the tubular and trabecular adenomas. Frequently, these canalicular tumours are cystic, often very largely so. The cystic space or spaces are lined by the cubical or columnar epithelium and frequently the cells proliferate to form small solid nodules of tumour tissue projecting into the cystic space (Fig. 106d, e). Nelson and Jacoway (1973) report on a series of 29 tumours, 26 of which were situated in or near the upper lip.

Papillary Cystadenoma. This uncommon tumour of the minor salivary glands occurs as a small circumscribed mass, mainly in the palate but also in the tongue, lip, buccal sulcus and third molar region. It takes the form of a cystic space or spaces lined by finely granular eosinophilic columnar cells with well stained oval nuclei. These cells also line papillary processes that project into the cystic space. The reported cases have been summarised by Brooks and colleagues (1956), Chaudhry, Vickers and Gorlin (1961), Calhoun, Cerine and Mathews (1965) and Wilson and MacEntee (1974). The tumour appears to be benign though in two reported cases there were

---

Fig. 106   **a,** monomorphic adenoma of the palate. The tumour presented as a palatal swelling of 12 months duration in a woman of 51 years. It was diagnosed clinically as pleomorphic adenoma. This low power view shows the circumscribed nature of the tumour and its uniform structure. × 12. **b,** higher magnification from **a,** showing the arrangement of the cells in an alveolar pattern. No myxoid change was present. × 200. **c,** a monomorphic adenoma of the parotid. The cells are arranged in a trabecular pattern, and many are of myoepithelial type. × 80. **d,** cystadenoma. The lesion presented as a lump in the upper lip in a man of 62 years. It had been present for 5 years, enlarging and diminishing in size from time to time in the same manner as a mucous cyst, which was the clinical diagnosis. The low power view shows the cystic nature of the lesion with proliferation at one point. Some other similar areas were present elsewhere. × 30. **e,** higher magnification from **d.** × 300.

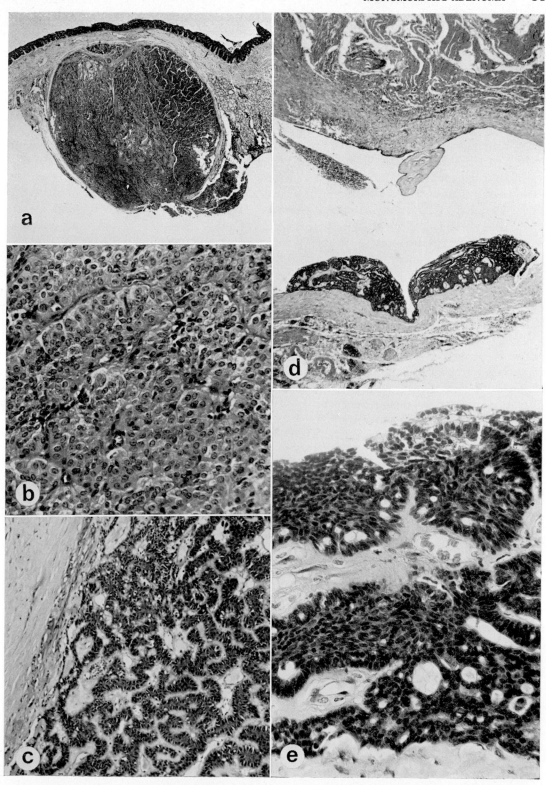

recurrences, possibly after incomplete removal. It is thought to arise from the intercalated ducts (Bauer and Bauer, 1953).

Basal Cell Adenoma. This was the first of the monomorphic adenomas (other than adeno-lymphoma and oxyphilic adenoma) to be recognised as an individual entity, by Kleinsasser and Klein (1967). Subsequently, a number of cases have been reported and it has been found that the tumour accounts for some 1·5 to 2 per cent of salivary gland neoplasms. The parotid is the usual site (Kleinsasser and Klein; Evans and Cruickshank, 1970; Batsakis, 1972). The tumour has also been reported in the lip (Bollinger and Hiatt, 1973), but there is some variation in the designations used by different authors. Some tumours reported as basal cell adenomas might be better classified as tubular or canalicular adenomas, but this is a detail of terminology where continuing experience with these lesions will doubtless lead to a concensus.

The predominating cells, which are small and darkly staining, do not resemble the myo-epithelial type of cell seen in the other adenomas. These small dark cells form solid sheets or masses, or sometimes they are arranged in branching columns or club-shaped processes resembling developing or regenerating salivary tissue. The cell masses may be bordered by a palisade layer, resulting in an appearance similar to basal cell carcinoma of the skin. In some areas the cell masses may show whorling, again reminiscent of some basal cell skin tumours (Fig. 107a).

The histochemistry of a basal cell tumour of the buccal mucosa has been fully investigated by Harrison (1974).

Clear Cell Adenoma. The dominant components of this type of adenoma are round or polygonal cells with abundant clear cytoplasm, in which glycogen can be demonstrated, if fixation is adequate. The tumour has therefore been described as glycogen-rich adenoma (Corridan, 1956; Feyrter, 1963; Goldman and Klein, 1972). The clear cells, which are arranged in rounded or cylindrical groupings surrounded by a delicate reticulin network, may make up the entire tumour, but frequently duct-like structures are also present, often in large numbers. They have a small central lumen bordered by cubical or low columnar cells, around which are the clear cells. It is generally considered that the clear cells are myoepithelial (Fig. 107b, c).

Sebaceous Adenoma and Sebaceous Lymphadenoma. The occurrence of sebaceous glands in the normal parotid, in pleomorphic adenoma and in adenolymphoma has already been noted (pp. 20, 304). These structures are also a feature of the rare sebaceous adenoma, which consists of rounded masses of sebaceous epithelium in a fibrous stroma (Albores-Saavedra and Morris, 1963; Barton, 1964; Epker and Henny, 1971). In the sebaceous lymphadenoma the sebaceous glands lie in a lymphoid stroma. In addition to the glands themselves, there may frequently be squamous cysts, and the stroma contains, as well as the lymphoid elements, fat cells, epithelioid histiocytes and occasional giant cells (Fig. 107d, e). Examples of this rare tumour have been reported by McGavran, Bauer and Ackerman (1960), Assor (1970), Wasan (1971) and Fleming and Morrice (1973). These authors cite the relevant literature.

Fig. 107   **a,** basal cell adenoma of the palate. The tumour is composed of small deeply staining cells with a bordering palisade layer. × 120. **b,** clear cell adenoma of parotid. The clear cells are the predominating element, but numerous duct-like structures are also present. × 50. **c,** higher magnification from **b.** × 120. **d,** sebaceous lymphadenoma of the parotid. Sebaceous glands and cysts lined by squamous epithelium lie in a lymphoid stroma. × 50. **e,** higher magnification from **d.** × 120.

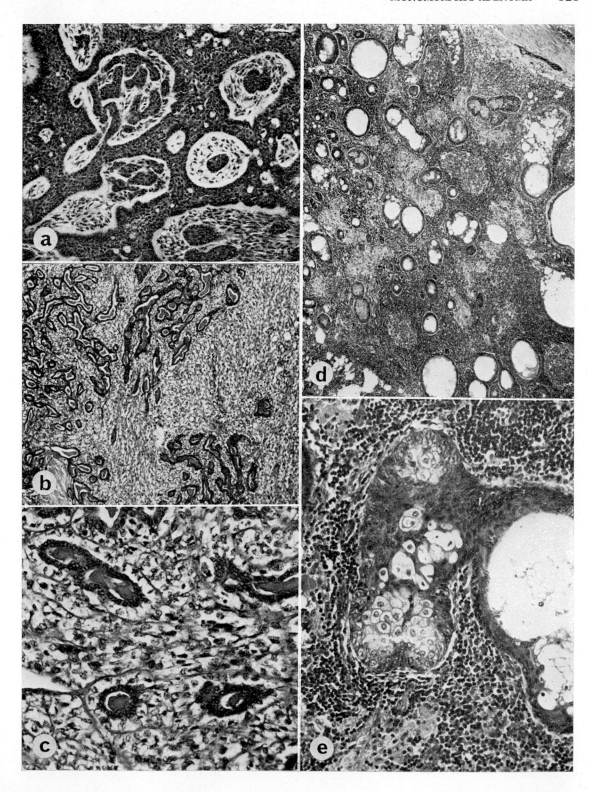

Histological Diagnosis

Although the adenomas often present characteristic histological pictures, difficulties in histological diagnosis can sometimes be encountered. The commonest problem is differentiation from pleomorphic adenoma. Small foci of any of the adenoma patterns may be seen in pleomorphic adenomas, but they do not usually cause much difficulty since the remainder of the tumour shows the obvious pleomorphic pattern. But occasionally much of a tumour may appear monomorphic and the pleomorphic areas may be overlooked; it is therefore necessary to examine all these tumours very fully before coming to a definitive diagnosis. Stromal degeneration in a monomorphic adenoma may suggest an erroneous diagnosis of pleomorphic adenoma. Although the stroma in most monomorphic adenomas is usually rather scanty, sometimes a type of mucoid change occurs which separates the epithelial elements quite widely and imparts to the stroma a basophilic homogeneous appearance that can closely resemble the myxochondroid of pleomorphic adenoma. This stromal mucoid differs from myxochondroid, however, in that it is sharply demarcated from the epithelium, whereas myxochondroid intermingles with epithelium in a rather characteristic manner, with the epithelial cells appearing to fray off and, as it were, melt into it. The only cells that are present in the mucoid stroma of monomorphic adenoma are connective tissue cells, and not epithelial.

Adenoid cystic carcinoma may be mimicked, sometimes quite closely, by monomorphic adenomas. Trabecular areas in adenoid cystic carcinoma may have a general pattern that is similar to that seen in trabecular adenomas, and the solid areas that are sometimes present can resemble basal cell adenoma. Since adenoid cystic carcinoma nearly always shows evidence of infiltrative activity and absence of encapsulation, the examination of sufficient material will enable the distinction to be made from the well-encapsulated adenomas.

Behaviour

The monomorphic adenomas are suitably treated when excised in the same way as pleomorphic adenoma. This is the usual treatment, since most monomorphic adenomas cannot be differentiated clinically from pleomorphic adenoma. The question of carcinomatous change in some of the adenomas is still open. Malignant types of sebaceous adenoma have been reported (Tsukada, de la Pava and Pickren, 1964) and also of clear cell adenoma (Goldman and Klein, 1972; Mohamed and Cherrick, 1975). The long-term behaviour of the other types of adenoma is not yet known with certainty. Undoubtedly, many of these tumours can be present for years, showing very little change, like pleomorphic adenoma, but whether a proportion of them eventually become malignant, again like pleomorphic adenoma, remains to be ascertained.

Mucoepidermoid Tumour

This tumour was first described as a distinctive entity by Stewart, Foote and Becker (1945), who reported 45 cases occurring in some 700 major and minor salivary gland tumours. Earlier accounts of individual cases had already been given, amongst others, by Masson and Berger (1924) who described the neoplasm as "épithelioma à double métaplasie" and by De and Tribedi (1939) who called it a mixed epidermoid and mucus-secreting carcinoma. The relatively recent recognition of tumours of this type as constituting a special group suggests that previously they had probably been diagnosed as squamous cell carcinomas or pleomorphic adenomas.

Stewart and his colleagues originally considered that benign and malignant varieties of the mucoepidermoid tumour could be recognised, but subsequently they felt that all tumours of this type bear malignant potentialities. A distinction, however, can be made in a very general way between tumours likely to be of a low grade of malignancy and those that will probably be of higher grade malignancy; many low grade tumours are locally invasive only and do not metastasize, and do not recur if adequately excised.

Clinical Features

Mucoepidermoid tumours occur at all ages, from childhood up to old age. The youngest patient appears to have been a one-year-old child (Hendrick, 1964). Most tumours, however, occur after middle life. Females are affected rather more frequently than males, and this appears to be so particularly with the tumours of the minor glands (Eversole, Rovin and Sabes, 1972; Melrose, Abrams and Howell, 1973).

Between 5 and 10 per cent of all tumours of the major salivary glands are of the mucoepidermoid type and nine-tenths of them occur in the parotid gland. The remainder occur in the submandibular gland. The incidence in the minor salivary glands is uncertain, various reports giving different figures. Rawson, Howard, Royster and Horn (1950) found 11 mucoepidermoid tumours (7 per cent) in their series of 160 tumours of the major and minor salivary glands. Nine of the tumours were from the parotid, the other two were from the tongue and the submandibular gland. Smith, Broadbent and Zavaleta (1954) found 7 mucoepidermoid tumours in their 32 oral mucous gland tumours, an incidence of over 20 per cent. In Chaudhry, Vickers and Gorlin's (1961) 94 tumours of the minor salivary glands there were 10 mucoepidermoid tumours (11 per cent), while in Ranger, Thackray and Lucas's (1956) cases there were 3 mucoepidermoid tumours in 80 tumours of the minor salivary and other mucous glands, just under 4 per cent.

Most mucoepidermoid tumours of the minor salivary glands occur in the palate; they also occur, less commonly, in connection with the other intraoral glands such as those of tongue, floor of mouth, gingiva, lip or cheek. Very occasionally, tumours occur as intraosseous growths, within the mandible or maxilla. Smith, Dahlin and Waite (1968) and Browand and Waldron (1975) review the literature. Some 50 cases have now been reported; they have occurred more often in females than in males, and twice as often in the mandible as in the maxilla. Most of the tumours were situated in the molar-premolar area. Radiologically, there was usually a multilocular radiolucency, similar to that produced by ameloblastoma.

Well-differentiated tumours present clinically in a similar manner to pleomorphic adenomas with, generally, a quite long history of a gradually enlarging painless mass. Occasionally, intraoral tumours may be fluctuant, from cyst formation, and palatal growths may be diagnosed as dental abscess. Tumours that are of a higher grade of malignancy grow rapidly and are often accompanied by pain and ulceration.

Pathology

Many mucoepidermoid tumours are similar in naked-eye appearance to pleomorphic adenomas. They may be partially encapsulated but sometimes there is no evidence of any capsule and the tumour is ill-defined and infiltrates adjacent tissues. Some tumours are solid but cyst formation is a common occurrence. The cysts contain clear mucus; sometimes it is thick and ropy and occasionally there has been haemorrhage. Tumours showing prominent cyst formation are less likely to be highly invasive and rapidly growing than the more solid growths. The intercystic tissue is greyish or yellowish white.

Microscopically, mucoepidermoid tumours are composed of mucus-secreting cells, cells of epidermoid type and an intermediate variety of cell, in varying proportions (Figs. 108 and 109). In tumours that are likely to be of a relatively low grade of malignancy mucus-secreting cells and epidermoid cells are most prominent. The mucous cells often line the cysts that are frequently present, either wholly or in part, and in single or multiple layers. These cells, with their large intracellular collections of mucin, are often quite obvious, but staining by mucicarmine frequently demonstrates small droplets of mucin not otherwise seen. Discharge of mucus into the cysts

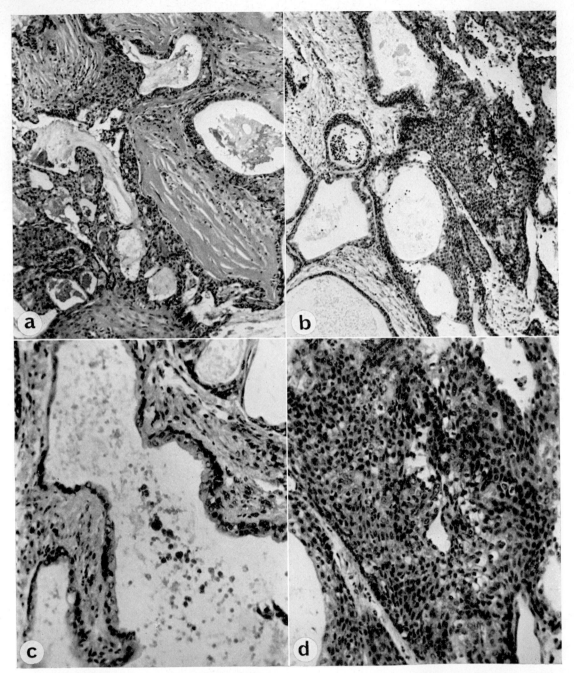

Fig. 108   Fields from a mucoepidermoid tumour of the parotid. **a,** masses of mucus-secreting cells in a fibrous stroma. Small irregular cystic spaces are present. × 80. **b,** larger cysts, lined mainly by mucus-secreting cells but also by epidermoid cells. × 80. **c,** the mucus-secreting cells are well seen in this higher power view. × 200. **d,** a sheet of epidermoid cells. × 200.

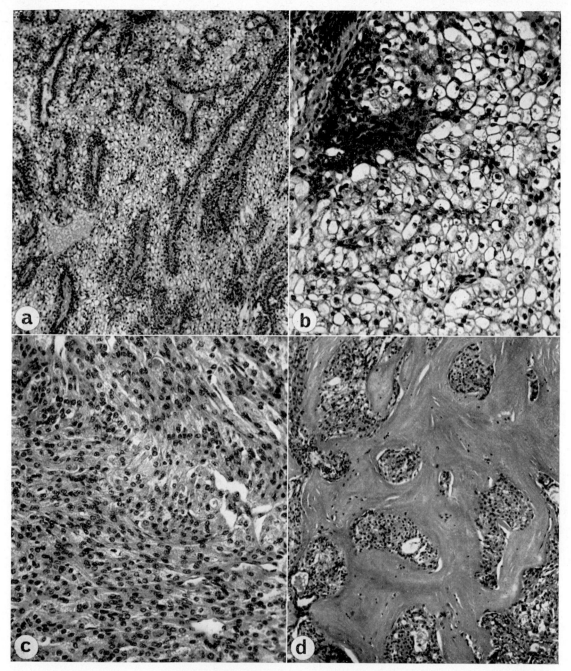

Fig. 109 **a, b,** a tumour of the mandibular gingiva in the retro-molar region. The tumour consists almost entirely of cells with abundant clear cytoplasm, though squamous areas and duct-like structures were also present. × 80 and × 200. **c,** an area of spindle cell growth in a palatal tumour. × 200. **d,** hyalinisation of the stroma in a palatal tumour. × 80.

leads to their distension and coalescence. Rupture of cysts is not uncommon, with escape of mucus into the stroma and consequent reactive changes. It is to be noted, however, that the myxoid stromal or intercellular changes so characteristic of the pleomorphic adenoma are never seen, though hyalinisation may occur. Epidermoid cells may also partially line the cysts, or form solid clumps. These cells are of squamous epithelial type, and may show evidence of keratinisation. The cells which Stewart, Foote and Becker have described as intermediate cells are smaller than either the epidermoid or the mucous cells and they often line cystic or duct-like spaces in a stratified arrangement. Cells with abundant clear cytoplasm are a prominent feature in some tumours. These clear cells do not stain with mucicarmine or fat stains. Areas of spindle cell growth may sometimes be present and, rarely, sebaceous cells may occur. Small foci of oncocytic cells may be seen occasionally. Much less commonly they may make up large areas.

Bhaskar and Bernier (1962) have described a histological variant in which the arrangement of cuboidal cells around large and small pools of homogeneous eosinophilic material produces an appearance resembling thyroid vesicles. In some of their cases, the similarity was so great that a mistaken diagnosis of metastatic thyroid carcinoma was made.

In tumours of a higher grade of malignancy there is cellular pleomorphism and nuclear hyperchromatism, and intermediate and epidermoid cells are more frequently seen than mucus-secreting cells. Mitoses, however, are not frequent. As already mentioned, infiltration at the edge of the tumour can be readily detected and lymphatic permeation is not infrequently seen. Metastatic deposits in regional lymph nodes and in viscera generally produce a picture similar to that of the primary growth, though sometimes mucous cells may be entirely absent. When this is the case, and the first specimen to be examined pathologically is the metastatic deposit, the histological diagnosis may well be squamous cell carcinoma.

The histochemistry of mucoepidermoid tumours has been investigated by Azzopardi and Smith (1959). They find that the mucus in the mucous cells and in the duct-like spaces is strongly PAS positive and shows moderate gamma-metachromasia, unaltered by hyaluronidase treatment. There is a variable amount of glycogen in the epidermoid cells, particularly in the hydropic cells which are often seen in low grade tumours.

Histogenesis

Mucoepidermoid tumours are considered to arise from the salivary ducts (Stewart, Foote and Becker, 1945). It is probable that they originate proximal to the lobules, since the eosinophilic cells that line the ducts distal to this are not found in the tumours (Foote and Frazell, 1954).

The histogenesis of the intraoral tumours has been discussed by a number of authors (Bhaskar, 1963; Brown and Lucchesi, 1966; Silverglade, Alvares and Olech, 1968; Smith, Dahlin and Waite, 1968). As has been noted previously (p. 299), salivary tissues may lie in an indentation of the mandible and it is possible that a tumour arising here may in time, with expansion and resorption of the adjacent bone, appear to be an intraosseous growth. However, for the genuine intraosseous tumour, with intact cortical plates, it is necessary to postulate intraosseous epithelium as the origin. Bhaskar (1963) suggested that this might be oral epithelium trapped within the developing mandible. The posterior position of the tumours also suggests that entrapped retromolar glands might sometimes be responsible. It is also possible that many tumours arise from odontogenic cysts. Mucous metaplasia is not uncommon in odontogenic cysts of various types, and it seems not unreasonable to assume that neoplasia can also occur on occasion. It is noteworthy that most of the intraosseous salivary tumours so far reported have been of the mucoepidermoid type. Other varieties are very rare. Recent reports include those of Alexander and colleagues (1974) and Marano and Hartman (1974).

Behaviour

In Foote and Frazell's series the local recurrence rate in 28 patients with low grade tumours was 15 per cent after 5 years, but in the patients with high grade tumours regional lymph node metastases were present in two-thirds after 5 years. Distant metastases, in bone, lung, brain and subcutaneous tissue, were present in about one-third. The five-year survival rate was just over 25 per cent. On the other hand, the figures from Bhaskar and Bernier's (1962) analysis of 144 cases of mucoepidermoid tumour indicate that many growths will not recur after adequate treatment. The five-year cure rate was 88 per cent, for all grades of tumour. In general, these authors found that the tumours usually described as low grade type—with mucus-containing cysts, epidermal cells and clear cells—did not recur or metastasize after wide excision. Tumours with much escape of mucin into the stroma, however, did tend to recur, but this was attributed more to the mechanical difficulties of complete removal than to inherent malignancy. Malignant tumours showed quite clear histological evidence of their sinister behaviour. In these tumours cyst formation is absent or inconspicuous, while the epidermal component approaches squamous cell carcinoma in appearance. Jakobsson, Blanck and Eneroth (1968) suggest that the distinction between high grade and low grade tumours is best made on evidence of invasive growth only, leaving aside other points of histology. They found a better prognosis for those tumours lacking evidence of invasive growth, although such tumours could on occasion also be fatal. In another recent report, however, it was thought that well differentiated, moderately differentiated and poorly differentiated tumours could be recognised and that these gradings of differentiation correlated with prognosis (Healey, Perzin and Smith, 1970).

It is apparent, therefore, that there is appreciable difference of opinion about the behaviour and prognosis of mucoepidermoid tumours. The foregoing remarks indicate the views of a few authors. Koblin and Koch (1974) cite many more, showing the variety of views held on this matter. The problem is discussed by Thackray and Lucas (1974), who point out that much of the variation in the published figures for prognosis is likely to be due to differences in diagnostic criteria. Since these criteria have become more precise and generally known, it is possible that the more recent reports give a reasonably accurate account of the occurrence and behaviour of the tumour. They conclude that the general consensus of opinion is that the majority of muco-epidermoid tumours neither metastasize nor recur if adequately treated. While a distinction between tumours that are likely to pursue a relatively benign course and those that are likely to grow more rapidly can be attempted on histological grounds, it has to be recognised that any mucoepidermoid tumour may metastasize, whatever its histological structure.

Acinic Cell Tumour

The acinic cell tumour is composed of cells resembling the serous cells of salivary glands. It was originally regarded as an adenoma but it was later recognised that despite the slow rate of growth this tumour could recur and might metastasize (Godwin and Colvin, 1948; Buxton and colleagues, 1953; and others).

The tumour occurs chiefly in the middle-aged and elderly, though it may be encountered at any age. It occurs two to three times more frequently in women than in men. In most cases the parotid gland is the site of growth, but the tumour also occurs, very uncommonly, in the sub-mandibular and sublingual glands (Fox, Remine and Woolner, 1963; Kauffman and Stout, 1963; Gorlin and Chaudhry, 1957) and in the minor salivary glands (Chaudhry, Vickers and Gorlin, 1961; Baden and Wallen, 1965; Wertheimer and Georgen, 1971). A tumour originating in a cervical lymph node has been reported by Bhaskar (1964). Bilateral parotid tumours have been reported (Eneroth, Hamberger and Jakobsson, 1966; Clarke, Hentz and Mahoney, 1969).

Y

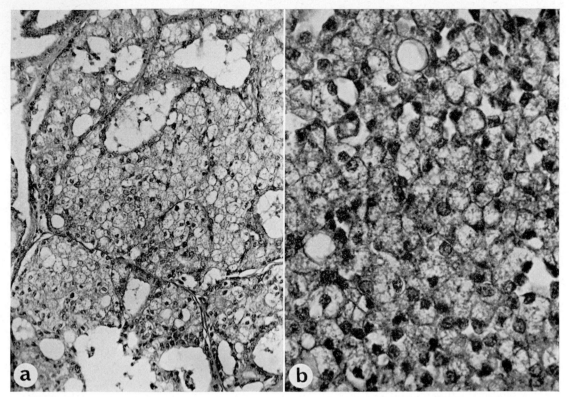

Fig. 110   Acinic cell tumour of the parotid. **a,** the tumour consists of sheets of cells showing evidence in some areas of ill-defined acinus formation. × 200. **b,** the cells are rounded or polygonal with granular cytoplasm and eccentrically placed nuclei. × 500.

In most cases the tumour presents in much the same way as does pleomorphic adenoma, as a slowly growing painless swelling, though cases have been reported in which pain and rapid growth have been features. Involvement of the facial nerve has also occurred. The tumour is usually encapsulated, although Angell and colleagues (1967) have found microscopic infiltration of the capsule to be common, and sometimes small foci of tumour may be found outside the capsule. These findings probably explain why recurrent tumours tend to be multinodular. The cut surface shows a homogeneous greyish-white appearance and areas of necrosis and cystic change are occasionally noted.

Microscopically, the principal cell type is the acinic cell, a relatively large rounded or polyhedral cell with basophilic cytoplasm, resembling the cells of normal serous acini. The cytoplasm is generally finely granular but the granules may be coarse enough to appear very similar to normal zymogen granules. Occasionally, the cytoplasm may be vacuolated or even completely clear. The eccentrically situated nucleus is small and stains darkly. Nucleoli are only occasionally obvious. Mitoses are rare. In the majority of cases the tumour grows as a solid mass of cells, though not infrequently the cells may be arranged in groups resembling salivary gland acini. However, no ducts or duct-like structures are seen though large vacuolated spaces may occur, into which papillary processes may protrude (Fig. 110). Presumably these spaces are due to the accumulation of secretion which cannot escape, because of the absence of a duct system. Abrams and colleagues (1965) have noted that in some cases some, or even the majority, of the tumour cells resemble those of salivary intercalated ducts. Such cells are cuboidal or low columnar, with eosinophilic cytoplasm and round, centrally placed nuclei with small distinct nucleoli. Transitions occur between these cells and the acinic type cells. These authors also noted, from their study of a series of 77 cases, that as well as the solid and papillary cystic types of growth a follicular pattern, resembling thyroid follicles, could occur. Here, the growth consisted of cuboidal or low columnar cells bordering follicular spaces containing homogeneous material. In two such cases the original diagnosis had been metastatic thyroid carcinoma.

The stroma in acinic cell tumour is generally very scanty but may be more abundant in some cases, with occasional hyalinisation of the collagenous connective tissue. Calcification, in the form of small round darkly staining calcospherites, may be present both in the stroma and in the epithelium. Lymphoid tissue may also be present, often abundantly (Eneroth, Jakobsson and Blanck, 1966). A patient with Sjögren's syndrome and a tumour of the parotid has also been reported (Delaney and Balogh, 1966).

Azzopardi and Smith (1959) have found that the histochemical reactions of the tumour cells are the same as those of normal parotid cells and Echevarria (1967), Kleinsasser and colleagues (1967) and Kay and Schatzki (1972) have shown that the fine structure of tumour and of normal serous cells is also similar. These findings, together with the absence of ductal elements and the formation of acinus-like structures, suggest that the tumour arises from serous cells.

On the other hand, Bhaskar (1964) and Abrams and colleagues (1965) favour ductal cells as the cells of origin. In normal development acinar cells originate from the ductal system and, in a variety of salivary gland lesions, the ductal cells give rise to replacement epithelium when regeneration takes place.

There is very often a long history of many years of slow growth in acinic cell tumour, but unless wide surgical excision is carried out local recurrence may be expected (Beahrs and colleagues, 1960; Grage, Lober and Arbelger, 1961). Metastases to regional lymph nodes and to distant sites may occur.

Adenoid Cystic Carcinoma

The tumour now generally known as *adenoid cystic carcinoma* appears to have been characterised first by Billroth (1859), who named it *cylindroma*. In Billroth's case the tumour was situated in the orbit, having probably arisen from mucous glands in a nasal sinus or possibly from the lacrimal gland. He used the name cylindroma because the epithelial and the connective tissue elements formed a system of intertwining cylinders. Malassez (1883) mentioned some earlier cases that appeared to fall into the same group. The term *basalioma* was used by Krompecher (1908), who considered this type of tumour to be of analogous nature to the basal cell growths of the skin. Ahlbom (1935) and Ringertz (1938) also used the term basalioma. The term most frequently used in the English language literature is *adenoid cystic carcinoma*, apparently introduced by Ewing (Foote and Frazell, 1954) and since generally adopted. Spies (1930), in reporting a series of cases under this name, emphasised that the neoplasm so designated should not be confused with the adenoid cystic epithelioma of Brooks and Fordyce, and that it was different from adenocarcinoma. Adenocarcinoma of cylindroma type has also been used as a designation (New and Childrey, 1931; Watson, 1935; Dockerty and Mayo, 1942, 1943; Quattlebaum, Dockerty and Mayo, 1946).

Tumours of the adenoid cystic carcinoma type were at first regarded simply as variants of the "benign salivary gland tumour," as it was then often called, and they were not considered to be essentially different from the majority of such tumours. Nevertheless, even some of the earliest reports had shown that these tumours were very prone to recur after removal (as in Billroth's case) and could even metastasize (Ribbert, 1907). Thus, tumours which behaved in a malignant manner were often reported as malignant mixed tumours rather than the adenoid cystic carcinomas that many of them undoubtedly were. Montanus (1938) and Mulligan (1943) review the earlier reports of metastasizing tumours of the salivary glands, many of which were certainly adenoid cystic carcinomas.

Clinical Features

Adenoid cystic carcinomas may occur at any age, though in most cases the patients are middle-aged or over. Rather more females than males are affected. Adenoid cystic carcinomas comprise some 5 per cent of all salivary tumours of the major glands and up to 25 per cent of tumours of the minor glands. In the major glands the parotid is most often affected, though nearly as many tumours occur in the submandibular gland. In the minor glands most of the tumours occur in the palate, with the tongue and floor of the mouth as the next most frequent sites. Occasional sites are the lip and peritonsillar region.

Adenoid cystic carcinomas grow slowly and the history is often similar to that in pleomorphic adenoma, the growth having been present for years in some cases. Ulceration of the mucosa in the case of intraoral tumours sometimes occurs, however, whereas this feature is very uncommon in pleomorphic adenoma. Pain is much commoner than in pleomorphic adenoma and there may be neurological symptoms from infiltration of nerves. Bone is frequently involved, but since the tumour tends to spread through the marrow spaces without at first destroying the trabecular pattern, there may be extensive involvement of bone in the absence of any radiological evidence.

Pathology

Adenoid cystic carcinomas usually resemble pleomorphic adenomas in their gross characteristics, except that infiltration of adjacent tissues is often an obvious feature. If there is any encapsulation, it is incomplete. On section, the cut surface is firm and greyish-white. Cyst formation and haemorrhage are very uncommon and the mucoid or almost gelatinous areas so commonly present in pleomorphic adenoma are not seen.

Microscopically, many adenoid cystic carcinomas show a readily recognisable pattern, consisting of rounded, ovoid or irregularly shaped masses of cells in a rather scanty connective tissue stroma. Numerous cystic or alveolar spaces are present in the cell masses, giving rise to the cribriform effect which is a very characteristic feature of this tumour (Fig. 111a). However, the cystic spaces are sometimes absent, the growth then being of solid type. As in pleomorphic adenoma, cells resembling myoepithelial cells and smaller cells, like those that line normal salivary ducts, are present. Ultrastructure studies confirm that these two types of cell occur in the tumour (Hoshino and Yamamoto, 1970). Sometimes the two cell types show an arrangement very similar to that which occurs in normal ducts, with the smaller cells forming an inner row around a lumen and the larger myoepithelial type of cells forming an outer row. The lumen frequently contains eosinophilic granular material, giving a strongly positive reaction with the PAS technique (Fig. 111b). In most tumours, however, ducts formed of two such regularly disposed rows of cells are not often seen, for one or other cell type usually preponderates, and quite complicated patterns may be produced (Fig. 111c, d, e).

Fig. 111 Varying patterns in adenoid cystic carcinoma. **a,** adenoid cystic carcinoma of the palate, showing the characteristic cribriform pattern. × 80. **b,** a duct-like structure lined by an outer row of cells of myoepithelial type and an inner row of smaller cells. × 500. **c,** adenoid cystic carcinoma of the parotid, in which the tumour tissue forms continuous interlacing strands enclosing cystic spaces, giving rise to a lace-like appearance. × 80. **d** and **e,** in some growths the tumour cells form small groups or elongated strands rather than larger cribriform patterns. × 80.

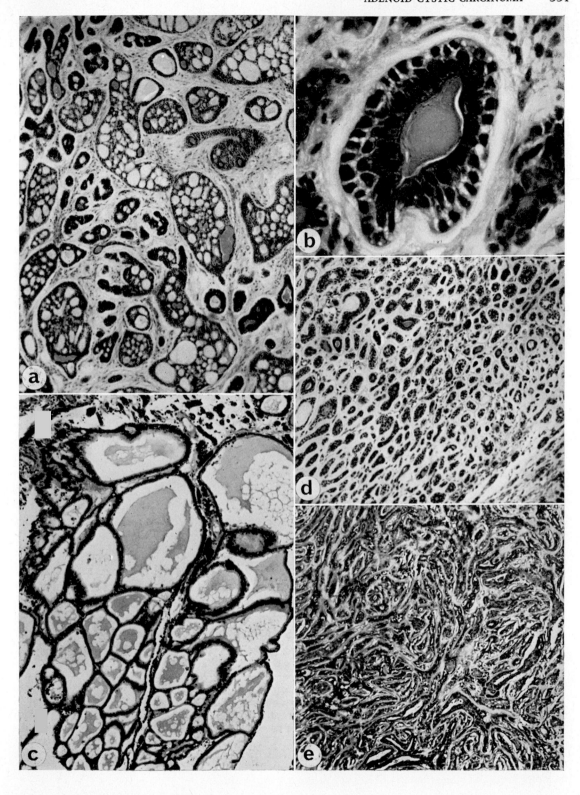

The cyst-like spaces may result from the enclavement of areas of stroma or of mucoid material which is produced by the tumour cells in proximity to the stroma. When such areas, because of the plane of section, appear to be entirely enclosed by epithelium the resemblance to an epithelial cyst is close. However, serial sections show that this appearance is due to the particular manner in which stroma and epithelium are juxtaposed.

These variations in histological pattern, with the differing modes of cyst formation, account for the apparent discrepancies in the staining reactions of the mucoid material in the cystic spaces which have been noted by a number of workers, both in adenoid cystic carcinomas of the salivary glands and in similar tumours of other mucous glands (Lemaitre, 1938; Kramer and Som, 1939; McDonald, Moersch and Tinney, 1945; Belsey and Valentine, 1951). However, Azzopardi and Smith (1959) and Thackray and Lucas (1960) have shown on histochemical and on histological grounds that the discrepancies are due not to variability in the properties of the mucin but to the fact that different mucins are present. Thus, the mucinous material in the duct-like structures that are lined by the cells which resemble those of the inner row of normal salivary ducts is eosinophilic and strongly PAS positive but is not metachromatic. On the other hand, the material in cysts lined entirely by myoepithelial type cells is weakly haematoxyphilic and only weakly PAS positive. It is strongly gamma-metachromatic and there is marked reduction of the metachromasia after incubation with hyaluronidase. The hyaline material which appears to be formed in the stroma is PAS positive to a moderate degree and is gamma-metachromatic, though less so than the material just mentioned. Methylene blue extinction confirms these differences.

Solid types of growth in adenoid cystic carcinoma are much less common than the cribriform pattern and usually a part only of the tumour shows such an appearance, most of it being of the more usual architecture. Occasionally, however, an almost completely solid type of growth is encountered, when the diagnosis may be difficult. Thorough examination, however, will generally reveal the presence of small areas exhibiting more characteristic traits. Compression of ductular structures may lead to a practically solid type of growth, but more often the appearances are due to the tumour cells forming continuous sheets or masses. Areas of necrosis tend to occur in solid growths (Fig. 112a). Mitotic figures are seldom seen in either solid or cystic tumours. Two unusual variants of the solid type of growth have been noted by Thackray and Lucas. In one, the cells were predominantly fusiform or spindle-shaped, often with a palisade arrangement of the nuclei (Fig. 112b). Parts of the growth thus had some resemblance to neurinoma. In the other variant most of the tumour was composed of acini of round or ovoid cells, myoepithelial cells being present in a few areas only at the edge of the tumour (Fig. 112c).

Stromal changes are often very prominent in adenoid cystic carcinoma. A rather scanty fibrous stroma is the commonest finding, but often the stroma is more abundant and frequently hyalin is present. The hyalin is either changed connective tissue of the stroma itself or it is a product of the tumour cells laid down in proximity to the stroma. Hyalinisation is often associated with a breaking-up of the cribriform pattern to form smaller cell groups. The deposition of mucinous material in proximity to the stroma, or the replacement of the stroma itself by mucoid,

Fig. 112   Further variations in pattern in adenoid cystic carcinoma. **a,** areas of solid growth may occur in discrete masses, showing, as in this palatal tumour, central necrosis. × 80. **b,** spindle cell growth with palisading of the nuclei may be seen, in small areas of some tumours or forming much of others. Parotid tumour. × 200. **c,** a parotid tumour, composed mainly of "lumenal" cells. × 200. **d,** a tumour of the floor of the mouth showing prominent mucoid change. Areas of this type closely resemble similar areas in pleomorphic adenomas. Cf. Fig. 100**b.** × 200. **e,** perineural infiltration is commonly seen in adenoid cystic carcinoma. From another tumour of the floor of the mouth. × 80.

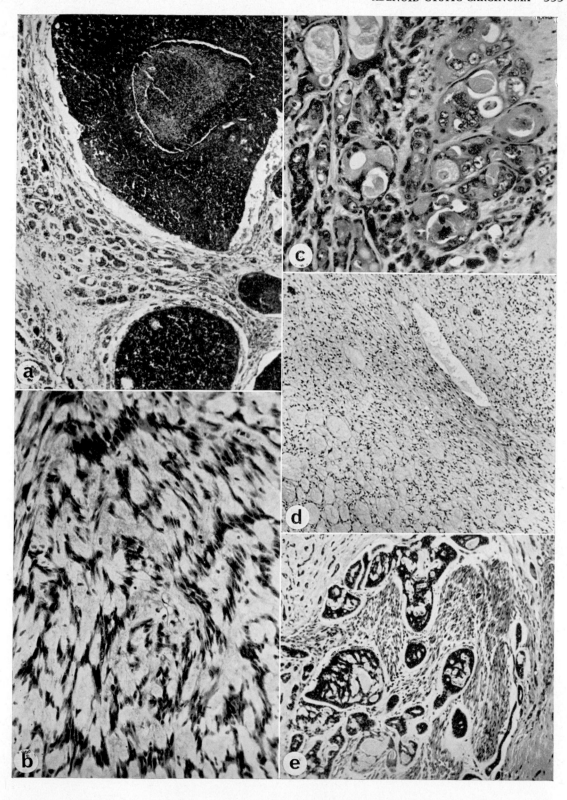

is also not uncommon. However, this change is generally strictly confined to the intercellular area, with a clear demarcation between the mucoid material and the cellular elements of the tumour. Only occasionally do the cells appear to "melt" into the mucoid intercellular material in the manner that is so frequently, and typically, seen in pleomorphic adenoma (Fig. 112d).

In most cases there is no difficulty in distinguishing between typical examples of adenoid cystic carcinoma and of pleomorphic adenoma. Occasionally, however, tumours are encountered in which the distinction is not so readily made. One source of possible difficulty is the mucoid change which is so typical a feature of the pleomorphic adenoma but may sometimes also occur in the adenoid cystic carcinoma. Here, however, the distinguishing feature, as already pointed out, is the clear demarcation of epithelial cells from mucoid intercellular material in adenoid cystic carcinoma, whereas in pleomorphic adenoma the cells often appear to blend with the mucin.

Generally, adenoid cystic carcinoma runs a fairly typical course, the histological picture remaining the same throughout. When metastases occur, they resemble the primary growth. In some cases, however, local recurrences or metastases may show quite a different picture, presenting as undifferentiated carcinoma from the histological point of view, and clinically assuming a more frankly carcinomatous course.

Histogenesis

Little is known about the exact mode of origin of adenoid cystic carcinoma. Krompecher (1908) thought that the tumour was a basal cell growth akin to basal cell carcinoma of the skin and others have also thought it to be of basal cell origin, arising from these cells in mucous membranes (Beck and Guttman, 1936). McDonald, Moersch and Tinney (1945) have seen tumour arising directly from mucous glands in the bronchial wall and Reid (1952) has seen the duct of a bronchial gland giving origin to tumour. Russell (1955) also favours mucous gland ducts as the site of origin and there is some histochemcial support for this view, Bruce and Wertheimer (1967) having shown that the enzyme activity pattern of the tumour resembles that of the ducts of normal salivary glands rather than the acini. Electron microscope investigations indicate that myoepithelial cells probably take part in the tumour formation (Eneroth and colleagues, 1968; Kleinsasser and colleagues, 1969).

Behaviour

Although an infiltrative and invasive tumour, the rate of growth of adenoid cystic carcinoma is slow and metastases do not usually develop until late in the disease. The prognosis for most patients is better, therefore, than it is in adenocarcinoma or squamous cell carcinoma. Recurrence after surgical excision has been relatively frequent in the cases reported in the literature (Quattlebaum, Dockerty and Mayo, 1946; Foote and Frazell, 1954; Ranger, Thackray and Lucas, 1956; Harrison, 1956; Moran and colleagues, 1961); this has probably been due, as in the case of pleomorphic adenoma, to inadequate appreciation of the ineffectiveness of local excision. Infiltration of adjacent tissues, including bone, is very characteristic of these growths and this is nearly always more extensive than appears to be the case on macroscopic inspection at operation. Thus, in the past, surgical procedures have probably been too conservative. Recurrent growths are always much more difficult to deal with than primary ones, and the prognosis is correspondingly worse. Blanck and colleagues (1967) have reported 5-year survival rates of about 70 per cent, but the 20-year rate drops to 13 per cent.

Perineural infiltration is not infrequently seen (Fig. 112e). Secondary deposits occur in the regional lymph nodes in about one-third of the cases and they are also found in distant sites, particularly bone, lung and liver. These metastases generally occur late in the disease, after there have been one or more local recurrences. Inadequate initial treatment probably predisposes to metastasis; Smith, Lane and Rankow (1965) have shown that the incidence of distant metastases is double where there has been treatment by inadequate surgery alone compared with treatment by radiotherapy alone. Radiotherapy, however, does not result in a permanent cure. Most tumours treated in this way have been recorded as ultimately recurring, but radiotherapy may offer a worthwhile degree of palliation for recurrent tumours and inoperable cases (Leafstedt, 1971; Eby, Johnson and Baker, 1972).

Chemotherapy may prove to be helpful. Potdar and Paymaster (1969) have found cyclophosphamide to show promise in controlling both primary and secondary growths, with relief of symptoms.

Adenocarcinoma, Squamous Cell Carcinoma and Undifferentiated Carcinoma

A small proportion of salivary gland tumours are carcinomas of the above types. Unlike most of the other salivary tumours, these carcinomas occur more often in men than in women; the average age of patients is 60 years.

Malignant tumours usually grow more rapidly than pleomorphic adenoma or the other benign tumours; there is therefore a shorter history and there is more likely to be complaint of pain. However, not infrequently there is little difference in presentation from pleomorphic adenoma and in a number of cases this is the preoperative diagnosis.

Adenocarcinomas consist of neoplastic ducts or tubules, often with areas of necrosis. Mucus production occurs in some tumours with, sometimes, the formation of large cystic spaces. Strands of cells may project into these spaces, giving a papillary appearance. Blanck, Eneroth and Jakobsson (1971) describe tumours of this type as mucus-producing adenopapillary carcinoma. Papillary growths of low grade malignancy occurring in the palate have been reported by Allen, Fitz-Hugh and Marsh (1974).

Squamous cell carcinomas resemble those seen elsewhere. They probably arise from metaplastic duct epithelium. Mucoepidermoid tumours in which the mucus-producing element is much less than the epidermoid may be confused with these carcinomas; it is desirable to make a distinction because the former are likely to behave less aggressively.

A number of carcinomas are undifferentiated; they show no evidence of tubule formation or of squamous appearance. These tumours are of spindle cell or spheroidal cell type, and show the usual cellular changes of malignancy—mitoses, hyperchromatism, pleomorphism and the like (Fig. 113).

All these tumours infiltrate locally and metastasize to regional nodes and to viscera. Squamous cell carcinomas are the most rapidly progressive, followed by undifferentiated growths.

MESENCHYMAL AND OTHER TUMOURS

Mesenchymal tumours occurring in the salivary glands are rare.

Haemangioma

This is a developmental lesion that is practically always detected in infants although, very rarely, it may be seen in older patients (Karabin, 1951; Bowerman and Rowe, 1970), and it is the commonest salivary gland tumour of infancy (Lane and Schwartz, 1958; Kauffman and Stout, 1963; Karlan and Snyder, 1968).

The lesion, which is commoner in females than males, generally occurs in the parotid gland though occasionally the submandibular may be affected. There is a swelling like that presented by a pleomorphic adenoma, but it may characteristically enlarge when the infant cries or strains and it may be pulsatile. In cavernous tumours thrombosis, with eventual calcification of the thrombus, may occur, leading to a radiological suspicion of calculi in the duct system.

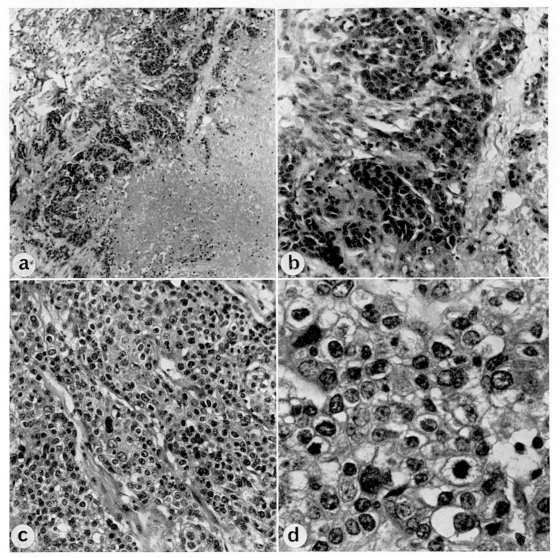

Fig. 113 **a,** carcinoma of the parotid, with the formation of cords of cells and areas of necrosis. × 80. **b,** detail from **a.** × 200. **c,** undifferentiated carcinoma of the parotid which metastasised to the regional lymph nodes. × 200. **d,** higher power view of another field from the same tumour. × 500.

Pathologically, the lesion presents usually as a capillary but occasionally as a cavernous haemangioma, with no unusual microscopic features. Its behaviour, however, may be very different from that of haemangioma elsewhere, for though the lesion generally grows slowly to begin with, it may at any time begin to enlarge more rapidly. This is associated with invasion of adjacent tissues and death may result from invasion or compression of vital structures. Excision is curative but it must remove the entire growth, otherwise there will be recurrences.

Malignant Melanoma

Malignant melanoma occurs, rarely, in the parotid gland. Primary tumours infiltrate the gland diffusely whereas secondary tumours occur either in the intraparotid lymph nodes or in the gland substance itself as circumscribed deposits. Greene and Bernier (1961) describe 5 cases of primary malignant melanoma of the parotid and discuss the difficulty in deciding whether the tumour is primary or secondary. They were able to demonstrate the presence of dopa-positive cells in the ducts and acini of normal human parotid glands, thus establishing a theoretical basis for the origin of primary tumours. It is also of interest to note that MacLennan and Shivas (1963) found marked pigmentation and nuclear hyperchromatism in the ducts and acini of the nearby mucous glands in a case of malignant melanoma of the oral mucosa.

Other Primary Tumours

Fibroma, fibrosarcoma, lipoma, neurilemmoma and lymphomas have been described, but are rare.

Metastatic Tumours

The salivary glands may be involved not only by the direct extension of neighbouring tumours but they may also be the site of haematogenous and lymphatic metastases. The primary tumour is usually situated in the head and neck region and it is usually a squamous cell carcinoma or a malignant melanoma. It is thus readily detected, but there do occur instances of metastic involvement of the salivary glands in which the primary tumour is not obvious and in which the metastasis is the first indication of disease, and may be diagnosed as a primary tumour of salivary gland. For example, adenocarcinoma of the stomach has metastasised to the parotid, to be initially diagnosed as a primary parotid carcinoma and metastic carcinoma of the kidney has appeared at first to be a clear-cell salivary tumour (Thackray and Lucas, 1974).

Most metastatic deposits occur in the parotid gland; the others are very rarely affected. Solomon, Rosen and Gardner (1975) report a case of metastatic breast carcinoma in the submandibular gland and give the literature of metastatic tumours in the salivary glands.

Fatty Infiltration of the Parotid Gland

Tumour-like enlargement of the parotid gland may be caused by the accumulation of fat. Apart from the separation of the parenchymal elements by fat cells there are no other changes. The condition appears to be harmless; it is likely to be diagnosed as salivary tumour. Descriptions are given by Gilman, Schwartz and Gilman (1956), Turner (1958) and Godwin and Dew (1958).

Benign Lymphoepithelial Lesion and Sjögren's Syndrome

The lesion of salivary glands now generally designated as benign lymphoepithelial lesion (Godwin, 1952) was first described by Mikulicz in 1888. Mikulicz considered the condition, characterised by bilateral enlargement of the lacrimal, parotid and submandibular glands, to be a chronic infection. Microscopically, there was replacement of the glandular tissue by small round cells, though normal acini could still be seen. Following Mikulicz's report many other cases were published, but though these cases resembled each other clinically it soon became apparent that the pathology underlying bilateral chronic enlargement of salivary glands could be very varied. Thus leukaemia, lymphosarcoma, syphilis, tuberculosis, gout and other conditions were found to be possible causes of salivary gland enlargement of the Mikulicz type. It seemed, therefore, appropriate to refer to Mikulicz's syndrome (Napp, 1907; Thursfield, 1913; Schaffer and Jacobsen, 1927). In addition to these known causes, however, there still remained the cases of unknown etiology that could be appropriately referred to as Mikulicz's disease and this was the designation used up to recent years. It became apparent, however, that the salivary gland enlargement might only be part of a widespread disorder of connective tissues, though all the manifestations of the condition were not in evidence in every case.

In 1933 Sjögren described a syndrome characterised by chronic inflammatory changes and hyposecretion of the lacrimal and salivary glands, resulting in conjunctivitis (keratoconjunctivitis sicca), rhinopharyngolaryngitis and xerostomia, and in which the lacrimal and the parotid, less frequently the submandibular, glands were enlarged. The histopathological changes in the salivary glands were subsequently found to be practically identical to those in Mikulicz's disease. In over half the patients with the condition there is evidence of a connective tissue disorder, usually rheumatoid arthritis, but polymyositis, scleroderma, systemic lupus erythematosus or polyarteritis nodosa may occur, though less frequently. The similarity between the changes in the salivary glands in this syndrome and those in the thyroid gland in Hashimoto's disease were noted by Morgan and Castlemen (1953). They were unable to find any cases in which thyroid and salivary gland disease coexisted, but it is now clear that a similarity does exist in that both conditions are believed to have a basis of disordered immunity mechanisms.

Clinical Features

As just mentioned, not all the possible manifestations of lymphoepithelial disorder are found in every case. If an isolated salivary gland lesion is the only manifestation, with no other symptoms, the term *benign lymphoepithelial lesion* is used. If there are ocular and salivary symptoms but no evidence of rheumatoid arthritis or other connective tissue disease, the condition is termed *sicca syndrome* or *sicca complex*, but if the triad of xerostomia, keratoconjunctivitis sicca and rheumatoid arthritis or other connective tissue disease is present, the diagnosis of *Sjögren's syndrome* is made. At present, it is not certain whether those patients who have salivary gland enlargement only are suffering from an early stage of Sjögren's syndrome. In some cases that have been followed for a long period the lymphoepithelial lesion in salivary gland has remained the only manifestation of disease. It is thus possible that lymphoepithelial lesion and Sjögren's syndrome are different diseases, although the salivary gland histopathology is apparently identical. Women are more often affected than men and middle age is the time of predilection, although children and adolescents have been affected.

When symptoms are present, xerostomia is the commonest presenting complaint. Salivary gland enlargement occurs in some 30 to 50 per cent of patients (Rauch, 1959; Bloch and colleagues, 1965). The parotids are the glands most commonly enlarged but any gland may be affected, unilaterally or bilaterally. The glandular enlargement is painless and occurs slowly, and there is often a history of some years duration. Occasionally the onset is associated with fever and there may be fluctuation in size of the swellings from time to time. Hypergammaglobulinaemia is present and various circulating autoantibodies can be demonstrated.

Pathology

The affected glands, which may or may not be enlarged, show either diffuse involvement by lesional tissue or the presence of discrete nodules. In either event, the normal lobular pattern is maintained. The consistency of an affected gland is rather rubbery and is whitish or yellowish-grey instead of showing the normal appearance of salivary glandular tissue. When the lesion is present as nodules these are well circumscribed, with normal gland tissue between them. Small cysts are occasionally seen. There is no capsular thickening.

Microscopically, a fully developed lesion consists of a mass of lymphoid tissue containing islands of epithelium (Fig. 114). The lymphoepithelial tissue has replaced almost all the normal gland parenchyma and it involves entire lobules of gland without, however, crossing the septa

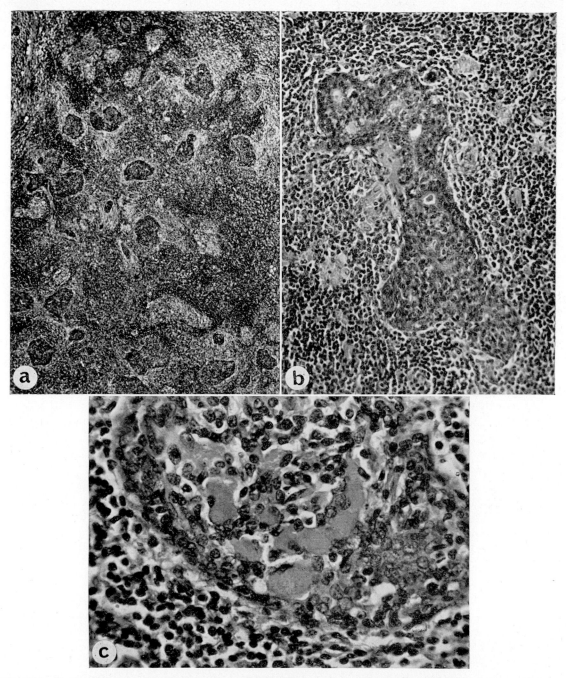

Fig. 114 Benign lymphoepithelial lesion. **a,** the parotid gland, showing complete replacement by lymphoid tissue containing epithelial islets. × 30. **b,** an epithelial islet, consisting of a closely packed mass of polyhedral cells. × 200. **c,** hyalin formation in an epithelial islet. × 500.

between lobules. The lymphoid component of the lesion consists of mature and immature lymphocytes, sometimes organised in lymphoid follicles and with germinal centres present, but often appearing simply as a diffuse infiltration.

The epithelial masses, which are distributed more or less evenly throughout the lymphoid tissue, are rounded, ovoid or rather irregular. They consist of spheroidal or polyhedral cells with vesicular nuclei, closely packed together to form solid masses. The cell walls may sometimes be ill-defined so that the mass is almost syncytial. Sometimes there is a lumen-like space in the cell mass, which may contain some amorphous eosinophilic material. Some cells may show hydropic changes and nuclear pyknosis. The presence of hyaline material between the cells, sometimes in quite large amounts, is not uncommon and it may ultimately replace the epithelium completely. Infiltration of the epithelial masses with lymphocytes is a constant feature.

The epithelial masses are referred to as epimyoepithelial islands, but convincing evidence of the participation of myoepithelial cells is not available. Recently, the fine structure of these cell islands was investigated by Boquist, Kumlien and Östberg (1970) but definite myoepithelial cells were not found and the authors suggest that the cell islands might be formed by proliferation and squamous metaplasia of duct cells.

Small cysts are sometimes seen. These are lined by epithelium, usually squamous but sometimes cuboidal or columnar.

The evolution of the lesion has been studied by Morgan and Castleman (1953) and Bernier and Bhaskar (1958). It commences as an infiltration of lymphocytes around the intralobular ducts, that gradually increases to replace the whole of the affected lobule. Concomitantly, the gland acini undergo progressive atrophy and finally disappear completely, but the ducts do not share in this disintegration of the parenchyma. On the contrary, they may show proliferative changes, first seen as basophilia of the normally eosinophilic lining cells, with nuclear enlargement and hyperchromatism. The cells then proliferate, leading to narrowing of the duct lumen and eventually to its complete disappearance. In this way the epithelial masses come to be formed from the ducts. Mitotic figures are quite often seen in those ducts that are still proliferating, but they are rare in the mature epithelial masses.

Morgan and Castleman consider that the primary lesion occurs in the ducts. The lymphocytic infiltration is a reaction to the ductal changes. Bernier and Bhaskar, on the other hand, believe that the lesion commences as a hyperplasia of the lymph nodes associated wth the salivary gland and that the lymphocytic elements then extend into glandular tissue along the ducts. These undergo proliferation and metaplastic changes and the lumenal occlusion that finally results leads to microcyst formation in the related acini.

Clinical involvement of the minor salivary glands is uncommon; cases have been reported by Calman and Reifman (1966), Cifarelli, Bennett and Zaino (1966), Cahn (1967) and Bertram (1967). Microscopic involvement, however, is not uncommon, and is the basis of a simple and useful aid to diagnosis, lip biopsy. Although focal lymphocytic deposits are present in the major salivary glands in a significant proportion of patients with rheumatoid arthritis and, indeed, of elderly persons dying of a variety of causes (Waterhouse, 1965; Waterhouse and Doniach, 1966; Chisholm, Waterhouse and Mason, 1970), Chisholm and Mason (1968) have shown that foci of lymphocytes do not normally occur in the minor salivary glands, but are present in Sjögren's syndrome in a high proportion of patients. A lip biopsy containing salivary glandular tissue will show these foci, and there is evidence to indicate that the severity of the disease is related to their number and size (Greenspan and colleagues, 1974). In mild cases there are relatively few foci, and they are small and contain large numbers of plasma cells. In severe cases the foci are more numerous and are larger, and they contain fewer plasma cells (Fig. 115). Lip biopsy has also been investigated by Tarpley, Anderson and White (1974) and Akin and colleagues (1975).

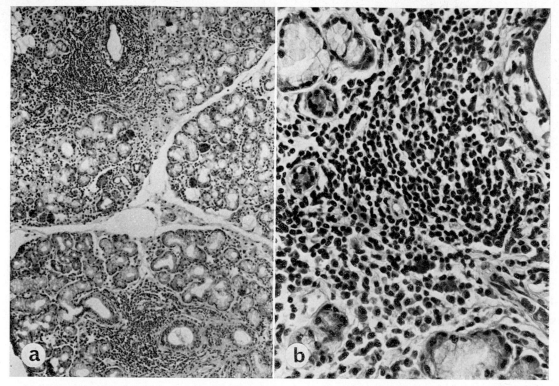

Fig. 115   Lip biopsy in Sjögren's syndrome. **a,** two foci of lymphocytic infiltration in labial salivary gland. × 30. **b,** higher magnification, showing that most of the cells are lymphocytes. Some plasma cells are also present. × 300.

Histological Diagnosis

The combination of lymphoid infiltration and epithelial hyperplasia, although distinctive, is not absolutely pathognomonic for the lymphoepithelial lesion. Epimyoepithelial islands have been seen in sarcoidosis and in calculous sialadenitis, and occasionally similar appearances have been noted in lymphomas (Maxwell, 1960; Hornbaker and colleagues, 1966). In sialadenitis the infiltration is, however, essentially inflammatory in character, with many more plasma cells and eosinophils, and fibrosis is common. This contrasts with the diffuse, almost purely lymphocytic infiltration of the lymphoepithelial lesion, in which fibrosis is absent. Moreover, the infiltrate in the lymphoepithelial lesion obscures all the normal features of the gland other than the proliferating ducts. In sialadenitis the ducts may show squamous metaplasia, and if islets resembling epimyoepithelial islands do form, they remain small. Also, the acini do not disintegrate completely. They may be infiltrated by inflammatory cells and show some distortion, but the general pattern of the remaining acini remains comparatively clear.

The diffuse infiltration of lymphoma resembles that seen in the lymphoepithelial lesion, but in the lymphomas the cellular infiltration passes from one lobule to another and the interlobular septa are obliterated. Also, the infiltrating cells show the features of a lymphoreticulosis rather than those of the mature lymphocytes of the lymphoepithelial lesion, although in lymphocytic types of lymphoma it may be difficult to make a distinction.

Pathogenesis

When Mikulicz first reported the condition he regarded it as a chronic inflammation due to low-grade infection and this was the generally accepted view for many years. It was also suggested that the lesion might be of benign neoplastic nature. However, Morgan and Castleman thought there might be some relationship between the condition and Hashimoto's disease, because of the histological similarities. They were unable to find any cases in which thyroid and salivary gland disease co-existed, but of course it is now clear that a similarity does exist in that both conditions are believed to have an autoimmune basis. The probable autoimmune nature of Sjögren's syndrome has been demonstrated by many workers, including Jones (1958), Heaton (1959, 1962), Bunim (1961), Sjögren (1961) and Anderson and colleagues (1961). Further support for this concept has been provided by the detection of a salivary duct autoantibody in a high proportion of patients with Sjögrens' syndrome (Bertram and Halberg, 1964; Feltkamp and von Rossum, 1968).

Lymphocytic sialadenitis has been produced in guinea pigs by immunisation with homologous salivary gland tissue incorporated in Freund's adjuvant (Chan, 1964). The lesions produced, however, differed from those in the salivary glands in lymphoepithelial lesion, in that epimyoepithelial islands were not present. It is of interest that Kessler (1968) has reported that lacrimal and salivary gland abnormalities, histologically identical to those of the human lesion, are found in some strains of mice that suffer spontaneously from autoimmune conditions. These abnormalities begin to appear about the fourth month, at the same time as other autoimmune phenomena are seen.

Behaviour

Apart from the xerostomia and possible glandular enlargement, the salivary lesions as such in Sjögren's syndrome are symptomless and the prognosis depends more on any associated connective tissue disorders. However, malignant lymphoma may complicate both the lymphoepithelial lesion occurring without any other manifestations and Sjögren's syndrome and the sicca complex. This occurs in some 6 to 7 per cent of cases. Reticulum cell sarcoma, Hodgkin's disease and follicular lymphoma have been reported (Talal and Bunim, 1964; Bloch and colleagues, 1965; Hornbaker and colleagues, 1966; Azzopardi and Evans, 1971). Waldenström's macroglobulinaemia has occurred in some patients (Pinkus and Dekker, 1970). Malignant change may, very rarely, occur in the epithelial component of the lesion, with squamous cell carcinoma or adenocarcinoma appearing (Hilderman and colleagues, 1962; Delaney and Balogh, 1966; Gravanis and Giansanti, 1970).

REFERENCES

Aboul-Nasr, A. L. (1961) Tumors of the minor salivary gland. *J. egypt. med. Ass.*, **44**, 464.

Abrams, A. M., Cornyn, J., Scofield, H. H., and Hansen, L. S. (1965) Acinic cell adenocarcinoma of the major salivary glands. A clinicopathologic study of 77 cases. *Cancer*, **18**, 1145.

Ackerman, L. V. (1943) Oncocytoma of the parotid gland. *Arch. Path.*, **36**, 508.

Ackerman, L. V., and Wheat, M. W. (1955) The implantation of cancer—an avoidable surgical risk? *Surgery*, **37**, 341.

Ahlbom, H. E. (1935) Mucous- and salivary-gland tumours. Clinical study with special reference to radiotherapy, based on 254 cases treated at Radiumhemmet, Stockholm. *Acta radiol.*, Suppl. **23**.

Akin, R. K., Kneller, A. J., Walters, P. J., and Trapani, J. S. (1975) Sjögren's syndrome. *J. oral Surg.*, **33**, 27.

Albores-Saavedra and Morris, A. W. (1963) Sebaceous adenoma of the submaxillary gland. *Arch. Otolaryngol.*, **77**, 500.

Albrecht, H., and Arzt, L. (1910) Beiträge zur Frage der Gewebsverirrung. I. Papilläre Cystadenome in Lymphdrüsen. *Frankfurt. Z. Path.*, **4,** 47.

Alexander, R. W., Dupuis, R. H., and Holton, H. (1974) Central mucoepidermoid tumor (carcinoma) of the mandible. *J. oral Surg.*, **32,** 541.

Allegra, S. R. (1971) Warthin's tumor: a hypersensitivity disease? Ultrastructural, light, and immuno-fluorescent study. *Hum. Path.*, **2,** 403.

Allen, M. S., Fitz-Hugh, G. S., and Marsh, W. L. (1974) Low-grade papillary adenocarcinoma of the palate. *Cancer,* **33,** 153.

Anderson, J. R., Gray, K. G., Beck, J. S., and Kinnear, W. F. (1961) Precipitating autoantibodies in Sjögren's disease. *Lancet,* **2,** 456.

Angell, D. C., Ousterhout, D., Hendrix, R. C., and French, A. J. (1967) Epithelial neoplasms of salivary gland: acinic-cell, mucous-cell, and duct-cell tumors. *Oral Surg.*, **23,** 362.

Assor, D. (1970) Sebaceous lymphadenoma of the parotid gland. A case report. *Amer. J. clin. Path.*, **53,** 100.

Azzopardi, J. G., and Evans, D. J. (1971) Malignant lymphoma of parotid associated with Mikulicz disease (benign lymphoepithelial lesion). *J. clin. Path.*, **24,** 744.

Azzopardi, J. G., and Hou, L. T. (1964) The genesis of adenolymphoma. *J. Path. Bact.*, **88,** 213.

Azzopardi, J. G., and Smith, O. D. (1959) Salivary gland tumours and their mucins. *J. Path. Bact.*, **77,** 131.

Azzopardi, J. G., and Zayid, I. (1972) Elastic tissue in tumours of salivary glands. *J. Path.*, **107,** 149.

Baden, E., and Wallen, N. G. (1965) Acinous cell tumor of the floor of the mouth: report of case. *J. oral Surg.*, **23,** 163.

Balogh, K., and Roth, S. I. (1965) Histochemical and electron microscopic studies of eosinophilic granular cells (oncocytes) in tumors of the parotid gland. *Lab. Invest.*, **14,** 310.

Bardwil, J. M. (1967) Tumors of the parotid gland. *Amer. J. Surg.*, **114,** 498.

Barton, R. T. (1964) Lymphoepithelial tumors of salivary gland with case report of sebaceous adenoma. *Amer. Surg.*, **30,** 411.

Batsakis, J. G. (1972) Basal cell adenoma of the parotid gland. *Cancer,* **29,** 226.

Bauer, W. H., and Bauer, J. D. (1953) Classification of glandular tumors of salivary glands. *Arch. Path.*, **55,** 328.

Bauer, W. H., and Fox, R. A. (1945) Adenomyoepithelioma (cylindroma) of palatal mucous glands. *Arch. Path.*, **39,** 96.

Bazaz-Malik, G., and Gupta, D. N. (1968) Metastasising (malignant) oncocytoma of the parotid gland. *Z. Krebsforsch.*, **70,** 193.

Beahrs, O. H., Woolner, L. B., Carveth, S. W., and Devine, K. D. (1960) Surgical management of parotid lesions. Review of seven hundred and sixty cases. *Arch. Surg.*, **80,** 899.

Beck, J. C., and Guttman, M. R. (1936) Basalioma or so-called cylindroma of the air passages. *Ann. Otol.*, **45,** 618.

Belsey, R. H. R., and Valentine, J. C. (1951) Cylindromatous mucous-gland tumours of the trachea and bronchi: a report of three cases. *J. Path. Bact.*, **63,** 377.

Bernier, J. L. (1946) Mixed tumors of the lip. *J. oral Surg.*, **4,** 193.

Bernier, J. L., and Bhaskar, S. N. (1958) Lymphoepithelial lesions of salivary glands. Histogenesis and classification based on 186 cases. *Cancer,* **11,** 1156.

Bertram, U. (1967) Xerostomia. Clinical aspects, pathology and pathogenesis. *Acta odont. scand.*, **25,** Suppl. **49.**

Bertram, U., and Halberg, P. (1964) A specific antibody against the epithelium of the salivary ducts in sera from patients with Sjögren's syndrome. *Acta Allergol.*, **19,** 458.

Bhaskar, S. N. (1963) Central mucoepidermoid tumors of the mandible. Report of 2 cases. *Cancer,* **16,** 721.

Bhaskar, S. N. (1964) Acinic-cell carcinoma of salivary glands. Report of twenty-one cases. *Oral Surg.*, **17,** 62.

Bhaskar, S. N., and Bernier, J. L. (1962) Mucoepidermoid tumors of major and minor salivary glands. Clinical features, histology, variations, natural history, and results of treatment for 144 cases. *Cancer,* **15,** 801.

Bhaskar, S. N., and Weinmann, J. P. (1955) Tumors of the minor salivary glands. A study of twenty-three cases. *Oral Surg.*, **8,** 1278.

Billroth, T. (1859) Beobachtungen über Geschwulste der Speicheldrüsen. *Virchows Arch.*, **17,** 357.

Blanck, C., Eneroth, C.-M., Jacobsson, F., and Jakobsson, P. Å. (1967) Adenoid cystic carcinoma of the parotid gland. *Acta radiol.*, **6,** 177.

z

Blanck, C., Eneroth, C.-M., and Jakobsson, P. Å. (1970) Oncocytoma of the parotid gland: neoplasm or nodular hyperplasia? *Cancer*, **25**, 919.

Blanck, C., Eneroth, C.-M., and Jakobsson, P. Å. (1971) Mucus-producing adenopapillary (non-epidermoid) carcinoma of the parotid gland. *Cancer*, **28**, 676.

Bloch, K. J., Buchanan, W. W., Wohl, M. J., and Bunim, J. J. (1965) Sjögren's syndrome: a clinical pathological and serological study of 62 cases. *Medicine*, **187**, 231.

Boley, J. O., and Robinson, D. W. (1954) Bilateral oxyphilic granular cell adenoma of parotid. Report of a case. *Arch. Path.*, **58**, 564.

Bollinger, T. E., and Hiatt, W. R. (1973) Basal-cell adenoma of the upper lip. Report of a case. *Oral Surg.*, **35**, 600.

Boquist, L., Kumlien and Östberg, Y. (1970) Ultrastructural findings in a case of benign lymphoepithelial lesion (Sjögren's Syndrome). *Acta otolaryngol.*, **70**, 216.

Bowerman, J. E., and Rowe, N. L. (1970) Haemangiomas involving the submandibular salivary gland. *Brit. J. oral Surg.*, **7**, 196.

Briggs, J., and Evans, J. N. G. (1967) Malignant oxyphilic granular-cell tumor (oncocytoma) of the palate. Review of the recent literature and report of a case. *Oral Surg.*, **23**, 796.

Brooks, H. W., Hiebert, A. E., Pullman, N. K., and Stofer, B. E. (1956) Papillary cystadenoma of the palate. A review of the literature and report of two new cases. *Oral Surg.*, **9**, 1047.

Browand, B. C., and Waldron, C. A. (1975) Central mucoepidermoid tumors of the jaws. Report of nine cases and review of the literature. *Oral Surg.*, **40**, 631.

Brown, R. L., Bishop, E. L., and Girardeau, H. S. (1959) Tumors of the minor salivary glands. *Cancer*, **12**, 40.

Brown, A. M., and Lucchesi, F. J. (1966) Central mucoepidermoid tumor of the mandible: report of case. *J. oral Surg.*, **24**, 356.

Bruce, R. A., and Wertheimer, F. W. (1967) Enzyme histochemistry of adenoid cystic carcinoma of minor salivary glands. *J. oral Surg.*, **25**, 30.

Bunim, J. J. (1961) A broader spectrum of Sjögren's syndrome and its pathogenetic implications. *Ann. rheum. Dis.*, **20**, 1.

Buxton, R. W., Maxwell, J. H., and French, A. J. (1953) Surgical treatment of epithelial tumors of the parotid gland. *Surg. Gynec. Obstet.*, **97**, 401.

Cahn, L. R. (1967) The role of the lymphatic apparatus in oral disease. *Brit. dent. J.*, **122**, 387.

Calhoun, N. R., Cerine, F. C., and Mathews, M. J. (1965) Papillary cystadenoma of the upper lip. Report of a case. *Oral Surg.*, **20**, 810.

Calman, H. I., and Reifman, S. (1966) Sjögren's syndrome. Report of a case. *Oral Surg.*, **21**, 158.

Chan, W. C. (1964) Experimental sialo-adenitis in guinea-pigs. *J. Path. Bact.*, **88**, 592.

Chaudhry, A. P., Vickers, R. A., and Gorlin, R. J. (1961) Intraoral minor salivary gland tumors. An analysis of 1,414 cases. *Oral Surg.*, **14**, 1194.

Chisholm, D. M., and Mason, D. K. (1968) Labial salivary gland biopsy in Sjögren's disease. *J. clin. Path.*, **21**, 656.

Chisholm, D. M., Waterhouse, J. P., Kraucunas, E., and Sciubba, J. J. (1974) Quantitative ultrastructural study of the pleomorphic adenoma (mixed tumor) of human minor salivary glands. *Cancer* **34**, 1631.

Chisholm, D. M., Waterhouse, J. P., and Mason, D. K. (1970) Lymphocytic sialadenitis in the major and minor glands: a correlation in postmortem subjects. *J. clin. Path.*, **23**, 690.

Christopherson, W. M. (1949) Oncocytoma of the parotid gland. *Arch. Path.*, **48**, 96.

Cifarelli, P. S., Bennett, M. J., and Zaino, E. C. (1966) Sjögren's syndrome. A case report with an additional diagnostic aid. *Arch. intern. Med.*, **117**, 429.

Clarke, J. S., Hentz, E. C., and Mahoney, W. D. (1969) Bilateral acinic cell carcinoma of the parotid gland. *Ann. Surg.*, **170**, 866.

Corridan, M. (1956) Glycogen-rich clear cell adenoma of the parotid gland. *J. Path. Bact.*, **72**, 623.

Cotchin, E. (1958) Mammary neoplasms of the bitch. *J. comp. Path.*, **68**, 1.

Davies, J. N. P., Dodge, O. G., and Burkitt, D. P. (1964) Salivary-gland tumors in Uganda. *Cancer*, **17**, 1310.

De, M. N., and Tribedi, B. P. (1939) A mixed epidermoid and mucus-secreting carcinoma of the parotid gland. *J. Path. Bact.*, **49**, 432.

Delaney, W. E., and Balogh, K. (1966) Carcinoma of the parotid gland associated with benign lymphoepithelial lesion (Mikulicz's disease) in Sjögren's syndrome. *Cancer*, **19**, 853.

Delarue, J. (1956) Les "tumeurs mixtes" plurifocales de la glande parotide. *Ann. Anat. path.*, **1**, 34.

Deppisch, L. M., and Toker, C. (1969) Mixed tumors of the parotid gland. An ultrastructural study. *Cancer*, **24**, 174.

D'Eramo, E. M., and Poidmore, S. J. (1975) Developmental submandibular gland defect of the mandible. Review of the literature and report of a case. *Oral Surg.*, **39,** 14.

Dockerty, M. B., and Mayo, C. W. (1942) Primary tumors of the submaxillary gland with special reference to mixed tumors. *Surg. Gynec. Obstet.*, **74,** 1033.

Dockerty, M. B., and Mayo, C. W. (1943) "Cylindroma" (Adenocarcinoma, cylindroma type). *Surgery,* **13,** 416.

Doyle, L. E., Lynn, J. A., Panopio, I. T., and Crass, G. (1968) Ultrastructure of the chondroid regions of benign mixed tumor of salivary gland. *Cancer*, **22,** 225.

Eby, L. S., Johnson, D. S., and Baker, H. W. (1972) Adenoid cystic carcinoma of the head and neck. *Cancer*, **29,** 1160.

Echevarria, R. A. (1967) Ultrastructure of the acinic cell carcinoma and clear cell carcinoma of the parotid gland. *Cancer*, **20,** 563.

Eggers, H. E. (1938) Mixed tumors of the lip. *Arch. Path.*, **26,** 348.

Eneroth, C.-M. (1964) Histological and clinical aspects of parotid tumours. *Acta otolaryngol.*, Suppl. **191.**

Eneroth, C.-M. (1971) Salivary gland tumors in the parotid gland, submandibular gland, and the palate region. *Cancer*, **27,** 1415.

Eneroth, C.-M., Hamberger, C. A., and Jakobsson, P. Å, (1966) Malignancy of acinic cell carcinoma. *Ann. Otol. Rhinol. Laryngol.*, **75,** 780.

Eneroth, C.-M., Hjertman, L., and Moberger, G. (1972) Salivary gland adenomas of the palate. *Acta Otolaryngol.*, **73,** 305.

Eneroth, C.-M., Hjertman, G., Moberger, G., and Wersäll, J. (1968) Ultrastructural characteristics of adenoid cystic carcinoma of salivary glands. *Arch. klin. exper. Ohren, Nasen und Kehlkopfheilk*, **192,** 358.

Eneroth, C.-M., Jakobsson, P. Å., and Blanck, C. (1966) Acinic cell carcinoma of the parotid gland. *Cancer*, **19,** 1761.

Epker, B. N., and Henny, F. A. (1971) Intra-oral sebaceous gland adenoma. *Cancer*, **27,** 987.

Erichsen, S. (1955) Connective-tissue mucin producing carcinoma of the canine mammary gland. *Acta path. microbiol. scand.*, **36,** 481.

Erichsen, S. (1955) A histochemical study on mixed tumours of the canine mammary gland. *Acta path. microbiol. scand.*, **36,** 490.

Evans, R. W., and Cruickshank, A. H. (1970) *Epithelial Tumours of the Salivary Glands.* Philadelphia. W. B. Saunders Company.

Eversole, L. R. (1970) Mucoepidermoid carcinoma: review of 815 reported cases. *J. oral Surg.*, **28,** 490.

Eversole, L. R., Rovin, S., and Sabes, W. R. (1972) Mucoepidermoid carcinoma of minor salivary glands: a report of 17 cases with follow-up. *J. oral Surg.*, **30,** 107.

Ewing, J. (1940) *Neoplastic Diseases.* 4th Edition. Philadelphia. W. B. Saunders Company.

Ewing, J. Cited by Martin and Ehrlich.

Feltkamp, T. E., and von Rossum, A. L. (1968) Antibodies to salivary duct cells and other autoantibodies in patients with Sjögren's syndrome and other idiopathic autoimmune diseases. *Clin. expl. Immunol.*, **3,** 1.

Feyrter, F. (1963) Über das glykogenreiche retikulierte Adenom der Speicheldrüsen. *Z. Krebsforsch.*, **65,** 446.

Fine, G., and Marshall, R. B. (1961) Malignant mixed tumor of parotid gland. *Amer. J. Surg.*, **102,** 86.

Fine, G., Marshall, R. B., and Horn, R. C. (1960) Tumors of the minor salivary glands. *Cancer*, **13,** 653.

Fleming, K. A., and Morrice, I. (1973) Sebaceous lymphadenoma of the parotid gland: a report of a case. *J. Path.*, **110,** 259.

Foote, F. W., and Frazell, E. L. (1953) Tumors of the major salivary glands. *Cancer*, **6,** 1065.

Foote, F. W., and Frazell, E. L. (1954) *Tumors of the Major Salivary Glands.* Atlas of Tumor Pathology. Section 4. Fascicle 11. Washington, D.C. Armed Forces Institute of Pathology.

Fox, N. M., Remine, W. H., and Woolner, L. B. (1963) Acinic cell carcinoma of the major salivary glands. *Amer. J. Surg.*, **106,** 860.

Frable, W. J., and Elzay, R. P. (1970) Tumors of minor salivary glands. A report of 73 cases. *Cancer*, **25,** 932.

Frazell, E. L. (1954) Clinical aspects of tumors of the major salivary glands. *Cancer*, **7,** 637.

Fry, R. M. (1928) The structure and origin of the "mixed" tumours of the salivary glands. *Brit. J. Surg.*, **15,** 291.

Fukushima, M. (1968) An electron microscopic study of human salivary gland tumors—pleomorphic adenoma and adenoid cystic carcinoma. *Bull. Tokyo med. dent. Univ.*, **15,** 387.

Gadient, S. E., and Kalfayan, B. (1975) Mucoepidermoid carcinoma arising within a Warthin's tumor. *Oral Surg.*, **40,** 391.

Gardner, A. F., Siegler, H. R., and Spire, E. D. (1964) A study of one hundred and seventy-three instances of pleomorphic adenomas of the salivary glands. *Amer. Surg.*, **30,** 539.

Gerughty, R. M., Scofield, H. H., Brown, F. M., and Hennigar, G. R. (1969) Malignant mixed tumors of salivary gland origin. *Cancer*, **24,** 471.

Gilman, R. A., Schwartz, M., and Gilman, J. S. (1956) Fatty infiltration of the parotid gland. Report of a case simulating a tumor. *J. Amer. med. Ass.*, **160,** 48.

Godwin, J. T., (1952) Benign lymphoepithelial lesion of the parotid gland (Adenolymphoma, chronic inflammation, lymphoepithelioma, lymphocytic tumor, Mikulicz disease). Report of eleven cases. *Cancer*, **5,** 1089.

Godwin, J. T., and Colvin, S. H., Jr. (1948) Adenoma of the parotid gland. *Arch. Path.*, **46,** 187.

Godwin, J. T., and Dew, J. H. (1958) Fatty infiltration of parotid glands. Report of a case. *Arch. Surg.*, **76,** 525.

Goldman, R. L., and Klein, H. Z. (1972) Glycogen-rich adenoma of the parotid gland. An uncommon benign clear-cell tumour resembling certain clear-cell carcinomas of salivary origin. *Cancer*, **30,** 749.

Gore, D. O., Annamunthodo, H., and Harland, A. (1964) Tumors of salivary gland origin. *Surg. Gynec. Obstet.*, **119,** 1.

Gorlin, R., and Chaudhry, A. (1957) Acinic cell tumor of the major and minor salivary glands. *J. oral Surg.* **15,** 304.

Grage, T. B., Lober, P. H., and Arbelger, S. W. (1961) Acinic cell carcinoma of the parotid gland. A clinicopathological review of eleven cases. *Amer. J. Surg.*, **102,** 765.

Gravanis, M. B., and Giansanti, J. S. (1970) Malignant histopathologic counterpart of the benign lympho-epithelial lesion. *Cancer*, **26,** 1332.

Greene, G. W., and Bernier, J. L. (1961) Primary malignant melanomas of the parotid gland. *Oral Surg.*, **14,** 108.

Greenspan, J. S., Daniels, T. E., Talal, N., and Sylvester, R. A. (1974) The histopathology of Sjögren's syndrome in labial salivary gland biopsies. *Oral Surg.*, **37,** 217.

Grishman, E. (1952) Histochemical analysis of mucopolysaccharides occurring in mucus-producing tumors. Mixed tumors of the parotid gland, colloid carcinomas of the breast, and myxomas. *Cancer*, **5,** 700.

Hamperl, H. (1931) Beiträge zur normalen pathologischen Histologie menschlicher Speicheldrüsen. *Zeit. mikr. Anat. Forsch.*, **27,** 1.

Hamperl, H. (1931) Onkocyten und Geschwülste der Speicheldrüsen. *Virchows Arch.*, **282,** 724.

Hamperl, H. (1936) Über das Vorkommen von Onkocyten in verschiedenen Organen und ihren Geschwülsten; (Mundspeicheldrüsen, Brauchspeicheldrüse, Epithelkorperchen, Hypophyse, Schilddrüse, Eileiter). *Virchows Arch.*, **298,** 327.

Hamperl, H. (1962) Benign and malignant oncocytoma. *Cancer*, **15,** 1019.

Harrison, J. D. (1974) Cystic adenoma of a minor salivary gland: a histochemical study. *J. Path.*, **114,** 29.

Harrison, K. (1956) A study of ectopic mixed salivary tumours. *Ann. roy. Coll. Surg. Engl.*, **18,** 99.

Hart, M. N., and Andrews, J. L. (1968) Papillary cystadenoma lymphomatosum arising in the oral cavity. *Oral Surg.*, **26,** 588.

Hartz, P. H. (1946) Development of sebaceous glands from intralobular ducts of the parotid gland. *Arch. Path.*, **41,** 651.

Harvey, W. F., Dawson, E. K., and Innes, J. R. M. (1938) Debatable tumours in human and animal pathology. IV. "Mixed tumours" of salivary glands. *Edin. med. J.*, **45,** 275.

Hayes, H. (1961) Aberrant submaxillary gland tissue presenting as a cyst of the jaw. *Oral Surg.*, **14,** 313.

Healey, W. V., Perzin, K. H., and Smith, L. (1970) Mucoepidermoid carcinoma of salivary gland origin. Classification, clinical–pathologic correlation, and results of treatment. *Cancer*, **26,** 368.

Heaton, J. M. (1959) Sjögren's syndrome and systemic lupus erythematosus. *Brit. med. J.*, **1,** 466.

Heaton, J. M. (1962) Sjögren's syndrome. *Proc. roy. Soc. Med.*, **55,** 479.

Hemplemann, L. H., Jr., and Womack, N. A. (1942) The pathogenesis of mixed tumors of the salivary gland type. *Ann. Surg.*, **116,** 34.

Hendrick, J. W. (1964) Mucoepidermoid cancer in the parotid gland in a one year old child. *Amer. J. Surg.*, **108,** 907.

Hilderman, W. C., Gordon, J. S., Large, H. L., and Carroll, C. F. (1962) Malignant lymphoepithelial lesion with carcinomatous component apparently arising in parotid gland. A malignant counterpart of benign lymphoepithelial lesion ? *Cancer*, **15,** 606.

Hornbaker, J. H., Foster, E. A., Williams, G. S., and Davis, J. S. (1966) Sjögren's syndrome and nodular reticulum cell sarcoma. *Arch. intern. Med.*, **118,** 449.

Hoshino, M., and Yamamoto, I. (1970) Ultrastructure of adenoid cystic carcinoma. *Cancer*, **25**, 186.

Howard, J. M., Rawson, A. J., Koop, C. E., Horn, R. C., and Royster, H. P. (1950) Parotid tumors in children. *Surg. Gynec. Obstet.*, **90**, 307.

Jacobs, M. H. (1955) The traumatic bone cyst. *Oral Surg.*, **8**, 940.

Jaffé, R. H. (1932) Adenolymphoma (onkocytoma) of the parotid gland. *Amer. J. Cancer*, **16**, 1415.

Jakobsson, P. Å., Blanck, C., and Eneroth, C.-M. (1968) Mucoepidermoid carcinoma of the parotid gland. *Cancer*, **22**, 111.

Jones, B. R. (1958) Lacrimal and salivary precipitating antibodies in Sjögren's syndrome. *Lancet*, **2**, 773.

Karabin, J. E. (1951) Cavernous hemangioma of the parotid gland. Report of a case. *Surgery*, **30**, 367.

Karlan, M. S., and Snyder, W. H. (1968) Salivary gland tumors and sialadenitis in children. Experience at Childrens Hospital of Los Angeles. *Calif. Med.*, **108**, 423.

Kauffman, S. L., and Stout, A. P. (1963) Tumors of the major salivary glands in children. *Cancer*, **16**, 1317.

Kay, S., and Schatzki, P. F. (1972) Ultrastructure of acinic cell carcinoma of the parotid salivary gland. *Cancer*, **29**, 235.

Kessler, H. S. (1968) A laboratory model for Sjögren's syndrome. *Amer. J. Path.*, **52**, 671.

Kleinsasser, O., Hübner, G., and Klein, H. J. (1967) Acinuszell-tumozen der Glandula parotis. *Arch. klin. exper. Ohren, Nasen und Kehlkopfheilk.*, **189**, 33.

Kleinsasser, O., Hübner, G., and Klein, H. J. (1969) Zur Histogenese der Cylindrome. *Arch. klin. exper. Ohren, Nasen und Kehlkopfheilk*, **195**, 192.

Kleinsasser, O., and Klein, H. J. (1967) Basalzelladenome der Speicheldrüsen. *Arch. klin. exper. Ohren, Nasen und Kehlkopfheilk.*, **189**, 302.

Kleinsasser, O., Klein, H. J., Steinbach, E., and Hübner, G. (1966) Onkocytäre adenomartige Hyperplasien, Adenolymphome und Onkocytome der Speicheldrüsen. *Arch. klin. exper. Ohren, Nasen und Kehlkopfheilk.*, **186**, 317.

Koblin, I., and Koch, H. (1974) On the nature of mucoepidermoid tumours of major and minor salivary glands. *J. max.-fac. Surg.*, **2**, 19.

Kondo, T., Muragishi, H., and Imaizumi, M. (1971) A cell line from a human salivary gland mixed tumor. *Cancer*, **27**, 403.

Kramer, R., and Som, M. L. (1939) Cylindroma of the upper air passages. A cylindromatous type of mixed tumor. *Arch. Otolaryngol.*, **29**, 356.

Krolls, S. O., and Hicks, J. L. (1973) Mixed tumors of the lower lip. *Oral Surg.*, **35**, 2.

Krompecher, E. (1908) Ueber die Beziehungen zwischen Epithel und Bindgewebe bei den Mischgeschwülsten der Hout und der Speicheldrüsen und über das Eustehen der Karzinosarkoma. *Beitr. path. Anat.*, **44**, 88.

Lane, S., and Schwarz, A. W. (1958) Infantile hemangioendothelioma of the parotid gland. *Amer. J. Surg.*, **96**, 784.

Lang, F. J. (1929) Cited by Martin and Ehrlich.

Leafstedt, S. W. (1971) Adenoid cystic carcinoma of major and minor salivary glands. *Amer. J. Surg.*, **122**, 756.

Lee, C. M. (1949) Intraparotid sebaceous glands. *Ann. Surg.*, **129**, 152.

Lemaitre, Y. (1938) Etude anatomo-clinique des tumeurs dites cylindromes. *Ann. Otolaryngol.*, **57**, 185.

Lennox, B., Pearse, A. G. E., and Richards, H. G. H. (1952) Mucin-secreting tumours of the skin: with special reference to the so-called mixed-salivary tumour of the skin and its relation to hidradenoma. *J. Path. Bact.*, **64**, 865.

Linhartova, A. (1974) Sebaceous glands in salivary gland tissue. *Arch. Path.*, **98**, 320.

Lumerman, H., Freedman, P., Caracciolo, P., and Remigio, P. S. (1975) Synchronous malignant mucoepidermoid tumor of the parotid gland and Warthin's tumor in adjacent lymph node. *Oral Surg.*, **39**, 953.

Luna, M. A., Mackay, B., and Gamez-Araujo, J. (1973) Myoepithelioma of the palate. Report of a case with histochemical and electron microscopic observations. *Cancer*, **32**, 1429.

Luna, M. A., Stimson, P. G., and Bardwil, J. M. (1968) Minor salivary gland tumors of the oral cavity. A review of sixty-eight cases. *Oral Surg.*, **25**, 71.

McDonald, J. R., Moersch, H. J., and Tinney, W. S. (1945) Cylindroma of the bronchus. *J. thorac. Surg.*, **14**, 445.

McFarland, J. (1926) Ninety tumors of the parotid region. In all of which the postoperative history was traced. *Amer. J. med. Sci.*, **172**, 804.

McFarland, J. (1927) Adenoma of the salivary glands. With a report of a possible case. *Amer. J. med. Sci.*, **174**, 362.

McFarland, J. (1936) Three hundred mixed tumors of the salivary glands, of which sixty-nine recurred. *Surg. Gynec. Obstet.*, **63**, 457.

McFarland, J. (1942) The histopathologic prognosis of salivary gland mixed tumors. *Amer. J. med. Sci.*, **203**, 502.

McFarland, J. (1943) The mysterious mixed tumors of the salivary glands. *Surg. Gynec. Obstet.*, **76**, 23.

McGavran, M. H., Bauer, W. C., and Ackerman, L. V. (1960) Sebaceous lymphoadenoma of the parotid salivary gland. *Cancer*, **13**, 1185.

MacLennan, W. D., and Shivas, A. A. (1963) "Melanogenic metaplasia" of mucous glands. *Brit. J. oral Surg.*, **1**, 50.

Malassez, L. (1883) Sur le "cylindrome" (épithéliome alvéolaire avec envahissement myxomateux). *Arch. Phys. norm. path.*, *3me série*, **1**, 186.

Marano, P. D., and Hartman, K. S. (1974) Central mucoepidermoid carcinoma arising in a maxillary odontogenic cyst. *J. oral Surg.*, **32**, 915.

Martin, H., and Ehrlich, H. E. (1944) Papillary cystadenoma lymphomatosum (Warthin's tumor) of the parotid salivary gland. *Surg. Gynec. Obstet.*, **79**, 611.

Marucci, L., Fontana, R., and Marcato, D. (1962) Gli oncocitomi della parotide (osservazione di un caso presentate caratteri di malignità). *Arch. ital. Otol.*, **73**, 756.

Masson, P., and Berger, L. (1924) Epithéliomas à double métaplasie de la parotide. *Bull. Ass. franç. Cancer*, **13**, 366.

Maxwell, J. H. (1960) Chronic lymphoepithelial sialadenopathy with sialodochiectasis. *Trans. amer. Acad. Ophthal. Otolaryngol.*, **64**, 225.

Melrose, R. J., Abrams, A. M., and Howell, F. V. (1973) Mucoepidermoid tumors of the intraoral minor salivary glands: a clinicopathologic study of 54 cases. *J. oral Path.*, **2**, 314.

Meza-Chávez, L. (1949) Sebaceous glands in normal and neoplastic parotid glands. *Amer. J. Path.*, **25**, 627.

Meza-Chávez, L. (1949) Oxyphilic granular cell adenoma of the parotid gland (oncocytoma). Report of five cases and study of oxyphilic granular cells (oncocytes) in normal parotid glands. *Amer. J. Path.*, **25**, 523.

Mikulicz, J. (1892) Ueber eine einartige symmetrische Erkrankung der Thränen- und Mundspeichel-drüsen. *Beitr. z. Chir. Festschr. f. Theodor Billroth*, p. 610.

Moberger, J. G., and Eneroth, C.-M. (1968) Malignant mixed tumours of the major salivary glands. Special reference to the histologic structure in metastases. *Cancer*, **21**, 1198.

Mohamed, A. H., and Cherrick, H. M. (1975) Glycogen-rich adenocarcinoma of minor salivary glands. A light and electron microscopic study. *Cancer*, **36**, 1057.

Montanus, W. P. (1938) Mixed tumor of the parotid gland with metastasis. A case report. *Surgery*, **4**, 423.

Moran, J. J., Becker, S. M., Brady, L. W., and Rambo, V. B. (1961) Adenoid cystic carcinoma. A clinico-pathological study. *Cancer*, **14**, 1235.

Morgan, W. S., and Castleman, B. (1953) A clinicopathologic study of "Mikulicz's disease." *Amer. J. Path.*, **29**, 471.

Morgan, M. N., and Mackenzie, D. H. (1968) Tumours of salivary glands. A review of 204 cases with 5-year follow-up. *Brit. J. Surg.*, **55**, 284.

Mulligan, R. M. (1943) Metastasis of mixed tumors of the salivary glands. *Arch. Path.*, **35**, 357.

Murata, I., and Miyaji, T. (1966) Histochemical evaluation of enzymatic activities in pleomorphic salivary adenoma. *Oral Surg.*, **22**, 82.

Mustard, R. A., and Anderson, W. (1964) Malignant tumors of the parotid. *Ann. Surg.*, **159**, 304.

Mylius, E. A. (1960) The identification and role of the myoepithelial cell in the salivary gland tumour. *Acta path. microbiol. scand.*, **50**, 1.

Napp, O. (1907) Ueber die Beziehungen der Mikuliczschen Erkrankung zur Tuberkulose. *Z. Augenheilk.*, **17**, 513.

Neisse, R. (1898) Über den Einschluss von Parotisläppchen in Lymphknoten. *Anat. Hefte Wiesb.*, **10**, 289.

Nelson, J. F., and Jacoway, J. R. (1973) Monomorphic adenoma (canalicular type). Report of 29 cases. *Cancer*, **31**, 1511.

New, G. B., and Childrey, J. H. (1931) Tumors of the tonsil and pharynx—Adenocarcinomas of the mixed type. *Arch. Otolaryngol.*, **14**, 669.

Nicholson, G. W. (1922) Studies on tumour formation. III. Tissue malformations. Anomalies of position and of blending. *Guy's Hosp. Rep.*, **72**, 333.

Nicholson, G. W. (1923) Studies on tumour formation. V. The importance of congenital malformations in tumour formation. *Guy's Hosp. Rep.*, **73**, 37.

Patey, D. H. (1931) The mixed tumours of the salivary glands. *Brit. J. Surg.*, **18**, 241.

Patey, D. H., and Thackray, A. C. (1958) The treatment of parotid tumours in the light of a pathological study of parotidectomy material. *Brit. J. Surg.*, **45**, 477.

Patey, D. H., and Thackray, A. C. (1970) Infected adenolymphoma: a new parotid syndrome. *Brit. J. Surg.*, **57**, 569.

Patey, D. H., Thackray, A. C., and Keeling, D. H. (1965) Malignant disease of the parotid. *Brit. J. Cancer*, **19**, 712.

de la Pava, S., Knutson, G. H., Mukhtar, F., and Pickren, J. W. (1965) Squamous cell carcinoma arising in Warthin's tumor of the parotid gland. First case report. *Cancer*, **18**, 790.

Pinkus, G. S., and Dekker, A. (1970) Benign lymphoepithelial lesion of the parotid glands associated with reticulum cell sarcoma. Report of a case and review of the literature. *Cancer*, **25**, 121.

Potdar, G. G., and Paymaster, J. C. (1969) Tumors of minor salivary glands. *Oral Surg.*, **28**, 310.

Praytor, R. B. (1966) Bilateral mixed tumors of the palate. *Oral Surg.*, **21**, 129.

Quattlebaum, F. W., Dockerty, M. B., and Mayo, C. W. (1946) Adenocarcinoma, cylindroma type, of the parotid gland. A clinical and pathologic study of twenty-one cases. *Surg. Gynec. Obstet.*, **82**, 342.

Ranger, D., Thackray, A. C., and Lucas, R. B. (1956) Mucous gland tumours. *Brit. J. Cancer*, **10**, 1.

Rauch, S. (1959) *"Die Speicheldrüsen des Menschen"*. Stuttgart. Georg Thieme Verlag.

Rawson, A. J., and Horn, R. C. (1950) Sebaceous glands and sebaceous gland-containing tumors of the parotid salivary gland. With a consideration of the histogenesis of papillary cystadenoma lymphomatosum. *Surgery*, **27**, 93.

Rawson, A. J., Howard, J. M., Royster, H. P., and Horn, R. C. (1950) Tumors of the salivary glands. A clinicopathological study of 160 cases. *Cancer*, **3**, 445.

Reid, J. D. (1952) Adenoid cystic carcinoma (cylindroma) of the bronchial tree. *Cancer*, **5**, 685.

Ribbert, M. W. H. (1907) Ueber das Zylindrom. *Dtsch. med. Wsch.*, **33**, 126.

Richard, E. L., and Ziskind, J. (1957) Aberrant salivary gland tissue in mandible. *Oral Surg.*, **10**, 1086.

Ringertz, N. (1938) Pathology of malignant tumours arising in the nasal and paranasal cavities and maxilla. *Acta otolaryngol.*, Suppl. **27**.

Ruebner, B., and Bramhall, J. L. (1960) Malignant papillary cystadenoma lymphomatosum. *Arch. Path.*, **69**, 110.

Russell, H. (1955) Adenomatous tumours of the anterior foregut region showing the cylindroma pattern. *Brit. J. Surg.*, **43**, 248.

Saksela, E., Tarkkanen, J., and Kohonen, A. (1970) The malignancy of mixed tumors of the parotid gland. A clinicopathological analysis of 70 cases. *Acta otolaryngol.*, **70**, 62.

Schaffer, A. J., and Jacobsen, A. W. (1927) Mikulicz's syndrome. A report of ten cases. *Amer. J. Dis. Child.*, **34**, 327.

Schiefer, H.-G., Hübner, G., and Kleinsasser, O. (1968) Riesenmitochondrien aus Onkocyten menschlicher Adenolymphome. Isolierung, morphologische und biochemische Untersuchungen. *Virchows Arch. (Zell Pathol.)*, **1**, 230.

Schulenberg, C. A. R. (1954) Salivary gland tumours. *S. Afr. med. J.*, **28**, 910.

Schwartz, I. S., and Feldman, M. (1969) Diffuse multinodular oncocytoma ("oncocytosis") of the parotid gland. *Cancer*, **23**, 636.

Seward, G. R. (1960) Salivary gland inclusions in the mandible. *Brit. dent. J.*, **108**, 321.

Sheldon, W. H. (1943) So-called mixed tumors of the salivary glands. *Arch. Path.*, **35**, 1.

Shklar, G., and Chauncey, H. H. (1965) Papillary cystadenoma lymphomatosum, a developmental malformation: histochemical evidence. *J. oral Surg.*, **23**, 222.

Sikorowa, L. (1973) Epithelial tumors of the salivary glands containing lymphoid tissue. *Patol. pol.*, **24**, 45.

Silverglade, L. B., Alvares, O. F., and Olech, E. (1968) Central mucoepidermoid tumors of the jaws. Review of the literature and case report. *Cancer*, **22**, 650.

Simpson, W. (1965) A Stafne's mandibular defect containing a pleomorphic adenoma: report of case. *J. oral Surg.*, **23**, 553.

Sjögren, H. (1933) Zur Kenntnis der Keratoconjunctivitis sicca (Keratitis filiformis bei Hypofunktion der Tränendrüsen). *Acta ophthal. Suppl.* 2.

Sjögren, H. (1961) Some new investigations concerning the sicca-syndrome. *Acta ophthal.*, **39**, 619.

Smith, A. G., Broadbent, T. R., and Zavaleta, A. A. (1954) Tumours of oral mucous glands. *Cancer*, **7**, 224.

Smith, L. C., Lane, N., and Rankow, R. M. (1965) Cylindroma (adenoid cystic carcinoma). A report of fifty-eight cases. *Amer. J. Surg.*, **110**, 519.

Smith, R. L., Dahlin, D. C., and Waite, D. E. (1968) Mucoepidermoid carcinomas of the jawbones. *J. oral Surg.*, **26**, 387.

Solomon, M. P., Rosen, Y., and Gardner, B. (1975) Metastatic malignancy in the submandibular gland. *Oral Surg.*, **39**, 469.

Spies, J. W. (1930) Adenoid cystic carcinoma. Generalized metastases in three cases of basal cell type. *Arch. Surg.*, **21**, 365.

Spiro, R. H., Koss, L. G., Hajdu, S. I., and Strong, E. W. (1973) Tumors of minor salivary glands. A clinicopathologic study of 492 cases. *Cancer*, **31**, 117.

Stein, I., and Geschickter, C. F. (1934) Tumours of the parotid gland. *Arch. Surg.*, **28**, 492.

Stewart, F. W., Foote, F. W., and Becker, W. F. (1945) Muco-epidermoid tumors of salivary glands. *Ann. Surg.*, **122**, 820.

Stuteville, O. H., and Corley, R. D. (1967) Surgical management of tumors of intraoral minor salivary glands. Report of eighty cases. *Cancer*, **20**, 1578.

Talal, N., and Bunim, J. J. (1964) The development of malignant lymphoma in the course of Sjögren's syndrome. *Amer. J. Med.*, **36**, 529.

Tarpley, T. M., Anderson, L. G., and White, C. L. (1974) Minor salivary gland involvement in Sjögren's syndrome. *Oral Surg.*, **37**, 64.

Thackray, A. C. (1957) Malignant tumours of the salivary glands, p. 154. In *Cancer*, Vol. 2. Ed. R. W. Raven. London. Butterworth & Co. Ltd.

Thackray, A. C., and Lucas, R. B. (1960) The histology of cylindroma of mucous gland origin. *Brit. J. Cancer*, **14**, 612.

Thackray, A. C., and Lucas, R. B. (1974) *Tumors of the Major Salivary Glands*. Atlas of Tumor Pathology, Second Series. Fascicle 10. Washington, D.C. Armed Forces Institute of Pathology.

Thackray, A. C., and Sobin, L. H. (1972) *International Histological Classification of Tumours. Histological Typing of Salivary Gland Tumours*. World Health Organization, Geneva.

Thomas, W. H., and Coppola, E. D. (1965) Distant metastases from mixed tumors of the salivary glands. *Amer. J. Surg.*, **109**, 724.

Thompson, A. S., and Bryant, H. C. (1950) Histogenesis of papillary cystadenoma lymphomatosum (Warthin's tumor) of the parotid salivary gland. *Amer. J. Path.*, **26**, 807.

Thursfield, H. (1913) Bilateral salivary swellings (Mikulicz's disease): a clinical review. *Quart. J. Med.*, **7**, 237.

Tsukada, Y., de la Pava, S., and Pickren, J. W. (1964) Sebaceous-cell carcinoma arising in mixed tumor of parotid salivary gland. Report of a case. *Oral Surg.*, **18**, 517.

Turner, D. D. (1958) Virchow's metamorphosis of the salivary glands. *Arch. Surg.*, **77**, 110.

Vellios, F., and Shafer, W. G. (1959) Tumors of the intraoral accessory salivary glands. *Surg. Gynec. Obstet.*, **108**, 450.

Veronesi, U., and Corbetta, L. (1960) Adenolymphoma of the lower lip. *Acta otolaryngol.*, **52**, 1.

Virchow, R. (1863) Cited by Ahlbom.

Warthin, A. S. (1929) Papillary cystadenoma lymphomatosum. A rare teratoid of the parotid region. *J. Cancer Res.*, **13**, 116.

Wasan, S. M. (1971) Sebaceous lymphadenoma of the parotid gland. *Cancer*, **28**, 1019.

Waterhouse, J. P. (1965) Inflammation in the salivary glands. *Brit. J. oral Surg.*, **3**, 161.

Waterhouse, J. P., and Doniach, I. (1966) Post-mortem prevalence of focal lymphocytic adenitis of the submandibular salivary gland. *J. Path. Bact.*, **91**, 53.

Watson, W. L. (1935) Adenocarcinoma of the oral cavity. *Amer. J. Roentgenol.*, **34**, 53.

Welsh, R. A., and Meyer, A. T. (1968) Mixed tumors of human salivary gland. Histogenesis. *Arch. Path.*, **85**, 433.

Wertheimer, F. W., and Georgen, G. J. (1971) Intraoral acinic cell adenocarcinoma. *Oral Surg.*, **32**, 923.

Willis, R. A. (1967) *Pathology of Tumours*. 4th Edition. London. Butterworth & Co. (Publishers) Ltd.

Wilson, D. F., and MacEntee, M. I. (1974) Papillary cystadenoma of ectopic minor salivary gland origin. *Oral Surg.*, **37**, 915.

Yates, P. O., and Paget, G. E. (1952) A mixed tumour of salivary gland showing bone formation, with a histochemical study of the tumour mucoids. *J. Path. Bact.*, **64**, 881.

Youngs, G. R., and Scheuer, P. J. (1973) Histologically benign mixed parotid tumour with hepatic metastasis. *J. Path.*, **109**, 171.

Zymbal, W. E. (1933) Histologische und experimentelle Untersuchungen über die Geschwülste der Speicheldrüsen. *Beitr. path. Anat.*, **91**, 193.

VIII
CYSTS OF THE ORAL TISSUES

31. Cysts of the Oral Tissues

Cysts of the oral tissues may be listed as follows:

INTRAOSSEOUS CYSTS

Non-odontogenic Developmental (Fissural) Cysts

1. Nasopalatine.
2. Median palatal.
3. Median mandibular.
4. Globulomaxillary.
5. Nasolabial.*

Odontogenic Cysts

1. Developmental.
   (*a*) Primordial.
   (*b*) Dentigerous.
2. Inflammatory.
      Radicular.

Non-epitheliated Bone Cysts

1. Solitary bone cyst.
2. Aneurysmal bone cyst.

CYSTS OF THE SOFT TISSUES

1. Salivary.
2. Gingival.†
3. Dermoid.
4. Branchial.
5. Thyroglossal.
6. Nasolabial (see above).

INTRAOSSEOUS CYSTS

NON-ODONTOGENIC DEVELOPMENTAL (FISSURAL) CYSTS

The lesions often collectively known as fissural cysts have generally been considered to arise from remnants of the epithelium that covered the developing facial processes in embryonic life. Klestadt (1921) postulated the origin of these cysts in epithelium remaining in the lines of closure

---

* This is a soft tissue lesion, but is conveniently considered with the other fissural cysts.
† These cysts are also of odontogenic origin.

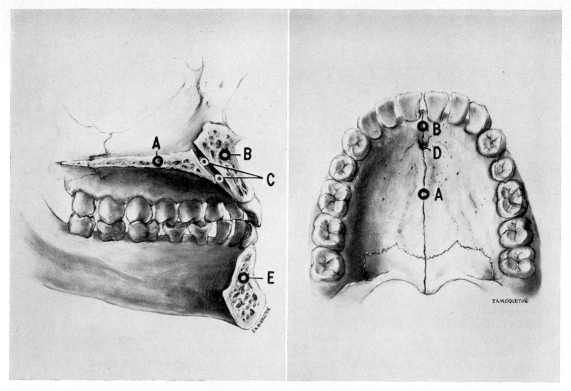

Fig. 116 Diagrammatic location of developmental cysts. A, B. Median palatal cyst. C. Nasopalatine cyst. D. Cyst of palatine papilla. E. Median mandibular cyst.

of the processes and Scott (1955) demonstrated the presence of microcysts in these areas in fetal material. Scott also suggested that in some cases the cysts may be forerunners of cleft palate and harelip. However, Ferenczy (1958) and others have pointed out that not all of these cysts are located in the lines of closure, and thus the term "fissural" cysts may be inaccurate. Indeed, the concept of the fusing of separate processes has itself been called into question. Nevertheless, the lesions form a well defined group, though they are not common, and it is convenient to use this generic name. The locations of those cysts that occur in bone are shown in Fig. 116.

Nasopalatine Cyst

The nasopalatine duct connects the oral and nasal cavities in many mammals, and in the embryo in man. Cyst formation may occur in the epithelial remnants of the ducts that normally persist in adult man, the cyst forming either in the region of the palatine papilla where the duct opens into the oral cavity or higher in the maxilla, in the incisive canal. Microcysts are very frequently present in the fetus, as Scott (1955) has shown, but in post-natal life the frequency of clinically obvious cysts is low. Radiological survey has shown that asymptomatic cysts are present in 1 per cent of persons (Stafne, Austin and Gardner, 1936), but lesions causing symptoms are less common. When they do occur, infection is the usual cause and there is a painful swelling in the palate and sometimes fistula formation with a sinus opening on or near the palatine papilla. Radiologically, there is a well defined translucent area situated apparently between or above

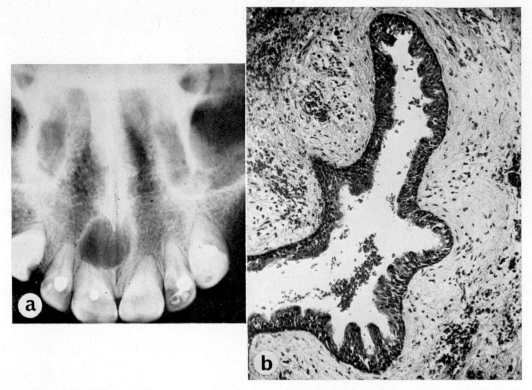

Fig. 117   Nasopalatine cyst. **a,** the cyst occurs in the region of the palatine papilla or in the incisive canal. When in the latter situation, the radiograph shows a heart-shaped translucency. **b,** the cyst lining consists mainly of squamous epithelium but in some areas it is of respiratory type. There is some chronic inflammatory infiltration in the subepithelial connective tissue. A few mucous gland acini were present, at some little distance beneath the cyst lining. $\times$ 120.

the roots of the maxillary central incisors. This may be bilateral and is characteristically heart-shaped, but may be round or oval (Fig. 117a).

The cyst is lined by stratified squamous epithelium, ciliated columnar epithelium or both types of epithelium may be present. Mucous glands are often present in the subepithelial connective tissue (Fig. 117b). Quite large blood vessels and nerve bundles are also often present, and this may be a helpful diagnostic feature.

A good review of the embryology, anatomy and pathology of the incisive canal and naso-palatine ducts is given by Abrams, Howell and Bullock (1963). Hatziotis (1966) gives the literature of clinical reports.

Median Palatal Cyst

The reported cases of the rare median palatal cyst are summarised by Courage, North and Hansen (1974). Some authorities do not consider that this type of cyst exists as an independent entity; they believe that the cysts which have been reported as such are really nasopalatine cysts that have extended, or are placed, posteriorly to an unusual extent. Those who do concede to the lesion the status of an independent entity believe that the cyst forms in epithelial remnants that have persisted in the line of fusion of the palatine processes of the maxilla. Thus these cysts may occur in the midline of the alveolus or the hard palate. However, it would seem very difficult, if

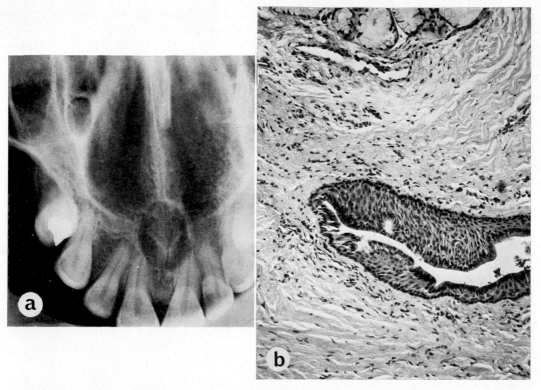

Fig. 118   Median palatal cyst. **a,** these cysts occur in the midline between the lateral palatal processes, either in the hard palate or more anteriorly in the incisor region, as in this example. **b,** the cyst is lined by stratified squamous epithelium. × 120.

not indeed impossible, to distinguish cysts in the former situation from cysts arising from odontogenic epithelium. The more posteriorly placed cysts would seem to be more readily identifiable.

Small cysts are frequently symptomless and discovered only on routine X-ray examination, which shows a well defined area of radiolucency (Fig. 118). A larger lesion can produce a palpable swelling. The cyst is lined by stratified squamous or ciliated columnar epithelium. There may be some chronic inflammatory infiltration in the subepithelial connective tissue.

Median Mandibular Cyst

Cysts that appear in the midline of the mandible have a varied etiology. Some are inflammatory, that is to say, they are radicular or residual cysts (p. 366), and they can usually be readily identified since the associated teeth, if still present, are non-vital and the cyst wall shows evidence of past or present inflammation. Cysts that are non-inflammatory may have formed as developmental anomalies from odontogenic epithelium. Many authorities believe that all cysts in the midline of the mandible fall into one or other of these categories. However, some consider that a non-odontogenic cyst can form in the mandibular midline from epithelial inclusions, but as Robinson (1961) and others have pointed out, since the bones uniting at the mandibular symphysis have their origin deep within mesenchyme, it seems unlikely that epithelial rests would be included. There is, therefore, considerable doubt as to the existence of a median mandibular cyst that is not odontogenic.

Those lesions that have been reported as median mandibular cyst show an area of radiolucency in the mental region (Fig. 119). They are usually lined by stratified squamous epithelium, but cysts lined partly by squamous and partly by columnar epithelium have been reported (Olech, 1957; Albers, 1973). The literature has been summarised by Buchner and Ramon (1974) and White, Lucas and Miller 1975).

Globulomaxillary Cyst

The globulomaxillary cyst occurs at the junction of the globular portion of the medial nasal process and the maxillary process. Generally symptomless, the cyst is usually discovered incidentally. It produces a well defined radiolucency, characteristically shaped like an inverted pear and situated between the roots of the lateral incisor and canine teeth, which are diverged. It is lined by stratified squamous or ciliated columnar epithelium (Fig. 119).

As with the other fissural cysts, there is controversy about the origin of the globulomaxillary cyst. Christ (1970) reviewed the literature and concluded that cysts of this type are odontogenic and do not arise from epithelium derived from the embryonic processes. Little and Jakobsen (1973), however, who describe the embryology of the region very fully, consider that the evidence available at present is inconclusive, and that neither the odontogenic nor the fissural hypothesis is proved or disproved.

Nasolabial Cyst (Nasoalveolar Cyst)

The nasolabial cyst occurs at the junction of the globular, the lateral nasal and the maxillary processes. Since the cyst occurs in soft tissue only, and not in the bone, it is not visible radiographically unless it has caused some resorption of the maxilla by pressure, as occasionally occurs. Clinically, there is a swelling in the nasolabial fold and in the nostril, with flaring of the alae nasi and fullness of the upper lip below the nasal vestibule. The lesion is usually unilateral but bilateral cysts may occur. The cyst is lined by stratified squamous or columnar epithelium (Boone, 1955; Atterbury, Vazirani and McNabb, 1961). A very full review of the literature and analysis of incidence and symptomatology is given by Roed-Petersen (1969).

Behaviour of Fissural Cysts

Fissural cysts are treated by simple enucleation and do not give rise to further trouble. An exceptional case reported by Aisenberg and Inman (1960) records the development of ameloblastoma in a globulomaxillary cyst, but the evidence presented is by no means conclusive.

ODONTOGENIC CYSTS

Cysts arising from odontogenic epithelium are of developmental origin or result from inflammation. The developmental cysts arise in the course of odontogenesis and vary in type according to the stage at which the cystic change has taken place. They may develop in the enamel organ itself, in the reduced enamel epithelium or in remnants of the odontogenic epithelium. The cause of cyst formation during odontogenesis is still unknown.

Fig. 119 **a,** median mandibular cyst. The radiograph shows an area of radiolucency in the mental region. The incisor teeth are vital and there is no evidence of periodontal disease. **b,** the cyst wall is lined by squamous epithelium. There is no inflammation. × 120. **c,** globulomaxillary cyst. There is a radiolucency between the roots of the lateral incisor and canine teeth, characteristically shaped like an inverted pear. **d,** the cyst is lined by squamous and by low columnar epithelium. × 120.

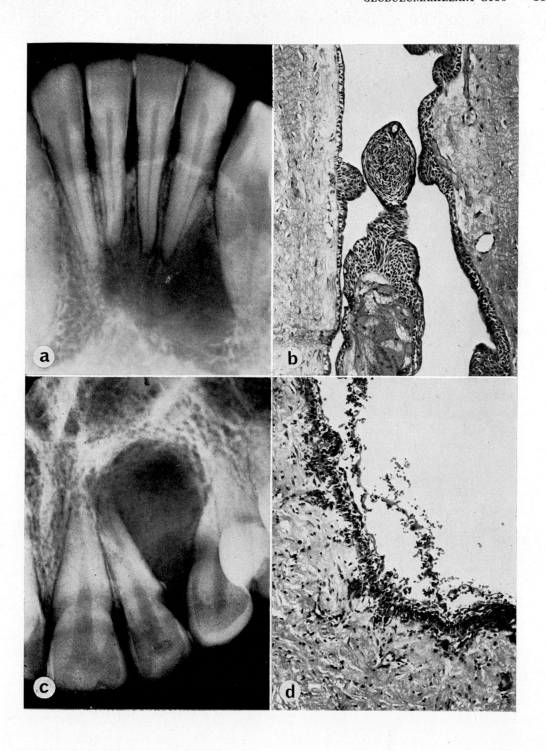

The inflammatory cysts are the result of infection extending from the pulp of a tooth into the periapical tissues.

DEVELOPMENTAL ODONTOGENIC CYSTS

Primordial Cyst (Odontogenic Keratocyst)

Cystic change may occur in the enamel organ at an early stage of its development, before enamel has begun to form. The stellate reticulum then disintegrates to leave a cystic space bounded by the inner and outer enamel epithelium, which becomes stratified squamous in type. Since a tooth cannot now develop, the primordial cyst takes the place of a missing tooth, often the mandibular third molar (Fig. 120). However, the normal complement of teeth may be present if the cyst arises from the primordium of a supernumerary tooth, or from the remnants of the dental lamina itself. Soskolne and Shear (1967) have illustrated very well the latter mode of origin, which is thought to be much the most frequent derivation of these cysts.

Clinical Features

Primordial cysts account for some 3 to 11 per cent of odontogenic cysts (Fickling, 1965; Killey and Kay, 1966; Toller, 1967). They are usually seen in young adults but may present in older patients because growth without bony expansion can continue for a long period, and until expansion does take place the condition is often symptomless. Eventually, the lesion may grow to large dimensions and, as Shear (1960) has noted, cysts in the mandibular third molar region may extend to involve practically the entire ramus of the mandible before bone expansion occurs. Although the eventual expansion of the bone is frequently the only symptom, some patients may complain of pain. This is likely to be due to infection, following perforation of the cortical bone. In Browne's (1970) series, perforation occurred in 41 per cent of cases. The extensive growth and ramification of these cysts, in the course of time, is a characteristic feature; no other jaw cysts enlarge to the extent seen in many of these cases. This propensity for progressive and extensive growth may be due to lytic substances in the cyst wall. Donoff, Harper and Guralnick (1972) have demonstrated collagenase activity in primordial cyst wall; it is absent from other cysts.

Seventy-five to eighty per cent of primordial cysts occur in the mandible and about two-thirds are located in the third molar region. Males and females have been equally affected in most series, although Panders and Hadders (1969) found a 3 to 1 male to female incidence and Radden and Reade (1973) 2 to 1.

Radiologically, there is a well defined area of radiolucency in the jaw (Fig. 120). If the cyst is large and irregular in shape the radiolucency may appear to be multiloculated and hence the appearances may suggest ameloblastoma. In some cases where there is an unerupted tooth, the appearances may be those of dentigerous cyst. Other odontogenic cysts or lesions may also give similar appearances. It is not usually possible, therefore, to arrive at a definitive diagnosis on clinical or radiological grounds alone. A useful adjunct to diagnosis has been worked out by Kramer and Toller (1973). Toller (1970) had shown that the cyst fluid in primordial cyst has a much lower soluble protein content than fluid from any other type of cyst. Kramer and Toller found that a concentration of 4·8 g per 100 ml. or less of soluble protein was suggestive of primordial cyst. In addition, they showed that cytological examination of the cyst fluid gives information as to keratinisation. The use of the two procedures gives helpful supportive evidence for the diagnosis.

Pathology

The cyst wall is composed of fibrous tissue with a lining of squamous epithelium. This is characteristically regular in width and rather narrow, thus contrasting with the epithelium in

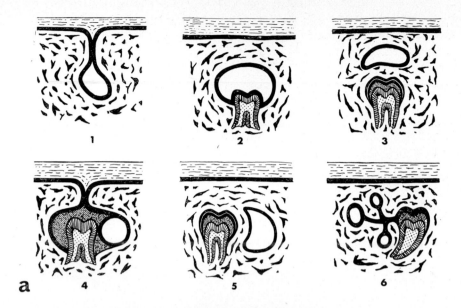

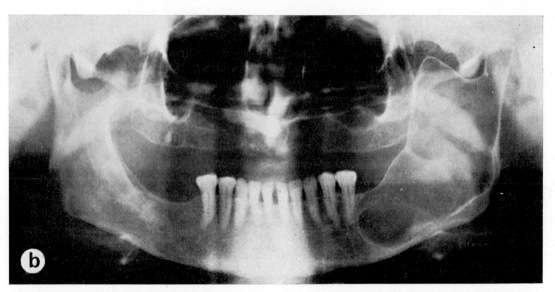

Fig. 120 **a,** diagrammatic representation of the mode of formation of the various types of developmental odontogenic cysts. 1. Cyst formation takes place in the enamel organ at an early stage, before the deposition of enamel. A primordial cyst results. 2. Cyst formation occurs in the enamel organ after the tooth has formed. A dentigerous cyst results. 3. A dentigerous cyst may, in some cases, result from cystic change in remnants of the dental lamina, with subsequent envelopment of the crown of the tooth in the cyst. 4. Cyst formation in the lateral part of the enamel organ produces a lateral dentigerous cyst. 5. A laterally situated cyst may also arise from cyst formation in epithelial rests. 6. Multiloculated cyst arising from cystification in buds forming from the enamel organ. (After Thoma and Goldman.) **b,** radiograph of primordial cyst. The lesion appears as a well defined multilocular radiolucency, extensively involving the body and ascending ramus of the mandible.

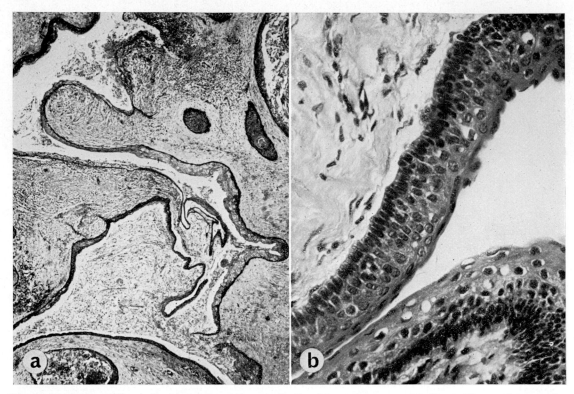

Fig. 121   Primordial cyst (keratocyst). **a,** the cyst is lined by squamous epithelium. The cavity contains keratin scales. × 30. **b,** the epithelium forms a layer of even width, with some vacuolation of the spinous cells and prominent basal cells. There is keratinisation. × 300.

infected dentigerous and radicular cysts, especially the latter, in which it frequently varies very considerably in width from field to field. Another rather characteristic feature is the wavy or folded appearance of the cyst lining. The stratum spinosum is usually no thicker than 6 to 9 cell rows; the cells often show vacuolation. The basal layer generally shows a very regular appearance without rete processes but sometimes the cells proliferate to form bud-like swellings. The basal cells themselves are columnar or cubical, and as the nuclei stain quite intensely the basal layer stands out distinctly. Some degree of keratinisation is nearly always present. There may be a layer of keratin, which is usually quite narrow; sometimes there is parakeratosis. Occasionally, keratin scales may fill the cyst cavity (Fig. 121). Mucous metaplasia, which is not uncommon in radicular and dentigerous cysts, is rare in the primordial cyst (Browne, 1972).

Groups of epithelial cells may be present, at some little distance from the main epithelial lining of the cyst. These cells are of odontogenic character and they may show microcystic change. The subepithelial connective tissue consists of rather thin and irregular collagen bundles; these contrast with the thick, well organised collagenous tissues of radicular and other cysts. As a result, the epithelium frequently separates from the underlying tissue in the preparation of sections. This artefactual cleavage indicates the weak attachment that exists naturally. There is generally no evidence of inflammation, but should the cyst have established a connection with the oral cavity this is present. Cholesterol clefts may then be found, as in radicular cysts, as may be hyaline bodies (p. 372) in the epithelium.

A striking feature of the primordial cyst is its propensity for recurrence. This has been brought out in all recent case reports, such as those of Pindborg and Hansen (1963), Fickling (1965), Toller (1967), Bramley and Browne (1967), Rud and Pindborg (1969) and Panders and Hadders (1969). The recurrence rate has varied widely, from around 6 to 60 per cent. Various suggestions have been made to account for this behaviour. One quite likely explanation for recurrence is the thin and comparatively delicate nature of the cyst wall, which might well result in portions being left behind during enucleation operations. Daughter or satellite cysts also would appear to occur quite frequently, possibly because adjacent areas of dental lamina undergo cystic change or, a less likely explanation, because multicystic change occurs in the enamel organ. Such daughter cysts might easily remain in the jaw after removal of the main cyst. In a recent series of 103 cysts, Payne (1972) found microcysts in the main cyst wall in 18 per cent of primordial cysts that had recurred, but in only 4 per cent of non-recurrent cysts. Browne (1971) did not find such associations; however, his material of recurrent cysts was smaller. It is also of interest to note that the epithelium of primordial cysts is much more active than that of other types of odontogenic cysts, as evidenced by mitotic counts (Main, 1970; Browne, 1971) or by thymidine uptake in cyst lining explants (Toller, 1971).

Pathogenesis

The term *odontogenic keratocyst*, widely used as a synonym for the primordial cyst, was introduced by Philipsen (1956) and Pindborg and Hansen (1963), these authors considering that a variety of cysts, including primordial, dentigerous, radicular and residual varieties, could show keratinisation. However, more recently it has been agreed that radicular cysts rarely keratinise (Hansen, 1967; Hjørting-Hansen, Andreasen and Robinson, 1969) and that those dentigerous cysts that have a keratinised lining occur mainly in the third molar region. In this area, as Shear (1960) has pointed out, cysts arising from extensions of the dental lamina might well envelop a third molar and assume the radiographic appearance of a dentigerous cyst. In Browne's (1970) series, also, nearly all the cysts that appeared radiologically as dentigerous cysts were shown to have a layer of fibrous tissue between the cyst cavity and the associated tooth. However, there would seem to occur at least some cysts of dentigerous type, developing from the dental follicle, that show the histological appearances described in the foregoing paragraphs. Because of the frequent presence of microcysts between the oral epithelium and the cysts proper, and for other reasons, Stoelinga and colleagues (1973, 1975) have suggested that the cysts originate from the basal layer of the oral epithleium.

Some authorities restrict the term *primordial* to those cysts that develop in place of a tooth, either one of the normal series or a supernumerary, but the World Health Organisation nomenclature uses the term primordial cyst to include all cysts that show the characteristic histology, and gives *keratocyst* as an alternative term. It seems likely that these cysts have a varied origin—from tooth germ, supernumerary tooth germ or from remnants of dental lamina. It has also been suggested that they may be derived from the oral mucosa (Stoelinga and Peters, 1973). However this may be, they form a distinctive clinicopathological entity. Their characteristic histology is never seen in radicular cysts or in residual cysts, using the latter term to denote radicular cysts that remain in the jaw after extraction of the associated tooth. It is seen in a minority only of dentigerous cysts, and this minority at least in part consists of cysts that are dentigerous only by reason of teeth becoming involved in an adjacent cyst of primordial origin.

Behaviour

The pronounced tendency to recurrence of primordial cysts has already been mentioned. Bramley (1974) makes the point that results in the future should be better than they have been to date because there is now a much greater appreciation of the nature and behaviour of these cysts, and modern operative procedures take this into account.

Toller (1967) suggested that carcinomatous change in primordial cysts, although rare, occurred more frequently than in other odontogenic cysts. This view awaits substantiation.

Dentigerous Cyst

The occurrence of cystic change in the enamel organ at a period prior to the deposition of enamel leads to the formation of a primordial cyst, as has been seen. More frequently, however, this change does not take place until the crown of the tooth has been formed. By this time, the enamel organ has become reduced to the few layers of epithelial cells that cover the crown of the tooth prior to eruption. The accumulation of fluid in these layers of epithelium, or between the epithelium and the crown of the tooth itself, results in the formation of a cyst into which the crown of the tooth protrudes, or which may be situated to one side of the crown. Hence a cyst of this type can be described as dentigerous. The term "follicular cyst" has also been used, since the cyst develops in connection with the dental follicle.

An intermediate stage between the primordial cyst and the dentigerous cyst as just described appears to be rare. That is to say, cyst formation in the enamel organ occurs either before the formation of the tooth, or after the enamel has been completely formed. As Robinson (1945) pointed out, if cyst formation occurred in the enamel organ while amelogenesis was still proceeding, there would be abnormalities of enamel formation. But in fact, the teeth in most dentigerous cysts have well formed crowns, indicating that amelogenesis has not been significantly interfered with.

Although it is generally accepted that most dentigerous cysts develop in the way just described, it is clear that cysts that do not originate in the enamel organ may also present as dentigerous cysts. As mentioned previously, this appears to occur in the case of some primordial cysts, which may grow to envelop a neighbouring tooth and thus become, literally, dentigerous. Similarly, a permanent tooth may "erupt" into a radicular cyst at the apex of its deciduous predecessor. Possibly as a result of extrafollicular development, a cyst may be situated at one side of a tooth rather than superficially to the crown. Cysts of this type are termed *lateral periodontal cysts*. However, some such cysts may be of inflammatory origin, representing radicular cysts in a lateral rather than apical position.

Clinical Features

Dentigerous cysts are generally detected in children or adolescents, though sometimes they are found in adults. Only permanent teeth are affected, particularly the mandibular third molar and the maxillary canine. There is progressive enlargement of the jaw, though this is generally painless. A considerable degree of deformity may result, as the lesion is capable of much enlargement with concomitant destruction of the bone, displacement of adjacent teeth and resorption of their roots as a result of pressure. Occasionally, very small cysts are found on teeth just about to erupt. These are termed *eruption cysts* and in some cases may be formed in the same way as dentigerous cysts, or they may form from epithelial remnants in the gingiva. They are fully described by Seward (1973).

Radiological examination of a dentigerous cyst shows a well defined translucency associated with the crown of an impacted or unerupted tooth. The radiolucency is generally unilocular, but a multilocular effect may be present when the cyst is of irregular shape. However, the cyst cavity itself is nearly always unicameral (Fig. 122a, b).

Pathology

Large cysts which have caused much expansion and thinning of the bone are often treated by marsupialisation, following which the associated tooth erupts and the cavity gradually closes,

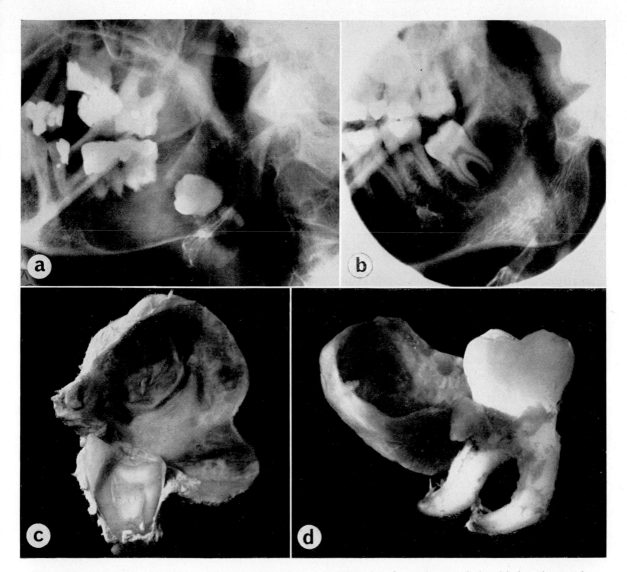

Fig. 122   Dentigerous cyst. **a,** this large cyst in the mandible has formed around the third molar tooth. **b,** in this case the cyst has formed laterally, on the distal side of the third molar tooth. **c,** gross specimen of dentigerous cyst. The cyst sac envelops the crown of the tooth. × 2. **d,** lateral dentigerous cyst situated at the side of the crown of the tooth. × 3.

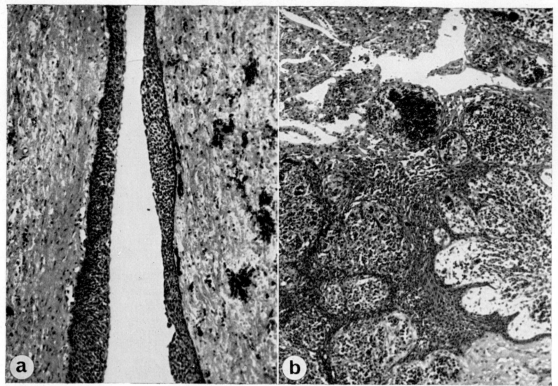

Fig 123   Wall of dentigerous cyst. **a,** in an area free from inflammation the squamous epithelial lining is relatively thin and quite regular × 80. **b,** another area from the same cyst, showing how the epithelial lining proliferates in an inflamed area. × 80.

with new bone formation. In these cases a portion of cyst lining only is generally available for pathological examination. Smaller lesions, however, are frequently excised completely, when the specimen available for examination consists of a tooth with a relatively thick walled cyst surrounding the crown or attached to it (Fig. 122c, d). The cyst wall should be carefully examined for localised thickenings or ingrowths, since it is thought that in some cases these may represent ameloblastomatous change.

The cyst contents consist of clear yellowish fluid, in which cholesterol crystals may be present, or purulent material if infection has occurred.

Dentigerous cysts are lined by stratified squamous epithelium, generally in a uniformly thin layer, a few cells in depth. If the cyst is sectioned with the tooth *in situ*, the cyst lining is seen to be continuous with the reduced enamel epithelium covering the crown. Occasionally the epithelium is cornified, with keratin scales in the cyst cavity. Mucous cells are sometimes present, interspersed amongst the squamous cells. Rarely, the lining may consist of ciliated columnar epithelium (Gorlin, 1957; Shear, 1960; Marsland and Browne, 1965; Small, 1967). Hyaline bodies may be seen. These are described in more detail below, in connection with radicular cysts.

In the subepithelial connective tissue islands of odontogenic epithelium are occasionally seen and sebaceous epithelium has been noted by Gorlin (1957) and Spouge (1966). Gorlin has also found lymphoid follicles with germinal centres in the walls of cysts.

No evidence of inflammation is seen in uncomplicated cysts (Fig. 123a), but where communication with the oral cavity has been established by incision or extraction of teeth chronic inflammatory infiltration is evident in the subepithelial connective tissue. If this has been of some duration the epithelial lining proliferates and shows prolongations like rete pegs extending into the subjacent connective tissue (Fig. 123b). Cholesterol clefts may be present in the cyst wall. Thus the infected dentigerous cyst shows appearances similar to those of the radicular cyst and microscopic differentiation between the two lesions is not possible.

Behaviour

It is widely held that ameloblastomas frequently arise in dentigerous cysts. This question is discussed in detail elsewhere (p. 48). Dentigerous cysts can be adequately treated by complete excision and curettage, or by marsupialisation. Recurrence is a possibility if some epithelium remains.

Multilocular Cysts

Most odontogenic cysts are unicameral lesions. Rarely, they may be multilocular, due possibly to cyst formation occurring in several adjacent tooth germs or to the formation of buds on a single enamel organ, with cystification occurring in the buds.

Multilocular cysts occur particularly in the mandibular third molar region and may form quite extensive lesions extending into the ramus of the mandible.

A tooth may or may not be present in this type of cyst according to the stage of odontogenesis at which cyst formation has occurred. The loculi in the mutilocular cyst may be completely separate, but in some cases the septa are partial.

Multiple Cysts

Odontogenic cysts generally occur as solitary lesions. Occasionally, however, more than one cyst may be present, and while this may not be due to any unusual circumstances, it is nevertheless important to consider the possibility of the basal cell carcinoma and jaw cyst syndrome, described in the following section. Multiple cysts have also been encountered in association with Marfan's syndrome (Smith, 1968; Oatis, Burch and Samuels, 1971).

Multiple Cysts and Basal Cell Carcinoma

The association of multiple cysts of the jaws with basal cell carcinoma was first emphasised by Binkley and Johnson (1951), though the syndrome was apparently first noticed by Jarisch (1894) and cases had been reported by Nomland (1932) and Straith (1939). It has since become clear, however, following Gorlin and Goltz's (1960) definitive description, that many other abnormalities can occur in what is now often referred to as the multiple naevoid basal cell carcinoma and jaw cyst syndrome (Gross, 1953; Boyer and Martin, 1958; Howell and Caro, 1959; Thoma, 1959; McKelvey, Albright and Prazak, 1960; Cawson and Kerr, 1964; Rayne, 1971; and others).

The condition appears in childhood and a family history is often obtained. The cystic lesions occur throughout the jaws, in close proximity to the teeth, giving rise to symptoms such as pain, swelling of the jaws or rupture with intraoral discharge in about half the cases. New cysts often continue to form and give rise to symptoms throughout life (Howell, Anderson and McClendon, 1966). Varying in size from millimetres to several centimetres in diameter, the cysts are unilocular or multilocular and are lined by squamous epithelium which may or may not form a layer of keratin, the general appearances being very similar to those of the primordial cyst. The epithelium generally forms a regular layer, though in some cases budding may be seen and in one instance (Gorlin, Yunis and Tuna, 1963) it was thought that an early ameloblastoma had formed. Maddox and colleagues (1964) found a typical ameloblastoma in one of their patients, but these cases seem to be exceptional. Some authors have described the cysts as dental or dentigerous, because of their proximity to the teeth, but it is clear that such descriptions indicate only an anatomical relationship. Moreover, cysts can occur in regions of the jaw that are not tooth-bearing or that do not normally contain odontogenic epithelium (Howell and colleagues, 1967). But even in such areas there may occur extensions of dental lamina, so that the primordial nature of the cysts need not be discounted.

The basal cell carcinomas are multiple and occur mostly on the face, trunk and arms, though the skin anywhere may be affected. Cystic, pigmented, cribriform and trichoepitheliomatous varieties occur. The lesions generally appear about the time of puberty and gradually increase in number and size. Thus, in younger patients, and even occasionally in some older ones, basal cell carcinomas may not yet have appeared, and this must be kept in mind in all cases of multiple jaw cysts.

Gorlin and colleagues (1963, 1965) have made careful analyses of the literature and show that of the lesions that occur in addition to the multiple jaw cysts and basal cell tumours, skeletal abnormalities and hyporesponsiveness to parathormone are the commonest. The skeletal anomalies include bifurcation, synostosis and partial agenesis of the ribs and a rather characteristic facies with frontal and parietal bossing, broadness of the nasal root and a mild degree of mandibular prognathism. The many other anomalies that may occur include palmar and plantar dyskeratosis, simple skin cysts and fibrous tumours, neurological conditions including mental retardation, hydrocephalus, calcification of the falx cerebri and medulloblastoma, eye anomalies, ovarian fibroma and other conditions.

The syndrome is transmitted as an autosomal dominant trait. Chromosome anomalies have been found in some cases but not in others (Yunis and Gorlin, 1963; Schønning and Visfeldt, 1964; Shear and Wilton, 1968).

INFLAMMATORY ODONTOGENIC CYSTS

Radicular Cyst

(Dental cyst, apical cyst, periodontal cyst)

This is the commonest of all cysts of odontogenic origin and indeed of all cysts of the oral region. It is the result of inflammation and is one of the end-results of dental caries.

When a carious lesion extends through the enamel and dentine of a tooth to the pulp, that tissue becomes inflamed. Extension of the inflammation by the root canal to the apical foramen and so into the periapical tissues is a frequent occurrence, and in these tissues at the root of the tooth there forms a localised mass of chronic inflammatory granulation tissue, the *apical granuloma*. The stimulus of inflammation causes the proliferation of the epithelial rests that are normally

Fig. 124   The apical granuloma, apical abscess and radicular cyst. **a,** two teeth *in situ* in the mandible, showing destruction of the crowns by caries. Infection had reached the periapical tissue of one tooth and here the bone has been resorbed, with replacement by a circumscribed chronic inflammatory mass, the apical granuloma. × 9. **b,** in this case an abscess has formed at the roots of a tooth. The tooth itself has a cavity in the crown, from which infection has extended into the pulp and thence to the periapical tissues. × 4. **c,** carious root, with attached radicular cyst. Cholesterol clefts are seen in the amorphous cyst contents. × 7·5. **d,** radiograph of radicular cyst. The lesion appears as a circumscribed radiolucency with a well defined outline at the apex of a tooth root.

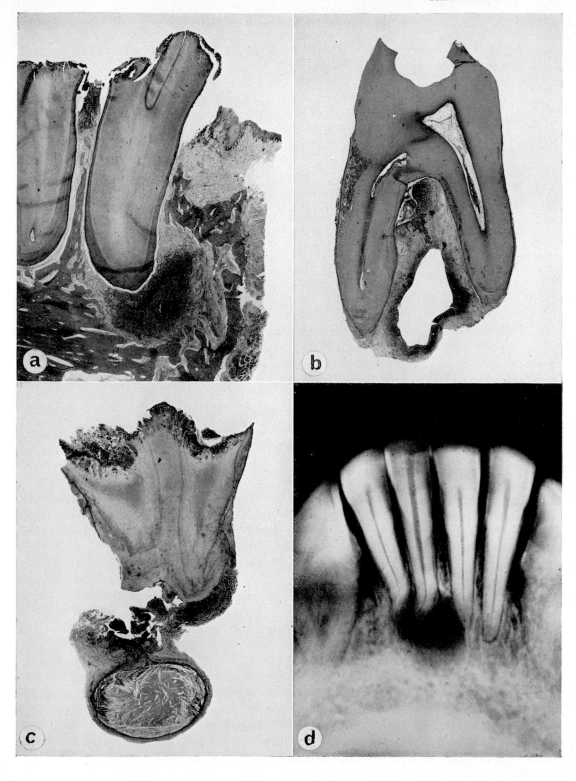

present around the roots of the teeth, and as a result strands of epithelium penetrate into the granuloma. Subsequently, cystification occurs in the epithelium so that ultimately the granuloma at the apex of the tooth becomes a cyst lined by squamous epithelium. Alternatively, chronic abscess formation occurs and the proliferating epithelium lines the abscess cavity (Main, 1970; Ten Cate, 1972; Summers, 1974).

Cyst formation is not an invariable sequel of apical granuloma, for the inflammatory lesion may remain static for long periods. Acute inflammatory exacerbations may also occur, with suppuration and spread of infection (Fig. 124a, b, c).

Clinical Features

Though the pulpitis that is the initial inflammatory process ultimately leading to the formation of a radicular cyst is often a painful condition, the cyst itself is very frequently symptomless. By the time the cyst has formed the pulp has already been dead for a considerable period. Thus, though a history of previous pain in connection with the affected tooth can be obtained, there is a subsequent symptom-free period and the presence of a cyst is often detected only on routine radiography. The tooth with which the cyst is associated is of course non-vital and it shows evidence of caries.

The majority of radicular cysts do not grow to large dimensions. In most cases there is very little, if any, expansion of the jaw. Unlike dentigerous cysts, which are found particularly in children and adolescents and affect especially certain teeth, radicular cysts may occur at any age and in connection with any tooth. *Residual cysts* are common. These are radicular cysts that have remained in the jaw, the related tooth having been extracted at some previous time. *Multiple cysts* occasionally occur in the same patient (Knight and Manley, 1955).

Radiographic evidence of extension of inflammation from the pulp into the periapical tissues is indicated by the presence of an area of translucency at the root apex. This is often well circumscribed, though in some cases it merges gradually into the surrounding normal bone (Fig. 124d). Whether or not cyst formation has taken place in the infected area at the apex cannot be determined from the radiographic appearance alone.

Pathology

In the precystic stages of periapical inflammation it may be possible to retain the affected tooth by apicectomy and root canal therapy. That is to say, the apex is excised, together with the adjacent infected periapical area, and a filling material is placed in the pulp cavity and root canal. The specimen in such cases consists of the apical end of the root of the tooth, with a small velvety pink nodule of perhaps 2 to 3 mm diameter attached to the tip. In other cases the tooth is extracted, and the whole tooth is submitted for examination, with the granuloma adherent to the apex. When cyst formation has taken place the tooth is extracted and the cyst removed. Again, the specimen may consist of the tooth with the cyst adherent to the apex or the tooth may have been extracted previously, and the cyst alone submitted for examination. Cysts are generally between 0·5 to 1·5 cm in diameter, with walls of variable thickness. The lining may be smooth or roughened and the contents consist of fluid that may shimmer owing to its cholesterol content, or of rather thick, cheesy material.

Microscopically, the precystic apical granuloma consists of a localised area of inflammatory infiltration at the apex of the tooth (Fig. 125a). At first this is small, but with the gradual increase in size of the focus there is concomitant resorption of alveolar bone. In the early stages there is both acute and chronic inflammatory infiltration and abscess formation may follow rapidly, with discharge of pus through the root canal of the tooth or through a sinus. Often, however, the inflammation remains in a chronic stage for long periods and it is during this stage that epithelial proliferation occurs. Serial sections of granulomas reveal the presence of epithelium in a high

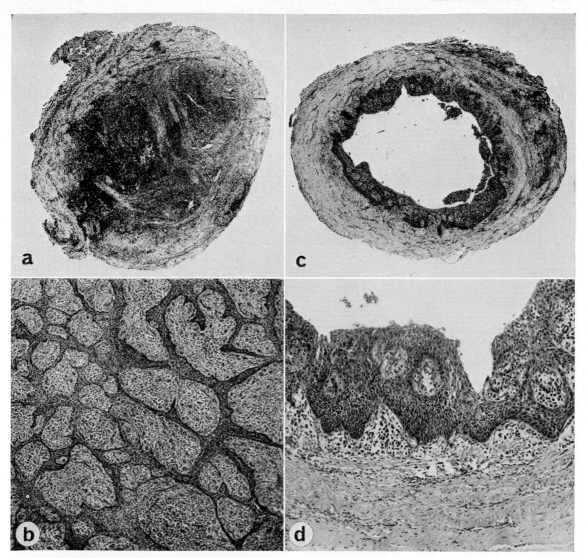

Fig. 125   **a,** apical granuloma. The lesion forms a circumscribed chronic inflammatory mass. × 15. **b,** higher magnification, showing permeation by a network of epithelial strands. × 40. **c,** radicular cyst. The cyst wall consists of fibrous tissue with a lining of squamous epithelium. A cyst of this type may result from cyst formation in the epithelium permeating a granuloma such as that shown in **b,** or epithelial rests may proliferate and line an abscess cavity like that shown in Fig. 106 **b.** × 15. **d,** radicular cyst wall. Higher magnification of the cyst in **c,** showing the squamous epithelial lining forming a relatively thick and irregular layer. Chronic inflammatory infiltration is a noticeable feature. × 80.

proportion of lesions, though it may not be detected in the usual one or two sections of routine work. It is generally accepted that the epithelium is derived from the epithelial rests of Malassez, though it is possible that in some cases it may come from the lining epithelium of the oral cavity by way of a sinus or a periodontal pocket (Ten Cate, 1972; Valderhaug, 1972). Rarely, it may be derived from the maxillary sinus in cases of granulomas of upper teeth that have extended to the sinus wall.

As the epithelium proliferates it permeates the granuloma in anastomosing cords, with the

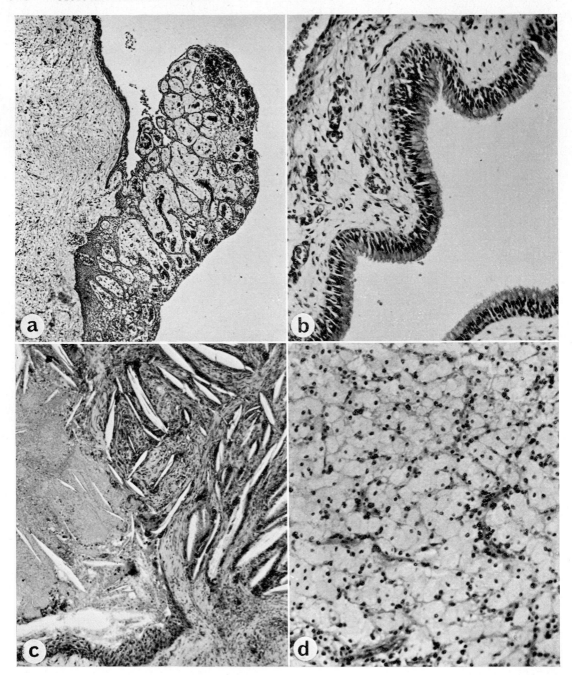

Fig. 126   **a,** another example of epithelial proliferation in the wall of a radicular cyst. Often, as here, the epithelial lining may be thin and compressed over large areas of the cyst wall, with other areas in which it proliferates and forms imterlacing strands in the connective tissue. × 30. **b,** rarely, in the case of maxillary radicular cysts, the lining may consist of columnar epithelium. × 200. **c,** cholesterol is frequently present in radicular cysts. The clefts can be seen both in the inspissated cyst contents and in the cyst wall, where foreign body giant cells are also often present. × 80. **d,** collections of foam cells are often seen, both in granulomas and in cyst walls. × 200.

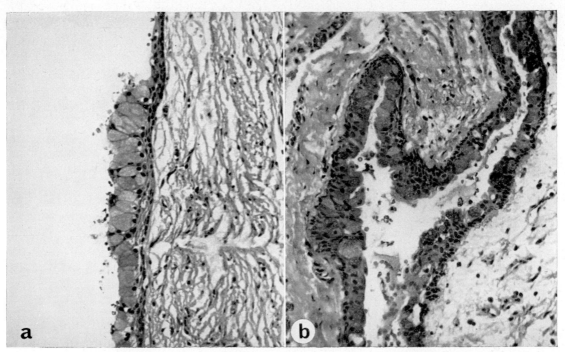

Fig. 127   **a, b,** mucous metaplasia in the lining of radicular cysts. The mucous cells may be scanty or they may occur in small groups or even, uncommonly, form much of the entire lining. × 200.

chronically inflamed connective tissue between the strands (Fig. 125b). Foam cells as well as lymphocytes and plasma cells are frequently seen and cholesterol clefts are often present, with foreign body giant cells in relation to them. Collagen fibres are laid down progressively around the granuloma as it ages, and in some cases where the tooth has been extracted or root canal therapy carried out, the whole lesion may heal by fibrosis.

However, in many cases, as has been seen, cyst formation occurs in the granuloma. The cyst is lined by squamous epithelium, but unlike the thin, regular layer in most uninfected dentigerous cysts, here the epithelium tends to form a relatively thick, irregular layer, with many processes penetrating into the underlying connective tissue. There is usually well marked chronic inflammatory infiltration of the cyst wall, and often it is heavy (Fig. 125c, d). The infiltration is present mainly in the subepithelial connective tissue but often it extends also into the epithelium, which shows oedema. Frequently the epithelial lining of the cyst is incomplete, with granulation tissue forming the cyst wall in the denuded areas. Dilated capillaries are often prominent in the granulation tissue and the epithelium tends to form interlacing cribriform patterns around them (Fig. 126a). In older cysts in which acute or subacute exacerbations of inflammation have become infrequent, the epithelial lining gradually becomes reduced in thickness and more regular, and thick acellular bands of collagen form in the subepithelial connective tissue. As noted, cysts may, rarely, be lined by columnar epithelium (Fig. 126b).

As in the apical granuloma, cholesterol clefts are frequently a very noticeable feature. They may be present in large numbers, usually in the subepithelial connective tissue but sometimes also in the inspissated contents of the cyst cavity. Foreign body giant cells are often seen close to the cholesterol clefts. Shear (1963) has found that the giant cells in some 6 per cent of cysts contain asteroid bodies of the type described by Cunningham (1951). He has also found Russell bodies in 50 per cent of cysts. Foam cells are often present in the cyst wall and trabeculae of woven bone and small foci of amorphous calcification are also quite often found (Fig. 126c, d).

Mucous cells may occur amongst the squamous cells of the cyst lining, in variable numbers (Fig. 127). Sometimes only a few are present but in other cases much of the lining epithelium may be mucus-secreting. Mucous cells occur as frequently in mandibular as in maxillary cysts, the incidence being 22 per cent in Hodson's (1956) series of odontogenic cysts of various types. The presence of these cells equally in mandibular cysts suggests that they arise by metaplasia rather than that they originate from the maxillary sinus, as might be thought were they to occur in the upper jaw alone. Browne (1972) has found that the incidence of mucous cells increases with increasing age of the patient. He gives a full account of this and other metaplastic changes.

Dewey (1918) noted the occurrence of hyaline bodies in the epithelium of radicular cysts and Rushton (1955) described these structures in more detail, finding them in about 4 per cent of radicular and dentigerous cysts. They generally occur in the epithelium lining the cyst, distributed here and there in patchy manner, but they may also be seen in the cyst cavity and occasionally in the connective tissue of the cyst wall. The bodies measure up to about 0·1 mm in length and are linear, straight or curved, often in a hairpin-like shape, and appear to fracture readily. Sometimes they are plate-like, or they may form irregular, circular or polycyclic agglomerations with a clear outer layer arranged around a core of granular material (Fig. 128). The clear material is eosinophilic, gives a positive Prussian blue reaction and stains selectively with aldehyde fuchsin. Rushton considered that it resembled the keratinised layer of the epithelial attachment of a tooth. The granular material enclosed by the clear outer layer is readily stained with most dyes but not aldehyde fuchsin, and it is not Prussian blue-positive. It might be degenerating cellular material. Molyneux (1957) thought that it could be the precursor of the hyaline bodies. Shear (1961) has investigated the histochemistry of the bodies and concludes that they are probably a form of keratin that contains cystine. It is not certain that the granular material contains keratohyalin, but it would seem to be related in some way to the clear bodies, since the association is so constant. Wertheimer, Fullmer and Hansen (1962) also find some histochemical similarities to keratin, but the correspondence is not complete. On the other hand, Medak and Weinmann (1960) suggested that the hyaline bodies may be cotton fibres, implanted at the time of an earlier surgical procedure. The absence of birefringence might be due to the action of oral organisms. But, as Shear points out, hyaline bodies have not been seen in cysts elsewhere in the body and there is no foreign body reaction, such as the presence of cotton fibres in the tissues elicits.

More recently, Bouyssou and Guilhem (1965) have concluded that the hyaline bodies are thrombi occurring in the venules of the connective tissue which have become varicose and encircled and strangled by epithelial "cuffs." The thrombi then shrink centrifugally and undergo splitting, or they may calcify. The large quantity of —SH and —S—S— groups in erythrocytes probably accounts for the reactions in the hyaline bodies which have been attributed by others to keratin. Dent and Wertheimer (1967) showed that the bodies react to several haemoglobin and iron stains but point out that histochemical reactions for haemoglobin are not specific. However, Sedano and Gorlin (1968) concur in the haematogenous origin of the bodies, on histochemical grounds. These findings are of interest in view of Hodson's (1966) demonstration that the dental cuticle reacts like denatured haemoglobin.

Another view, put forward by Morgan and Johnson (1974) and based on histochemistry and ultrastructure, is that the hyaline bodies are a secretory product of the epithelium which is deposited on particulate matter such as cell debris or cholesterol crystals. This process might be considered analogous to the way in which dental cuticle is deposited on the unerupted portions of enamel surfaces. Jensen and Erickson (1974) have also investigated the ultrastructure of the hyaline

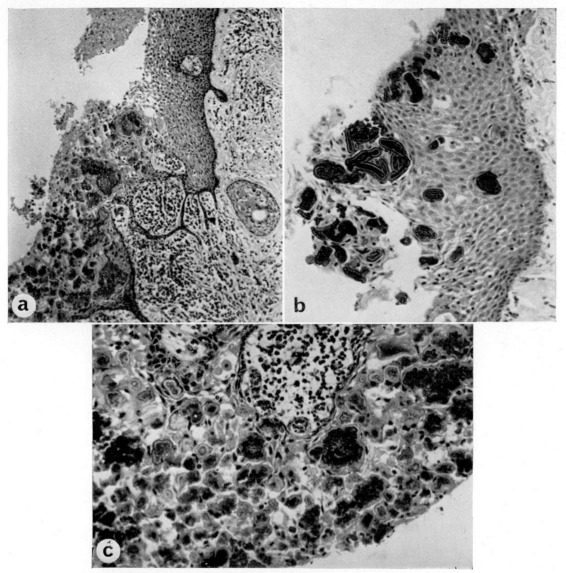

Fig. 128   Hyaline bodies in the epithelium of radicular cysts. **a,** the bodies form irregular agglomerations with a clear outer layer and an inner core of granular material. × 80. **b,** in some cases the bodies are linear and straight, curved or hairpin-shaped. × 200. **c,** higher magnification of a field from the same specimen as in **a.** × 200.

bodies and conclude that although it cannot be determined which of the two major hypotheses— epithelial cell production or haematogenous origin—is likely to be correct, the bodies are not composed of keratin.

The mechanisms controlling the growth of radicular cysts have been investigated by a number of workers. Toller (1967, 1970) has shown that there is a difference in osmolality between cyst fluid and plasma, creating an expansile hydrostatic force. The proteins in cyst fluid have been fully investigated by Skaug (1973, 1974) and Skaug and Hofstadt (1973). In addition to the pressure from within, there is evidence to indicate a diminution of resistance from without.

Harris and colleagues (1973) have shown that explants of radicular cysts in tissue culture with mouse calvaria resorbed the bone, and that the resorption factor is possibly a prostaglandin.

NON-EPITHELIATED BONE CYSTS

Solitary Bone Cyst

(Traumatic cyst, haemorrhagic cyst)

Though solitary bone cysts occur most often in the humerus and other long bones they are seen from time to time in the mandible.

Clinical Features

As is the case with this lesion in other bones, jaw lesions occur particularly in children and adolescents. There is often a history of trauma to the jaw though this is not always recent. The condition is generally painless and may be discovered by the patient only if there is swelling of the jaw. However, expansion of the bone is not common in the earlier stages and the lesion is frequently symptomless, being discovered only on routine radiological examination.

Males are affected more often than females. The lesion occurs usually in the subapical region of the posterior portion of the mandible, from the canine area to the ramus. This is the area in which is situated the marrow cavity in young persons. The incisor region may also be affected, though less frequently. The lesion occurs rarely in the maxilla.

Radiologically, there is a well defined translucency that has a very characteristic scalloped appearance where it extends between the roots of teeth (Fig. 129a).

Pathology

Solitary bone cysts of the jaw are very rarely obtained as complete lesions, since surgical intervention is normally undertaken on the basis of the clinical and radiological features to obtain a biopsy specimen. When the surgeon enters the lesion for this purpose he finds a space in the bone that contains a little clear or perhaps blood-stained fluid only, and which is lined by a very thin connective tissue membrane. There is no dissectable cyst sac. If the cavity is posterior to the mental foramen the mandibular vessels and nerve may be found freely exposed within it. These findings being sufficiently characteristic of solitary bone cyst the cavity is evacuated and packed, or curetted. Accordingly, the material available for pathological examination comprises simply a mass of bone fragments, blood clot and small scraps of soft tissue.

There is little to note on microscopic examination other than the presence of some bone fragments with a thin connective tissue lining that may be no more than a few cells in thickness (Fig. 129b). Haemosiderin may be present in the connective tissue. Fragments of fibrin with red cells and perhaps some multinucleated giant cells in its meshes, are to be noted.

Specimens obtained with the cyst intact as in Waldron's (1954) case, show a space in the bone containing some clear yellowish or blood-stained fluid and lined by a thin layer of connective tissue. The lining may be rather more abundant in some areas, and consist of granulation tissue. The surrounding bone may show evidence of osteoclastic resorption and may be more vascular than normal.

Pathogenesis

The cause and mode of formation of solitary bone cyst are still unknown. It is commonly believed that there is a relationship to trauma, but it is not clear how trauma produces a cyst, or why cysts are not associated at least with some traumatic fractures if trauma is the cause. Pommer (1919) considered that trauma insufficient to cause a fracture produced intramedullary haemorrhage. Subsequent resorption of the clot, instead of organisation, leaves a space in the bone,

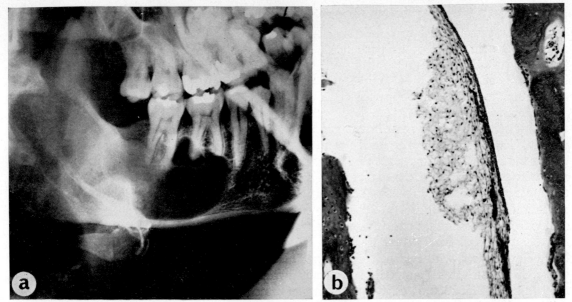

Fig. 129   Solitary bone cyst in a man of 25 years. There had been some pain, though not severe, in the mandible for a few weeks. There was no history of trauma. **a,** the radiograph shows a well defined area of radiolucency in the posterior region of the right side of the mandible, extending upwards into the interdental space between the molar teeth. **b,** the cavity was curetted; it contained only a little blood and some fine strands of tissue. Microscopically, the cyst wall consists of bone, with a thin lining of connective tissue. × 80.

which continues to enlarge because of increased intracystic pressure resulting from deficient venous drainage (Blum, 1932; Olech, Sicher and Weinmann, 1951). Whinery (1955), however, adduced arguments to show that increased pressure in these cysts is most unlikely and notes, as do other authors, that though a history of trauma can often be obtained its time of incidence does not always agree with the estimated duration of the cyst.

Other theories of origin include cystic degeneration in giant cell or other tumours or in areas of low-grade infection, disturbed calcium metabolism and ischaemic marrow necrosis, but there is little positive evidence to support them. Jaffe (1953) considers that the traumatic theory is untenable for jaw cysts as well as for cysts in other bones, particularly when the frequency with which the mandible is subjected to trauma is considered. He suggests that cysts in all locations represent the results of an aberration in the development and growth of the local osseous tissue. Howe (1965) gives a very full discussion of the theories of pathogenesis and a review of the literature. More recent cases are collated by Huebner and Turlington (1971) and Hansen, Sapone and Sproat (1974) report on a series of 66 cases.

Behaviour

Jaffe (1958) has divided the solitary bone cysts of the long bones into two groups, active and latent. Active cysts are those which extend to the epiphyseal cartilage plate and are to be regarded as still having growth potentialities. Latent cysts are those that have moved away from the plate. Between the cyst and the plate there is now a reconstructed area of shaft and growth activity has ceased. The cyst may remain in this latent state for years.

The solitary bone cyst of the mandible, like that of the long bones, is treated by evacuation of the cyst contents. Curettage is sometimes also carried out. Healing readily follows, with filling in of the defect by new bone.

Aneurysmal Bone Cyst

The aneurysmal bone cyst, characterised as such by Jaffe and Lichtenstein (1942), Jaffe (1950) and Lichtenstein (1950), occurs particularly in the long bones and vertebral column. It may occur also in other bones, but is rare in the jaws. The jaw lesions in the literature have been reviewed by Gruskin and Dahlin (1968) and Daugherty and Eversole (1971). Ellis and Walters (1972) and Oliver (1973) have also reported cases.

Patients with jaw lesions, as are those with lesions in other bones, are young and there is often a history of trauma. The mandible is generally affected, but the lesion may also occur in the maxilla. There is a firm enlargement of the jaw that may be tender. Radiologically, there is a unilocular or multilocular translucency that may show the characteristic ballooned-out appearance with expansion of the cortex that Jaffe has described as a subperiosteal "blowout." However, the appearances in the jaws tend to be less characteristic than in the long bones (Fig. 130a). When the lesion is entered it is found to contain blood and reddish-brown tissue, and further bleeding occurs from the wall of the cavity, though this is in the nature of a welling-up of blood rather than free haemorrhage. Microscopically, there are numerous capillaries and intercommunicating blood-filled spaces, with evidence of fresh and older haemorrhage in the intervening connective tissue. Multinucleated giant cells are usually much in evidence, particularly around foci of haemorrhage (Fig. 130b, c, d). Irregular areas of osteoid are also generally present.

The cause of aneurysmal bone cyst is unknown. Even though a history of trauma is often obtained it is not certain that it can be directly related to the development of the lesion. The lesion has no relationship to the solitary bone cyst and although it may occur in bone that has previously been apparently normal, it is frequently associated with other lesions. In Biesecker and colleagues' (1970) series of 66 cases of aneurysmal bone cyst, for example, 32 per cent were associated with other lesions, including giant cell granuloma, chondroblastoma, fibroma and fibrous dysplasia. Buraczewski and Dabska (1971), Oliver (1973) and others have also noted its association with fibrous dysplasia. In the jaws, aneurysmal bone cyst has been associated with giant cell granuloma. Bernier and Bhaskar (1958) suggested that the two lesions were related, and other authors who have reported jaw lesions have noted the similarities between them. The nature of aneurysmal bone cyst is thus obscure; clearly it can occur as a solitary and apparently independent lesion, but often it seems to be associated with other lesions, possibly as an unusual type of vascular reaction.

No jaw lesions have yet been noted to recur, although in other bones there have been recurrence rates of up to 59 per cent, following curettage. Malignant forms have been reported (Clough and Price, 1968; Hirst and colleagues, 1970), but not in the jaws.

CYSTS OF THE SOFT TISSUES

Salivary Cyst

Small cysts arising in connection with the minor salivary glands are very common, and may be found anywhere in the oral submucosa. Favourite sites are the lower lip (the upper is rarely

Fig. 130 Aneurysmal bone cyst of mandible in a man of 29 years. The patient became aware of a swelling in the mandible following a recent blow on the chin. It had been increasing in size since. After curettage, which was accompanied by much bleeding, the lesion healed uneventfully. Three years later he was well, with no recurrence. **a,** radiograph, showing a large, ill-defined, finely trabeculated translucency pushing apart the roots of the central and lateral incisor teeth. **b,** the curettings consist of connective tissue with numerous capillaries and blood-containing spaces. × 80. **c,** higher magnification, showing numerous giant cells. × 200. **d,** in some areas hyalinisation is prominent. × 90.

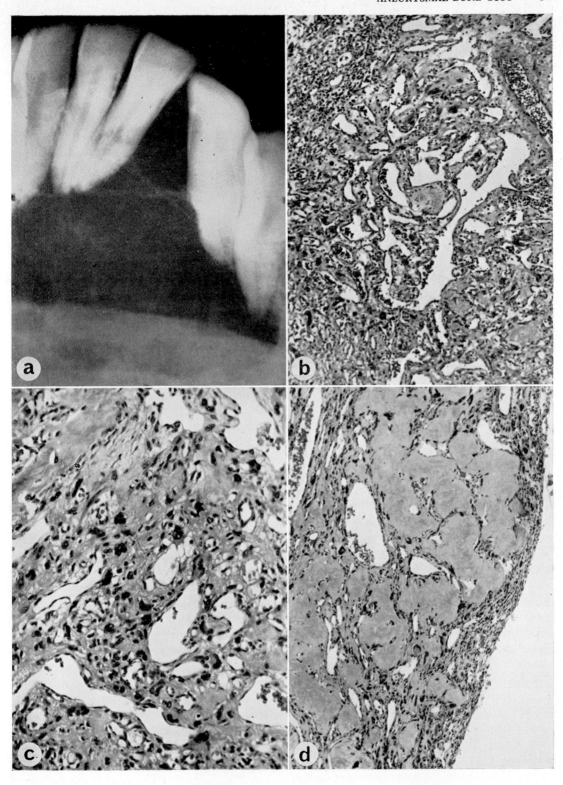

affected), the cheeks, the under surface of the tip of the tongue and the floor of the mouth (ranula). When superficial, the cyst presents as a firm circumscribed bluish-white swelling that feels to the patient like a small shot beneath the mucosa, though not infrequently larger lesions are seen, up to 0·5 cm in diameter or more. Spontaneous rupture often occurs, with the liberation of viscous fluid. However, in the course of a few weeks or perhaps longer, more fluid accumulates and the lesion reappears. This cycle of rupture, collapse of the cyst and refilling may be repeated indefinitely.

Microscopically, the lesion consists of a cyst-like space or spaces in connective tissue containing mucus and lined by a thin layer of flattened cells that may resemble an epithelial lining, but which are in fact compressed connective tissue cells. In many cases even this lining is absent, only granulation tissue being seen. As well as mucus the cystic space also contains histiocytes, polymorphs and lymphocytes, and there is usually a moderate degree of chronic inflammatory infiltration in the surrounding tissues. The adjacent salivary gland acini also show some chronic inflammatory changes and their ducts are often dilated (Fig. 131a, b, c). In a few cases the cyst does have a lining of squamous epithelium but this is rarely complete.

It is possible that some of the deep, burrowing types of ranula in the floor of the mouth may not be of salivary origin (Mandel and Baurmash, 1957). However, in most cases the ranula is a mucous extravasation cyst, arising from the sublingual gland. Unlike the small cysts that are found immediately beneath the epithelium and that are lined by granulation tissue, some of these larger and deeper cysts have a lining of squamous or cuboidal epithelium, though this may later be lost.

The pathogenesis of mucous cysts is not altogether clear. It was formerly assumed that duct obstruction led to dilatation and hence ultimately to cyst formation, but Bhaskar, Bolden and Weinmann (1956) showed in mice and rats that it was not possible to produce a lesion resembling human mucous cyst by duct ligation. On the other hand, if a duct were cut, permitting escape of saliva into the tissues, a cyst was formed and the lesion corresponded in appearance to that found in man, that is, a mucus-containing space lined by connective or granulation tissue. This suggested that mucous cyst formation results from trauma, and also seemed to explain the absence of an epithelial lining in so many cases. Standish and Shafer (1957) took a similar view on histological grounds. More recently, however, Robinson and Hjørting-Hansen (1964) have examined a large series of mucous cysts in serial section and have found a higher proportion of lesions with epithelial linings than has been reported hitherto. They conclude that obstruction is, therefore, an important factor in the pathogenesis of the lesion.

It may well be that both mechanisms operate. The absence of lesions following experimental duct ligation cannot be regarded as conclusive, since if cyst formation does result from duct obstruction, it may be expected to do so in most cases as a result of incomplete blockage and not total obstruction, which would usually lead to atrophy. However, it is possible that complete, or very nearly complete, occlusion of ducts may on occasion lead to cystic dilatation, as indicated by Harrison and Garrett (1972).

Harrison (1975) has examined a series of naturally occurring cysts and concludes that there are two types, extravasation and retention. The former occur most often in younger patients and in the lower lip. The retention type occurs most often in older patients, and elsewhere in the mouth.

Fig. 131 **a,** salivary cyst of the lower lip in a man of 44 years. The lesion formed a small blue swelling that had been present for some time, intermittently enlarging and decreasing in size. The photomicrograph shows the superficial situation of the cyst and its relation to a group of salivary glands. × 12·5. **b,** the cyst wall, with lining of connective tissue. × 80. **c,** another example of salivary cyst wall. Note the absence of epithelium. × 80. **d,** gingival cyst. The cyst, which lies just beneath the surface epithelium, is lined by squamous epithelium. × 80.

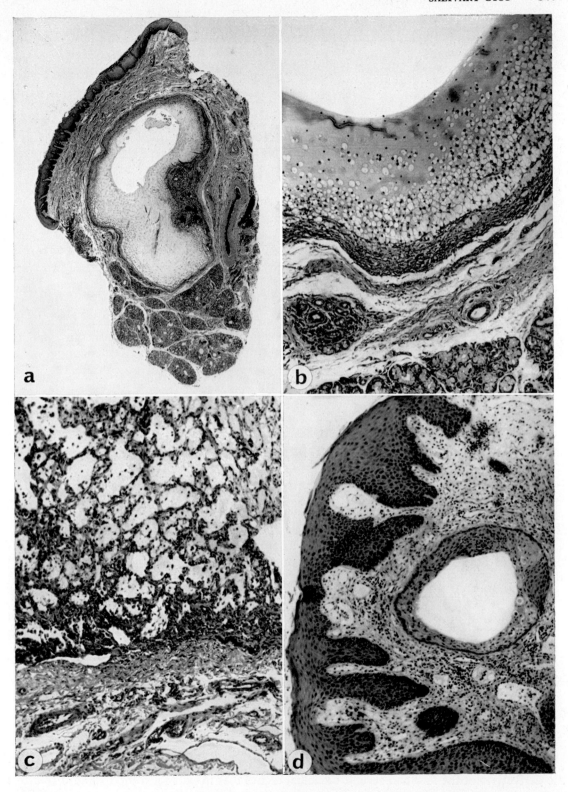

A very much rarer cause of salivary cyst formation is congenital anomaly. Cyst-like lesions in the floor of the mouth in infants, due to imperforate submandibular ducts, are reported by Hoggins and Hutton (1974).

Mucous cysts are treated by excision, together with the associated salivary tissue. If excision is incomplete, the lesion may recur.

Gingival Cyst

Ritchey and Orban (1953) have drawn attention to the presence of asymptomatic microcysts in the gingivae. These small cysts, which are of infrequent occurrence, are lined by squamous epithelium (Fig. 131d). Ritchey and Orban suggest a number of possibilities for their origin. Though salivary glandular tissue does not normally occur in the gingivae heterotopic glands may occasionally do so, and Traeger (1961) has reported a gingival cyst which clearly arose from such a source. Gingival cysts may also arise from remnants of the dental lamina or enamel organ and other possibilities are degeneration in a downgrowth of surface epithelium or traumatic implantation. Occasionally, larger lesions may occur (Bhaskar and Laskin, 1955; Standish and Shafer, 1958; Rickles and Everett, 1961). Other reports are listed by Alexander and Griffith (1966).

Dermoid Cyst

Dermoid cysts in the oral region occur in the floor of the mouth and the submandibular and sublingual regions. They are thought to arise from epithelial rests persisting in the midline after fusion of the mandibular and hyoid branchial arches. However, this view is not accepted by all authorities; Seward (1965) discusses alternative views and also gives a good account of the growth and development of these lesions.

Cysts in the floor of the mouth above the geniohyoid may be large enough to elevate the tongue and cause difficulty in mastication and speech. Cysts situated between the geniohyoid and the mylohyoid produce a submental swelling. Microscopically, dermoid cysts are lined by squamous epithelium and contain keratin scales and sebaceous material. Sebaceous glands, sweat glands and hair follicles may be present in the cyst wall and occasionally other structures such as muscle, bone and respiratory or alimentary epithelium may be found (Fig. 132a). Some cysts contain keratin only and may be due to implantation of epithelium, as in the case of epidermoid cysts of the skin. Cysts of this type have been reported in the tongue (Quinn, 1960; Rise, 1964), floor of mouth (Kelln, 1965; Kinnman and Suh, 1968) and lip (Ettinger and Manderson, 1973). Gorlin and Jirasek (1970) review the reported cases of cysts lined by gastric or intestinal mucosa occurring in the floor of the mouth and in the tongue.

Branchial Cyst

Rarely, a branchial cyst may occur in the floor of the mouth. Its structure in this situation is the same as when it occurs in its customary site in the neck—a lining of stratified squamous epithelium with subjacent lymphoid tissue (Fig. 132b). The origin and development of these cysts are well discussed by Wilson (1955) and Willis (1958). For case reports see Acevedo and Nelson (1971), Merchant (1972) and Giunta and Cataldo (1973).

Carcinomatous change may rarely occur in the cystic epithelium. A possible case of a tumour of this type in the posterior part of the mouth has been reported by Stockdale (1960).

Thyroglossal Cyst

The thyroid gland rudiment appears during the 4th embryonic week in the midline between the derivatives of the first and second branchial arches that in part form the tongue. From this

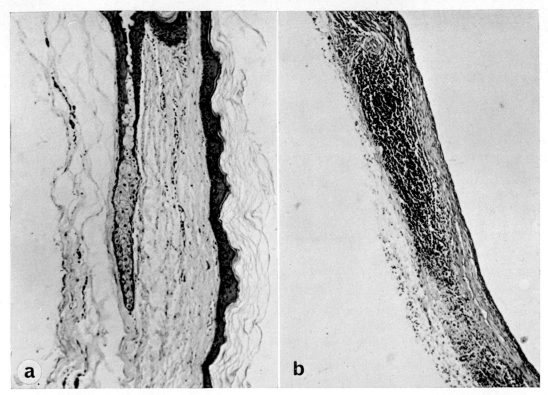

Fig. 132 **a,** dermoid cyst of the floor of the mouth in a man of 22 years. The lesion caused a swelling beneath the tongue which had been increasing in size for the past 3 years. The cyst is lined by squamous epithelium and contains keratin scales. Sebaceous glands are present in the wall. × 80. **b,** branchial cyst in the floor of the mouth in a man aged 27 years. The cyst is lined by squamous epithelium and the wall contains lymphoid tissue. × 80.

point, which will later become the foramen caecum, the gland grows downwards to its permanent situation. Its hollow stalk, the thyroglossal duct, thus extends from the foramen caecum in the base of the tongue down through the neck to the gland itself, but this duct breaks up and disappears by about the 10th week. Cysts may form from the residues of the duct at any point, the commonest area being close to the hyoid bone. In the oral tissues, cysts occur in the posterior part of the tongue at the foramen caecum and in the floor of the mouth.

Cysts occurring above the level of the hyoid bone are often lined by stratified squamous epithelium and those below this level by ciliated respiratory type or columnar epithelium. However, the arrangement is variable and a single cyst may show different types of epithelium from area to area.

Rarely, carcinoma may arise in remnants of the thyroglossal duct. The tumour usually presents as a papillary adenocarcinoma; the reported cases have been collected by Snedecor and Groshong (1965) and further cases have been recorded by Falkinburg, Hoey and Stuart (1966), Kalderon and Cohn (1966) and Butler and colleagues (1969).

It is convenient here to mention the occurrence of lingual thyroid tissue. Erdheim (1904) and Schilder (1911) noted the presence of cysts lined by squamous and ciliated columnar epithelium in the base of the tongue in cases of cretinism. In these cases the cervical thyroid gland was absent but some non-functioning thyroid vesicles were present in the cyst walls. Willis (1958) noted that many cases of sporadic cretinism show the combination of aplasia or hypoplasia of the cervical thyroid gland and functionless lingual thyroid.

Functioning lingual thyroid tissue may form a tumour-like mass if cervical thyroid insufficiency induces its hyperplasia. Sicher (1953) notes that the thyroid insufficiency may arise when a special stress exists, for instance puberty, pregnancy, lactation or the menopause, and in the total absence of a cervical thyroid gland. Most lingual thyroids have resembled normal thyroid tissue but when enlargement occurs the changes of colloid goitre are seen. Sometimes adenoma or carcinoma may develop (Fish and Moore, 1963). Myerson and Smith (1966) review the literature and an extensive discussion of the subject is given by Baughman (1972).

Aberrant thyroid tissue has also been found in the floor of the mouth (Knoblich, 1965).

REFERENCES

Abrams, A. M., Howell, F. V., and Bullock, W. K. (1963) Nasopalatine cysts. *Oral Surg.*, **16**, 306.

Acevedo, A., and Nelson, J. F. (1971) Lymphoepithelial cysts of the oral cavity. Report of nine cases. *Oral Surg.*, **31**, 632.

Aisenberg, M. S., and Inman, B. W. (1960) Ameloblastoma arising within a globulomaxillary cyst. *Oral Surg.*, **13**, 1352.

Albers, D. D. (1973) Median mandibular cyst partially lined with pseudostratified columnar epithelium. Report of a case. *Oral Surg.*, **36**, 11.

Alexander, W. N., and Griffith, J. G. (1966) Gingival cysts: report of two cases. *J. oral Surg.*, **24**, 338.

Atterbury, R. A., Vazirani, S. J., and McNabb, W. J. (1961) Nasoalveolar cyst. *Oral Surg.*, **14**, 769.

Baughman, R. A. (1972) Lingual thyroid and lingual thyroglossal tract remnants. A clinical and histopathologic study with review of the literature. *Oral Surg.*, **34**, 781.

Bernier, J. L., and Bhaskar, S. N. (1958) Aneurysmal bone cysts of the mandible. *Oral Surg.*, **11**, 1018.

Bhaskar, S. N., Bernier, J. L., and Godby, F. (1959) Aneurysmal bone cyst and other giant cell lesions of the jaws: report of 104 cases. *J. oral Surg.*, **17**, 30.

Bhaskar, S. N., Bolden, T. E., and Weinmann, J. P. (1956) Experimental obstructive adenitis in the mouse. *J. dent. Res.*, **35**, 852.

Bhaskar, S. N., Bolden, T. E., and Weinmann, J. P. (1956) Pathogenesis of mucoceles. *J. dent. Res.*, **35**, 863.

Bhaskar, S. N., and Laskin, D. M. (1955) Gingival cysts. Report of three cases. *Oral Surg.*, **8**, 803.

Biesecker, J. L., Marcove, R. C., Huvos, A. G., and Miké, V. (1970) Aneurysmal bone cysts. A clinicopathologic study of 66 cases. *Cancer*, **26**, 615.

Binkley, G. W., and Johnson, H. H. (1951) Epithelioma adenoides cysticum: basal cell nevi, agenesis of the corpus callosum and dental cysts. *Arch. Dermat. Syph.*, **63**, 73.

Blair, V. P. (1923) Ranula. *Ann. Surg.*, **77**, 681.

Blair, A. E., and Wadsworth, W. (1968) Median mandibular developmental cyst: report of case. *J. oral Surg.*, **26**, 735.

Blum, T. (1932) Unusual bone cavities in the mandible: a report of three cases of traumatic bone cysts. *J. amer. dent. Ass.*, **19**, 281.

Blum, T. (1955) An additional report on traumatic bone cysts. Also a discussion of Dr. John G. Whinery's paper, "Progressive Bone Cavities of the Mandible." *Oral Surg.*, **8**, 917.

Bolden, T. E. (1957) Pathogenesis of mucoceles. Report of a case. *Oral Surg.*, **10**, 310.

Boone, C. G. (1955) Nasoalveolar cyst. *Oral Surg.*, **8**, 40.

Bouyssou, M., and Guilhem, A. (1965) Recherches morphologiques et histochemiques sur les corps hyalins intrakystiques de Rushton. *Bull. Group. int. Rech. sc. Stomat.*, **8**, 81.

Boyer, B. E., and Martin, M. M. (1958) Marfan's syndrome: Report of a case manifesting giant bone cyst of mandible and multiple (110) basal cell carcinoma. *Plast. reconstr. Surg.*, **22**, 257.

Bramley, P. (1974) The odontogenic keratocyst—an approach to treatment. *Internat. J. oral Surg.*, **3**, 337.

Bramley, P. A., and Browne, R. M. (1967) Recurring odontogenic cysts. *Brit. J. oral Surg.*, **5**, 106.

Brown, P. R. H. (1967) An unusual case of globulomaxillary cyst. *Oral Surg.*, **24**, 719.

Browne, R. M. (1970) The odontogenic keratocyst. Clinical aspects. *Brit. dent. J.*, **128**, 225.

Browne, R. M. (1971) The odontogenic keratocyst. Histological features and their correlation with clinical behaviour. *Brit. dent. J.*, **131**, 249.

Browne, R. M. (1972) Metaplasia and degeneration in odontogenic cysts in man. *J. oral Path.*, **1**, 145.

Buchner, A., and Ramon, Y. (1974) Median mandibular cyst—a rare lesion of debatable origin. *Oral Surg.*, **37**, 431.

Buraczewski, J., and Dabska, M. (1971) Pathogenesis of aneurysmal bone cyst. Relationship between the aneurysmal bone cyst and fibrous dysplasia of bone. *Cancer*, **28**, 597.

Butler, E. C., Dickey, J. R., Shill, O. S., and Shalak, E. (1969) Carcinoma of the thyroglossal duct remnant. *Laryngoscope*, **79**, 264.

Carp, L. (1921) Ranula of branchial origin. *Surg. Gynec. Obstet.*, **31**, 182.

Cawson, R. A., and Kerr, G. A. (1964) The syndrome of jaw cysts, basal cell tumours and skeletal anomalies. *Proc. roy. Soc. Med.*, **57**, 799.

Christ, T. F. (1970) The globulomaxillary cyst; an embryologic misconception. *Oral Surg.*, **30**, 515.

Clough, J. R., and Price, C. H. G. (1968) Aneurysmal bone cysts, review of twelve cases. *J. Bone Jt. Surg.*, **50B**, 116.

Counsell, A. C. (1932) The pathology of dental cysts. *Brit. dent. J.*, **53**, i, 69.

Courage, G. R., North, A. F., and Hansen, L. S. (1974) Median palatine cysts. Review of the literature and report of a case. *Oral Surg.*, **37**, 745.

Cunningham, J. A. (1951) Characteristics of stellate inclusions in giant cells and the associated tissue reactions. *Amer. J. Path.*, **27**, 761.

Daugherty, J. W., and Eversole, L. R. (1971) Aneurysmal bone cyst of the mandible. Report of a case. *J. oral Surg.*, **29**, 737.

Dent, R. J., and Wertheimer, F. W. (1967) Hyaline bodies in odontogenic cysts: a histochemical study for hemoglobin. *J. dent. Res.*, **46**, 629.

Dewey, K. W. (1918) Cysts of the dental system. *Dent. Cosmos*, **60**, 555.

Donoff, R. B., Harper, E., and Guralnick, W. C. (1972) Collagenolytic activity in keratocysts. *J. oral Surg.*, **30**, 879.

Ebling, J., and Wagner, J. E. (1964) Aneurysmal bone cyst of the mandible. *Oral Surg.*, **18**, 646.

Ellis, D. J., and Walters, P. J. (1972) Aneurysmal bone cyst of the maxilla. *Oral Surg.*, **34**, 26.

Erdheim, J. (1904) I. Über Schilddrüsenaplasie. II. Geschwülste des Ductus Thyreoglossus. III. Über einige menschliche Kiemenderivate. *Beitr. path. Anat.*, **35**, 366.

Ettinger, R. L., and Manderson, R. D. (1973) Implantation keratinizing epidermoid cysts. A review and case history. *Oral Surg.*, **36**, 225.

Falkinburg, L. W., Hoey, W. O., and Stuart, J. R. (1966) Papillary adenocarcinoma arising in a thyroglossal duct cyst. *Oral Surg.*, **21**, 358.

Ferenczy, K. (1958) The relationship of globulomaxillary cysts to the fusion of embryonal processes and to cleft palates. *Oral Surg.*, **11**, 1388.

Fickling, B. W. (1965) Cysts of the jaw: a long-term survey of types and treatment. *Proc. roy. Soc. Med.*, **58**, 847.

Fish, J., and Moore, R. M. (1963) Ectopic thyroid tissue and ectopic thyroid carcinoma—a review of the literature and report of a case. *Ann. Surg.*, **157**, 212.

Giunta, J., and Cataldo, E. (1973) Lymphoepithelial cysts of the oral mucosa. *Oral Surg.*, **35**, 77.

Gorlin, R. J. (1957) Potentialities of oral epithelium manifest by mandibular dentigerous cysts. *Oral Surg.*, **10**, 271.

Gorlin, R. J., and Goltz, R. W. (1960) Multiple nevoid basal cell epithelioma, jaw cysts, and bifid rib. A syndrome. *New Engl. J. Med.*, **262**, 908.

Gorlin, R. J., Yunis, J. J., and Tuna, N. (1963) Multiple nevoid basal cell carcinoma, odontogenic keratocysts and skeletal anomalies. A syndrome. *Acta Derm. Venereol.*, **43**, 39.

Gorlin, R. J., Vickers, R. A., Kelln, E., and Williamson, J. J. (1965) The multiple basal-cell nevi syndrome. An analysis of a syndrome consisting of multiple nevoid basal-cell carcinoma, jaw cysts, skeletal anomalies, medulloblastoma, and hyporesponsiveness to parathormone. *Cancer*, **18**, 89.

Gorlin, R. J., and Jirasek, J. E. (1970) Oral cysts containing gastric or intestinal mucosa: unusual embryologic accident or heterotopia. *J. oral Surg.*, **28**, 9.

Gross, P. P. (1953) Epithelioma adenoides cysticum with follicular cysts of maxilla and mandible: report of case. *J. oral Surg.*, **11**, 160.

Gruskin, S. E., and Dahlin, D. C. (1968) Aneurysmal bone cysts of the jaws. *J. oral Surg.*, **26**, 523.

Hansen, J. (1967) Keratocysts in the jaws. *Trans. 2nd Congr. internat. Assoc. oral Surg.*, Copenhagen. Munksgaard.

Hansen, L. S., Sapone, J., and Sproat, R. C. (1974) Traumatic bone cysts of jaws. Report of sixty-six cases. *Oral Surg.*, **37**, 899.

Harris, M., and Goldhaber, P. (1973) The production of a bone resorbing factor by dental cysts in vitro. *Brit. J. oral Surg.*, **10**, 334.

Harris, M., Jenkins, M. V., Bennett, A., and Wills, M. R. (1973) Prostaglandin production and bone resorption by dental cysts. *Nature*, **245**, 213.

Harrison, J. D. (1975) Salivary mucoceles. *Oral Surg.*, **39**, 268.

Harrison, J. D., and Garrett, J. R. (1972) Mucocele formation in cats by glandular ligation. *Arch. oral Biol.*, **17**, 1403.

Hatziotis, J. (1966) Median palatine cyst: report of case. *J. oral Surg.*, **24**, 343.

Hertz, J. (1963) Globulomaxillary cyst invading the maxillary sinus. *Oral Surg.*, **16**, 392.

Hirst, E., McKellar, C. C., Ellis, J. M., and Smith, V. K. (1970) Malignant aneurysmal bone cyst. *J. Bone Jt. Surg.*, **53B**, 791.

Hjørting-Hansen, E., Andreasen, J. O., and Robinson, L. H. (1969) A study of odontogenic cysts, with special reference to location of keratocysts. *Brit. J. oral Surg.*, **7**, 15.

Hodson, J. J. (1956) Muco-epidermoid odontogenic cysts of the jaws with special reference to those in the mandible. *Proc. roy. Soc. Med.*, **49**, 637.

Hodson, J. J. (1966) Origin and nature of the cuticula dentis. *Nature*, **209**, 990.

Hoggins, G. S., and Hutton, J. B. (1974) Congenital sublingual cystic swellings due to imperforate salivary ducts. Two case reports. *Oral Surg.*, **37**, 370.

Hoppe, W. (1968) An aneurysmal bone cyst of the mandible. Report of a case. *Oral Surg.*, **25**, 1.

Howe, G. L. (1965) Haemorrhagic cysts of the mandible. *Brit. J. oral Surg.*, **3**, 55.

Howell, J. B., and Caro, M. R. (1959) Basal cell nevus: its relationship to multiple cutaneous cancers and associated anomalies of development. *Arch. Dermatol.*, **79**, 67.

Howell, J. B., Anderson, D. E., and McClendon, J. L. (1966) Multiple cutaneous cancers in children: the nevoid basal cell carcinoma syndrome. *J. Pediat.*, **69**, 97.

Howell, J. B., Byrd, L., McClendon, J. L., and Anderson, D. E. (1967) Identification and treatment of jaw cysts in the nevoid basal cell carcinoma syndrome. *J. oral Surg.*, **25**, 129.

Huebner, G. R., and Turlington, E. G. (1971) So-called traumatic (hemorrhagic) bone cysts of the jaws. Review of the literature and report of two unusual cases. *Oral Surg.*, **21**, 354.

Jaffe, H. L. (1950) Aneurysmal bone cyst. *Bull. Hosp. Joint Dis.*, **11**, 3.

Jaffe, H. L. (1953) Giant-cell reparative granuloma, traumatic bone cyst, and fibrous (fibro-osseous) dysplasia of the jawbones. *Oral Surg.*, **6**, 159.

Jaffe, H. L. (1958) *Tumors and Tumorous Conditions of the Bones and Joints.* London. Henry Kimpton.

Jaffe, H. L., and Lichtenstein, L. (1942) Solitary unicameral bone cyst with emphasis on the roentgen picture, the pathologic appearance and the pathogenesis. *Arch. Surg.*, **44**, 1004.

James, W. W., and Counsell, A. (1932) A histologic study of the epithelium associated with chronic apical infection of the teeth. *Brit. dent. J.*, **53**, ii, 463.

Jarisch (1894) Cited by Gorlin and colleagues (1965).

Jensen, J. L., and Erickson, J. O. (1974) Hyaline bodies in odontogenic cysts: electron microscopic observations. *J. oral Path.*, **3**, 1.

Kalderon, A. E., and Cohn, J. D. (1966) Papillary adenocarcinoma in a thyroglossal cyst. Case report and review of the literature. *Cancer*, **19**, 839.

Kelln, E. E. (1965) Oral epidermal cysts and probable histogenesis. Report of a case. *Oral Surg.*, **19**, 359.

Killey, H. C., and Kay, L. W. (1966) *Benign Cystic Lesions of the Jaws: their Diagnosis and Treatment.* Edinburgh and London. E. & S. Livingstone Ltd.

Kinnman, J., and Suh, K. W. (1968) Dermoid cysts of the floor of the mouth: report of three cases. *J. oral Surg.*, **26**, 190.

Klestadt, W. (1921) Embryologische und literarische Studie zur Genese der Gesichtsspaltensysten und ähnlicher Gebilde. *Zeit. f. Ohrenh.*, **81**, 330.

Knight, J. S., and Manley, E. B. (1955) The formation of multiple dental cysts. *Brit. dent. J.*, **99**, 419.

Knoblich, R. (1965) Accessory thyroid in the lateral floor of the mouth. Report of a case, with embryologic considerations. *Oral Surg.*, **19**, 234.

Kramer, I. R. H., and Toller, P. A. (1973) The use of exfoliative cytology and protein estimations in preoperative diagnosis of odontogenic keratocysts. *Internat. J. oral Surg.*, **2**, 143.

Lichtenstein, L. (1950) Aneurysmal bone cyst. A pathological entity commonly mistaken for giant-cell tumor and occasionally for hemangioma and osteogenic sarcoma. *Cancer*, **3**, 279.

Little, J. W., and Jakobsen, J. (1973) Origin of the globulomaxillary cyst. *J. oral Surg.*, **31**, 188.

Lucchesi, F. J., and Topazian, D. S. (1961) Multilocular median developmental cyst of the mandible: report of a case. *J. oral Surg.*, **19**, 336.

Maddox, W. D., Winkelmann, R. K., Harrison, E. G., Devine, K. D., and Gibilisco, J. A. (1964) Multiple nevoid basal cell epitheliomas, jaw cysts, and skeletal defects. *J. amer. med. Ass.*, **188**, 106.

Main, D. M. G. (1970) The enlargement of epithelial jaw cysts. *Odont. Revy.*, **21**, 29.

Main, D. M. G. (1970) Epithelial jaw cysts: a clinicopathological reappraisal. *Brit. J. oral Surg.*, **8**, 114.

Mandel, L., and Baurmash, H. (1957) Ranulae. *Oral Surg.*, **10**, 567.

Marsland, E. A., and Browne, R. M. (1965) Two odontogenic cysts, partially lined with ciliated epithelium. *Oral Surg.*, **19**, 502.

McKelvey, L. E., Albright, C. R., and Prazak, G. (1960) Multiple hereditary familial epithelial cysts of the jaws with the associated anomaly of trichoepithelioma. *Oral Surg.*, **13**, 111.

Medak, H., and Weinmann, J. P. (1960) Hyaline bodies in dental cysts. *Brit. dent. J.*, **109**, 312.

Melhado, R. M., Rulli, M. A., and Martinelli, C. (1973) the etiopathogenesis of gingival cysts. A histochemical study of three cases. *Oral Surg.*, **35**, 510.

Merchant, N. E. (1972) Lympho-epithelial cyst of the floor of the mouth. A case report. *Brit. dent. J.*, **132**, 271.

Meyer, I. (1957) Developmental median cyst of the mandible. Report of a case. *Oral Surg.*, **10**, 75.

Molyneux, G. (1957) Hyaline bodies in the wall of dental cysts. *Aust. dent. J.*, **2**, 155.

Morgan, P. R., and Johnson, N. W. (1974) Histological, histochemical and ultrastructural studies on the nature of hyalin bodies in odontogenic cysts. *J. oral Path.*, **3**, 127.

Myerson, M., and Smith, H. W. (1966) Lingual thyroid—a review. *Conn. Med.*, **30**, 341.

Nomland, R. (1932) Multiple basal cell epitheliomas originating from congenital pigmented basal cell nevi. *Arch. Derm.*, **25**, 1002.

Oatis, G. W., Burch, M. S., and Samuels, H. S. (1971) Marfan's syndrome with multiple maxillary and mandibular cysts: report of case. *J. oral Surg.*, **29**, 515.

Olech, E. (1957) Median mandibular cysts. A clinical and histological report of two cases. *Oral Surg.*, **10**, 69.

Olech, E., Sicher, H., and Weinmann, J. P. (1951) Traumatic mandibular bone cysts. *Oral Surg.*, **4**, 1160.

Oliver, L. P. (1973) Aneurysmal bone cyst. Report of a case. *Oral Surg.*, **35**, 67.

Panders, A. K., and Hadders, H. N. (1969) Solitary keratocysts of the jaws. *J. oral Surg.*, **27**, 931.

Payne, T. F. (1972) An analysis of the clinical and histopathologic parameters of the odontogenic keratocyst. *Oral Surg.*, **33**, 538.

Philipsen, H. P. (1956) Cited by Rud and Pindborg.

Pindborg, J. J., and Hansen, J. (1963) Studies on odontogenic cyst epithelium. 2. Clinical and roentgenological aspects of odontogenic keratocysts. *Acta path. microbiol. scand.*, **58**, 283.

Pommer, G. (1919) Zur Kenntniss der progressiven Hämatom- und Phlegmasieveränderungen der Röhrenknochen auf Grund der mikroskopischen Befunde im neuen Knochenzystenfalle H. v. Haberers. *Arch. f. Orth.*, **17**, 17.

Quinn, J. H. (1960) Congenital epidermoid cyst of anterior half of tongue. *Oral Surg.*, **13**, 1283.

Radden, B. G., and Reade, P. C. (1973) Odontogenic keratocysts. *Pathology*, **5**, 325.

Rayne, J. (1971) The multiple basal cell naevi syndrome. *Brit. J. oral Surg.*, **9**, 65.

Rickles, N. H., and Everett, F. G. (1961) Gingival and lateral periodontal cysts. Report of two cases. *Paradont.*, **14**, 41.

Rise, E. N. (1964) Dermoid cysts of the tongue and floor of the mouth. *Arch. Otolaryngol.*, **80**, 12.

Ritchey, B., and Orban, B. (1953) Cysts of the gingiva. *Oral Surg.*, **6**, 765.

Robinson, H. B. G. (1945) Classification of cysts of the jaws. *Amer. J. Orthodont. (Oral Surg. Sect.)*, **31**, 370.

Robinson, H. B. G. in Archer, W. H. (1961) *Manual of Oral Surgery*. 3rd Edition. Philadelphia. W. B. Saunders Co.

Robinson, L., and Hjørting-Hansen, E. (1964) Pathologic changes associated with mucous retention cysts of minor salivary glands. *Oral Surg.*, **18**, 191.

Roed-Petersen, B. (1969) Nasolabial cysts. A presentation of five patients with a review of the literature. *Brit. J. oral Surg.*, **7**, 84.

Rud, J., and Pindborg, J. J. (1969) Odontogenic keratocysts: a follow-up study of 21 cases. *J. oral Surg.*, **27**, 323.

Rushton, M. A. (1946) Solitary bone cysts in the mandible. *Brit. dent. J.*, **81**, 37.

Rushton, M. A. (1955) Hyaline bodies in the epithelium of dental cysts. *Proc. roy. Soc. Med.*, **48**, 407.

Schilder, P. (1911) Über Missbildungen der Schilddruse. *Virchows Arch.*, **203**, 246.

Schønning, L., and Visfeldt, J. (1964) The syndrome of jaw cysts—basal cell carcinomas—skeletal anomalies. Clinical study with chromosomal analyses of a family. *Acta Derm. Venereol.*, **44**, 437.

Scott, J. H. (1955) The early development of oral cysts in man. *Brit. dent. J.*, **98**, 109.

Sedano, H. O., and Gorlin, R. J. (1968) Hyaline bodies of Rushton. Some histochemical considerations concerning their etiology. *Oral Surg.*, **26**, 198.

Seward, G. R. (1965) Dermoid cysts of the floor of the mouth. *Brit. J. oral Surg.*, **3**, 36.

Seward, M. H. (1973) Eruption cyst: an analysis of its clinical features. *J. oral Surg.*, **31**, 31.

Shear, M. (1960) Primordial cysts. *J. dent. Ass. S. Africa*, **15**, 211.

Shear, M. (1960) Secretory epithelium in the lining of dental cysts. *J. dent. Ass. S. Africa*, **15**, 117.

Shear, M. (1961) The hyaline and granular bodies in dental cysts. *Brit. dent. J.*, **110**, 301.

Shear, M. (1961) Clinical statistics of dental cysts. *J. dent. Ass. S. Africa*, **16**, 360.

Shear, M. (1963) The microscopic features of the fibrous walls of dental cysts. *Diastema*, **1**, 9.

Shear, M., and Wilton, E. (1968) Cytogenetic studies of the basal cell carcinoma syndrome. *J. dent. Ass. S. Africa*, **23**, 99.

Sicher, K. (1953) Lingual thyroid. *Brit. med. J.*, **2**, 186.

Skaug, N. (1973) Proteins in fluid from non-keratinizing jaw cysts. *J. oral Path.*, **3**, 47.

Skaug, N. (1974) Proteins in fluid from non-keratinizing jaw cysts. *J. oral Path.*, **2**, 280, 326.

Skaug, N., and Hofstadt, T. (1973) Proteins in fluid from non-keratinizing jaw cysts. *J. oral Path.*, **2**, 112.

Small, E. W. (1967) Ciliated epithelium lining a mandibular dentigerous cyst: report of case. *J. oral Surg.*, **25**, 260.

Smith, N. H. H. (1968) Multiple dentigerous cysts associated with arachnodactyly and other skeletal defects. Report of a case. *Oral Surg.*, **25**, 99.

Snedecor, P. A., and Groshong, L. E. (1965) Carcinoma of the thyroglossal duct. *Surgery*, **58**, 969.

Soskolne, W. A., and Shear, M. (1967) Observations on the pathogenesis of primordial cysts. *Brit. dent. J.*, **123**, 321.

Spouge, J. D. (1966) Sebaceous metaplasia in the oral cavity occurring in association with dentigerous cyst epithelium. Report of a case. *Oral Surg.*, **21**, 492.

Stafne, E. C. (1942) Bone cavities situated near the angle of the mandible. *J. amer. dent. Ass.*, **29**, 1969.

Stafne, E. C., Austin, L. T., and Gardner, B. S. (1936) Median anterior maxillary cysts. *J. amer. dent. Ass.*, **23**, 801.

Standish, S. M., and Shafer, W. G. (1957) Serial histologic effects of rat submaxillary and sublingual salivary gland duct and blood vessel ligation. *J. dent. Res.*, **36**, 866.

Standish, S. M., and Shafer, W. G. (1958) The lateral periodontal cyst. *J. Periodont.*, **29**, 27.

Stockdale, C. R. (1960) Branchial carcinoma. Report of a case. *Oral Surg.*, **13**, 136.

Stoelinga, P. J. W., Cohen, M. M., and Morgan, A. F. (1975) The origin of keratocysts in the basal cell nevus syndrome. *J. oral Surg.*, **33**, 659.

Stoelinga, P. J. W., and Peters, J. H. (1973) A note on the origin of keratocysts of the jaws. *Internat. J. oral Surg.*, **2**, 37.

Stoelinga, P. J. W., Peters, J. H., van de Staak, W. J. B., and Cohen, M. M. (1973) Some new findings in the basal cell nevus syndrome. *Oral Surg.*, **36**, 686.

Straith, F. E. (1939) Hereditary epidermoid cysts of the jaws. *Amer. J. Orthodont.*, **25**, 673.

Summers, L. (1974) The incidence of epithelium in periapical granulomas and the mechanism of cavitation in apical dental cysts in man. *Arch. oral Biol.*, **19**, 1177.

Ten Cate, A. R. (1972) The epithelial cell rests of Malassez and the genesis of the dental cyst. *Oral Surg.*, **34**, 956.

Thoma, K. H. (1959) Polycystoma. *Oral Surg.*, **12**, 484.

Thompson, J. (1920) Surgery and embryology. *Surg. Gynec. Obstet.*, **31**, 18.

Thompson, J. (1920) The relationship between ranula and branchiogenetic cysts. *Ann. Surg.*, **72**, 164.

Toller, P. A. (1966) Epithelial discontinuities in cysts of the jaws. *Brit. dent. J.*, **120**, 74.

Toller, P. A. (1967) Origin and growth of cysts of the jaws. *Ann. roy. Coll. Surg. Engl.*, **40**, 306.

Toller, P. A. (1970) The osmolality of fluids from cysts of the jaws. *Brit. dent. J.*, **129**, 275.

Toller, P. A. (1971) Autoradiography of explants from odontogenic cysts. *Brit. dent. J.*, **131**, 57.

Traeger, K. A. (1961) Cyst of the gingiva (mucocele). *Oral Surg.*, **14**, 243.

Valderhaug, J. (1972) A histologic study of experimentally induced radicular cysts. *Int. J. oral Surg.*, **1**, 137.

Vianna, M. R. (1962) Aneurysmal bone cyst in the maxilla. *J. oral Surg.*, **20,** 432.

Waldron, C. A. (1954) Solitary (hemorrhagic) cyst of the mandible. *Oral Surg.*, **7,** 88.

Wang, S. Y. (1960) An aneurysmal bone cyst in the maxilla. *Plast. reconstr. Surg.*, **25,** 62.

Wertheimer, F. W., Fullmer, H. M., and Hansen, L. S. (1962) A histochemical study of hyaline bodies in odontogenic cysts and a comparison to the human secondary dental cuticle. *Oral Surg.*, **15,** 1466.

Whinery, J. G. (1955) Progressive bone cavities of the mandible. A review of the so-called traumatic bone cyst and a report of three cases. *Oral Surg.*, **8,** 903.

White, D. K., Lucas, R. M., and Miller, A. S. (1975) Median mandibular cyst: review of the literature and report of two cases. *J. oral Surg.*, **33,** 372.

Willis, R. A. (1958) *The Borderland of Embryology and Pathology*. London. Butterworth & Co. (Publishers) Ltd.

Wilson, C. P. (1955) Lateral cysts and fistulae of the neck of developmental origin. *Ann. roy. Coll. Surg. Engl.*, **17,** 1.

Yunis, J. J., and Gorlin, R. J. (1963) Chromosomal study in patients with cysts of the jaw, multiple nevoid basal cell carcinoma and bifid rib syndrome. *Chromosome*, **14,** 146.

IX
DYSPLASIAS OF BONE

32. Fibrous Dysplasia of Bone and Ossifying Fibroma

Many pathologists and surgeons include in the general category of fibrous dysplasia all lesions of the jaws in which normal bone is replaced by fibrous tissue from which new calcified tissue subsequently forms by metaplasia. These include, as well as the typical lesions of fibrous dysplasia, other lesions that have been described as ossifying fibroma, fibro-osteoma, fibrocementoma and under other designations. The lesions that have long been known as cancellous and ivory osteoma have also been gathered in by some. The familial condition, cherubism, has also been included on occasion. Here, these lesions are considered as separate entities.

FIBROUS DYSPLASIA

Fibrous dysplasia of bone may affect the jaws as a monostotic lesion, as one of the lesions of polyostotic disease affecting several or many bones, or as one of the lesions of Albright's syndrome, in which the polyostotic lesions are accompanied by such manifestations as cutaneous pigmentation, endocrine disorders and precocious puberty and premature skeletal maturation.

Lesions in the jaws, as in other bones, were until quite recently classified as types of osteitis fibrosa or as benign tumours of bone, for it is only within the past thirty to forty years that the concept of fibrous dysplasia of bone has emerged as a distinctive clinical and pathological entity. The recognition of osteitis fibrosa dates from von Recklinghausen's (1891) description of a series of cases that appeared to fall into the same group, but which in fact represented more than one condition, as is now known. In the following years the diagnosis of osteitis fibrosa came to be applied freely to a variety of conditions, though experimental work was beginning to indicate the relationship of the parathyroid glands to bone physiology and pathology. With the first parathyroidectomy in a case of generalised osteitis fibrosa by Mandl (1926) the picture was clarified to some extent. Nevertheless, there still remained fibro-osseous lesions demonstrably not due to hyperparathyroidism, including the cases termed by Hunter and Turnbull (1931) diffuse osteitis fibrosa in multiple foci, in contrast to the lesions of hyperparathyroidism, or osteitis fibrosa cystica generalisata. Thus the fibro-osseous lesions of non-endocrine origin still continued to be classified as types of osteitis fibrosa. Some of these lesions, it was known, were accompanied by cutaneous pigmentation and other extraskeletal manifestations. Weil (1922) was apparently the first to record a case of this type, and subsequently a number of others were noted. These were reviewed in detail by McCune and Bruch (1937). In 1937 Albright, Butler, Hampton and Smith, described fully further cases, and subsequently the condition has been referred to as Albright's syndrome. In this syndrome the patients were generally children with lesions in several or many bones and skeletal deformities in severe cases, areas of light yellow or yellowish-brown pigmentation of the skin and sexual precocity, particularly in girls. Precocious skeletal maturation could also occur and various other manifestations such as hyperthyroidism and diabetes mellitus were described from time to time. The serum calcium and phosphorus levels were always within normal limits in these cases, though the alkaline phosphatase might be elevated. Shortly after Albright's description Lichtenstein (1938) recognised that the bone lesions were the essential feature of Albright's syndrome, and that they could, and in fact often did, occur in the absence of the extra-skeletal manifestations. He therefore introduced the term polyostotic fibrous dysplasia as a more appropriate designation for the condition. Further study (Lichtenstein and Jaffe, 1942), however, showed that only one bone might be affected, so that a more suitable designation appeared to be simply fibrous dysplasia of bone, occurring in a polyostotic or a monostotic form.

Distribution of Lesions and Incidence

In polyostotic fibrous dysplasia the lesions often occur in the bones of one limb, particularly the lower. When the upper limb is affected there may also be lesions in one or more skull bones. Or both arm and leg may be affected on one side of the body together with some bones of one or both limbs on the other side. The vertebrae, pelvis and ribs are also often involved, either alone or together with limb bones and skull bones. With regard to the skull in particular, Windholz (1947) estimated that in about one-half of the cases with a moderate degree of skeletal involvement there will also be changes in the skull, while in severe cases the skull is constantly involved. Fairbank (1950) found that the skull was involved in one-third of the cases without cutaneous pigmentation and in two-thirds of those with pigmentation. Thus almost any combination of lesions may occur, but there is a well marked tendency for the lesions to occur segmentally, with localisation in one limb or on one side of the body.

In monostotic cases practically any bone may be involved, but most often a limb bone, a rib or a cranial bone, particularly a jaw bone. Windholz found that skull lesions accounted for about 10 per cent of the cases of monostotic fibrous dysplasia, and in Schlumberger's (1946) series of 67 monostotic lesions there were 9 maxillary and mandibular lesions.

With regard to incidence, the fully developed case of polyostotic fibrous dysplasia accompanied by extra-skeletal lesions is comparatively rare, but cases with involvement of a few bones only, and monostotic cases, are not uncommon. Jaffe (1945) has estimated that for every case of the fully developed type there occur 20 to 30 cases in which only one bone or at most only a small number of bones are affected. In most cases the lesions are noted in childhood or adolescence, particularly when they are of any degree of severity, but solitary lesions may not be noted till adult life, and may even then be discovered accidentally.

There is a definite sex predilection, two to three times as many females being affected as males.

Distribution and incidence of jaw lesions. In most cases of fibrous dysplasia in which the jaws are involved the lesion is a solitary one, occurring rather more often in the maxilla than in the mandible. Less frequently there may be multiple jaw lesions, for example, a lesion in each side of the mandible or a lesion in both maxillae or in the maxilla and mandible of one side. One or more jaw lesions may also be accompanied by lesions in the facial and cranial bones. Least common are jaw lesions in association with lesions of the trunk and limb bones. Only 1 out of 69 patients with jaw lesions in Zimmerman, Dahlin and Stafne's (1958) series had polyostotic fibrous dysplasia, and of 13 patients with polyostotic lesions only 2 had jaw lesions. In 12 cases of polyostotic disease Sherman and Glauser (1958) found only 2 cases of jaw involvement and in one of these the changes were questionable.

Clinical Features

Patients with polyostotic disease affecting more than a few bones are practically always seen first as children, since the deformities and pathological fractures that follow on the weakening of bone as a result of replacement of osseous by fibrous or fibro-osseous tissue call attention to the condition at an early stage. In cases with only a few, or solitary, lesions symptoms are of course less severe, and though most of the patients with this type of disease are first seen in childhood or adolescence, occasionally the lesion is noted first in adult life. Sometimes patients who seek advice for the first time as adults are aware that they have had a lesion or lesions that have been quiescent for many years but have recently shown growth activity.

In the jaws specifically, symptoms are often slight. Gradually increasing facial asymmetry in a child or adolescent may be first noticed by the parents. Very often this does not cause a great deal of deformity by the time the lesion ceases to be active, which is generally at cessation of normal bone growth. However, in some cases growth is more rapid and more extensive, and in a comparatively short time there may develop a large mandibular swelling or a maxillary lesion that may extend to cause marked swelling of the cheek, exophthalmos and proptosis or nasal obstruction. It is probable that many of the cases formerly diagnosed as "leontiasis ossea" were examples of fibrous dysplasia (or of Paget's disease or other lesions) affecting the facial bones and giving rise to the fancied leonine appearance.

Pain is not a feature of the jaw lesions, though it may occasionally occur. There is seldom disturbance of function, though sometimes teeth may be displaced and occlusion interfered with. In children, teeth implicated by the lesion may fail to erupt.

Both maxillary and mandibular lesions occur as bony hard swellings that expand the jaw and are not tender on palpation. Maxillary lesions generally involve the maxillary sinus and may displace the orbital contents. Mandibular lesions occur most frequently in the premolar and molar regions, but may occur anywhere or even involve almost the entire bone.

As is the case with solitary lesions in extracranial bones, jaw lesions are not accompanied by the non-osseous manifestations of fibrous dysplasia, except very occasionally for pigmentation. This is of minimal degree, consisting of one or two small yellowish patches, perhaps on the trunk but occurring anywhere, and has been reported in cases where cranial as well as jaw lesions were present. Gorlin and Chaudhry (1957) reported a case in which there was pigmentation of the oral mucosa as well as of the skin. Another case of oral pigmentation was reported by Bowerman (1969).

The blood chemistry shows no abnormalities in jaw lesions, except for the serum alkaline phosphatase level, which may sometimes be raised.

Radiologically, there is expansion of the affected bone, with either a translucent cystic appearance with mottled areas or an opaque appearance that is generally likened to ground glass. The loculated or cystic appearance may sometimes be due in part to the presence of cysts in the dysplastic tissue but is more often the result of ridges of bone forming on the inner aspect of the cortex. The tissue in these cases also is more fibrous than osseous, whereas the ground glass type of appearance is seen in those lesions that contain a large proportion of osseous tissue. The outlines of the lesion are often ill-defined, blending gradually into adjacent normal bone, though sometimes they are quite clearly demarcated. Periosteal new bone formation is not seen. Gibson and Middlemiss (1971) report on the radiology in a series of 55 cases; 46 monostotic and 9 polyostotic. They found that while certain radiological features were common to both forms, the monostotic lesions generally had a well defined and often sclerotic border whereas the polyostotic lesions tended to merge gradually with normal bone.

In the jaws, the radiological appearances are in general similar to those seen in other bones. Both translucent and ground glass appearances are seen, the latter being commoner in the mandible than in the maxilla. A very characteristic pattern, resembling orange peel, is seen in intraoral films of those areas that show the ground glass appearance in ordinary extraoral radiographs. Lesions of the translucent cyst-like type may occasionally appear unilocular, particularly in the mandible, and sometimes there is a clearly demarcated osteosclerotic outline. Diffuse lesions in the maxilla and facial bones may extend up to, and distort, the suture lines, but do not cross them (Fig. 133). Skull radiographs in jaw cases frequently show that there is increased density at the

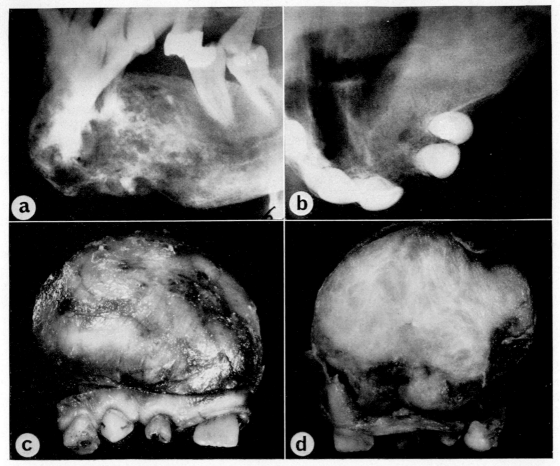

Fig. 133. **a,** radiograph of a fibrous dysplasia lesion in the mandible of a man of 41 years. The patient was unaware of this extensive lesion prior to 3 weeks before reporting to hospital. There had then been pain, swelling and mental anaesthesia, all of which subsided on antibiotic treatment. At operation there was a cavity in the bone, partly filled with soft tissue and partly with fluid. The radiograph shows an area of diffuse radiopacity, with scattered masses of highly calcified tissue. **b,** radiograph of a maxillary lesion from another patient. There is expansion of the maxilla by a diffuse radiopacity. **c, d,** maxillary lesion in an African girl of 12 years. The swelling had been present for the past 5 years, gradually enlarging. At operation, the lower part of the tumour, which extended into the hard palate, was clearly demarcated, but the upper part extending into and displacing the infraorbital margin, was ill-defined. The resected specimen shows the outer and cut surfaces of the tumour. The latter displayed a whorled appearance like that of a fibroma, and was of similar consistency, but some patchy areas of hard tissue were also present. The histology is shown in Fig. 134 **b, c, d.** × $1\frac{1}{2}$.

base of the skull. Harris, Dudley and Barry (1962) and others have shown that this is a very characteristic finding in fibrous dysplasia.

Pathology

In most cases the material available for pathological examination consists of the relatively small portions of tissue removed at biopsy, or of a larger mass of tissue when surgery is undertaken to correct deformity. The tissue is of yellowish or greyish-white appearance and imparts a gritty sensation to the knife when cut. If a lesion is obtained intact in the jaw it will be seen that the bone is expanded, resulting in a rounded or fusiform swelling that may or may not be clearly demarcated (Fig. 133c, d). Occasionally, multicentric lesions may be present. On section, the normal bone is replaced by firm yellowish-white tissue that may be homogeneous throughout, or cysts may be present, although this is rare in jaw lesions (Obwegeser and colleagues, 1973).

Microscopically, the lesion consists of fibrous tissue that replaces the normal bone and gives rise to osseous trabeculae by metaplasia (Fig. 134). The proportion of fibrous to bony tissue varies from case to case and in different areas in the same lesion. It has been suggested that the proportion of fibrous tissue diminishes with the increasing age of a lesion, while calcification increases, but this is no more than a trend and is by no means a regular occurrence. The fibrous element of the lesion may be notably cellular, consisting of spindle cells arranged in a whorled manner, with little intervening collagen, or alternatively thick interlacing strands of collagen may be the principal feature, with a relative paucity of cells.

The trabeculae, consisting of immature bone, are most plentiful in those areas where the fibrous tissue is cellular, but tend to be scantier in the collagenous areas. They are irregular in size and shape though generally rather slender. Many have a rather characteristic V- or W-shape. The trabeculae consist at first of osteoid, later becoming well calcified, and rows of osteoblasts are very occasionally seen lining their margins. Evidence of osteoclastic activity may also be seen in connection with the trabeculae, but osteoclast-like giant cells are quite often present in the fibrous tissue, at some distance from bone. Lamellar bone may be evident, although some workers consider that its presence negatives a diagnosis of fibrous dysplasia. They consider that fibrous dysplasia is due to a failure of bone maturation and that therefore the bone in the lesion does not develop beyond the immature, woven stage (Reed, 1963; Reed and Hagy, 1965). On the other hand, Waldron and Giansanti (1973) have shown in serial biopsies that lamellar maturation does occur, and that those lesions that contain appreciable quantities of lamellar bone always come from older patients. Similarly, Dahlgren and colleagues (1969) found lamellar bone in patients over the age of 40, and they also were able to show that maturation from immature to lamellar bone takes place (Fig. 135).

Microcyst formation due to focal degeneration of the fibrous tissue may occur, particularly in the more collagenous areas, and confluence of these small cysts leads to the formation of the cystic spaces noted macroscopically. Although cartilage occurs in the lesions in polyostotic cases it is rare in monostotic lesions and has not been reported in jaw lesions. Collections of foam cells may occasionally be seen. They are generally related to areas of degeneration and haemorrhage (Fig. 136).

The appearances just described may be observed in polyostotic or monostotic lesions in any bone, including the jaws, but in the jaws there are often additional features to be seen. As a rule, jaw lesions are more heavily ossified than are lesions in other bones, and thus the bony trabeculae tend to be thicker and blunter than the slender trabeculae of the trunk or limb bone lesions. Spheroidal calcifications, described in more detail on p. 399, may be present (Figs. 135 and 136).

Etiology

The nature and etiology of fibrous dysplasia are unknown. Various theories have been put forward, including maldevelopment, liver damage, glandular dysfunction and infection; these

FIG. 134. a, low power view of an area of fibrous dysplasia of the maxilla, showing the replacement of the normal bony architecture by a fibrocellular tissue in which new bony trabeculae are being laid down. × 8. b, c, d, from the lesion shown in Fig. 133 c, d. b and c show the cellular fibrous tissue that replaces normal bone in the fibrous dysplasia lesion, with the development in it of slender bony trabeculae. × 80. d shows how these trabeculae arise directly from the fibrous tissue by metaplasia. × 200.

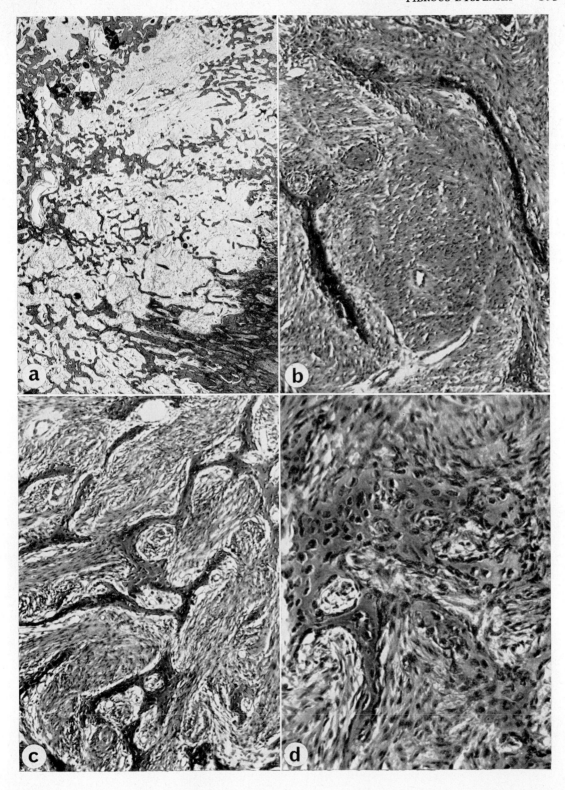

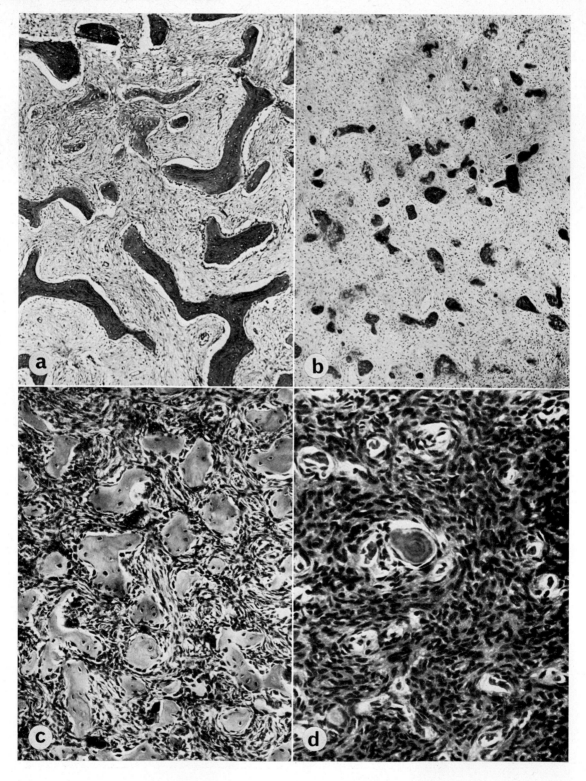

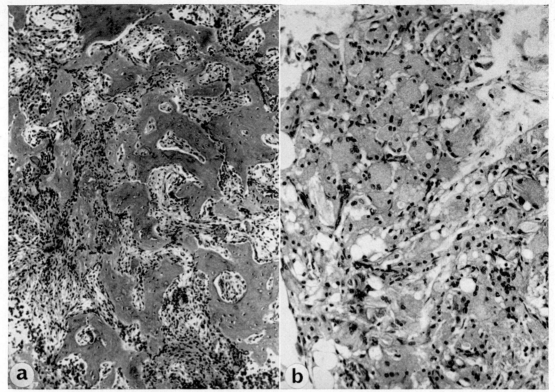

Fig. 136. **a,** in jaw lesions of fibrous dysplasia the bony trabeculae are often, as shown in this maxillary lesion, more plentiful and blunter than in lesions in other bones. × 80. **b,** foam cells in a mandibular lesion of fibrous dysplasia. × 200.

are discussed at some length by Dockerty, Ghormley, Kennedy and Pugh (1945). The view of Thannhauser (1944) and others that the condition is a type of neurofibromatosis gained some prominence, but Jaffe (1945) and Valls, Polak and Schajowicz (1950) have demonstrated that this cannot be accepted. Snapper (1949) interpreted the changes as an expression of lipoid granulomatosis, on the basis of the presence of the foam cells that are often seen in the lesions, but it is now generally agreed that these are merely lipid-laden phagocytes, related to areas of haemorrhage and degeneration (Fig. 136).

The consensus of opinion at present regards fibrous dysplasia as a developmental defect. This is supported by the strikingly segmental distribution of the lesions in many cases, as well as by the age incidence and the natural history of the disease. As noted, the condition is usually detected in children, and even infants, while in older patients there is often evidence that the lesions have been present for a long time. However, the disease is neither familial nor hereditary. There is no evidence to suggest that the lesions are neoplastic. On the contrary, they do not exhibit persistence of growth but tend instead to become inactive or stabilised after the normal period of skeletal growth has come to an end.

Fig. 135. Varying features in fibrous dysplasia. **a,** lamellar bone may be present. Osteoblast rimming is sometimes also seen. × 50. **b,** the hard tissue may appear as rather lumpy masses or curvilinear formations rather than slender trabeculae. × 50. **c,** the fibrous element may be notably cellular. × 120. **d,** cellular fibrous element and spheroidal calcifications. × 120.

Most observers are agreed that the lesions in polyostotic and in monostotic disease are histologically identical (except for the absence of cartilage in monostotic lesions) but some have maintained that while the polyostotic lesions represent a developmental anomaly the monostotic lesions are reparative reactions to trauma (Schlumberger, 1946).

Little is known about the histogenesis of the condition. Lichtenstein (1938) considered that there is perverted activity of the specific bone-forming mesenchyme. Falconer, Cope and Robb-Smith (1942) suggested that the primary change is marrow fibrosis with subsequent absorption of the laminated trabeculae, followed by new formation of fibre bone. Changus (1957) has demonstrated a high alkaline phosphatase activity in the osteoblasts and stromal fibroblasts of the lesion, which suggests to him that the basic abnormality is a hyperplasia or exaggerated response of osteoblasts to stimuli of unknown nature.

Behaviour

The lesions of fibrous dysplasia tend towards stabilisation with the completion of normal skeletal growth, though they do not necessarily show continuous growth up to that time. Thus lesions in a child may grow actively for a period and then become quiescent, well before skeletal growth has been completed. On the other hand, lesions that have been quiescent for some time may undergo a phase of renewed growth. This may occur in adults, who may be aware that a quiescent lesion has been present since childhood, or the presence of such a lesion may not have been previously detected. Occasionally, reactivation of lesions may occur in pregnancy (Henry, 1969).

Normally, conservative surgical treatment is satisfactory, with removal of small lesions in their entirety or sufficient of large masses to reduce deformity. Since in children and adolescents further post-operative growth may occur, surgical treatment may be postponed till adult life, though even then there may be post-operative growth in some cases. The lesion is not radio-sensitive and, though the risk is small, the possibility of postradiation sarcoma exists.

Rarely, malignant change may occur in a bone with a fibrous dysplasia lesion and fibrosarcoma, osteosarcoma and chondrosarcoma have been reported (Coley and Stewart, 1945; Dustin and Ley, 1950; Sutro, 1951; Perkinson and Higinbotham, 1955; Jaffe, 1958; Kiehn, DesPrez and Harris, 1961; Schwartz and Alpert, 1964; Riddell, 1964; Bell and Hinds, 1967; Smith and Belcher, 1969). There is some doubt as to whether the sarcoma does not arise coincidentally, rather than from the fibrous dysplasia lesion. However, there is no doubt that malignant change may occur, rarely, in a fibrous dysplasia lesion following radiation. In the facial and jaw bones cases of this type have been reported by Cahan and colleagues (1948), Sabanas and colleagues (1956), Tanner, Dahlin and Childs (1961). Slow, Stern and Friedman (1971) give the literature.

OSSIFYING FIBROMA

Before the emergence of fibrous dysplasia as a clinical and pathological entity, most fibro-osseous lesions in the jaws were regarded as focal examples of osteitis fibrosa or as benign neoplasms. Montgomery (1927) appears to have been the first to designate jaw lesions of this type as ossifying fibromas and further reports from Phemister and Grimson (1937), Eden (1939), Scarff and Walker (1948) and others classified the lesions as osteitis resulting from infection, fibrous osteoma, osteofibroma, ossifying fibroma or osteofibrosis. Probably, too, a number of cases reported as giant cell tumours of the jaws really fell into the fibro-osseous group. Schlumberger's (1946) report on monostotic lesions in fibrous dysplasia drew attention to the fibro-osseous jaw lesions as possible examples of this condition and subsequent reports showed a general acceptance that at least some of these lesions were really monostotic manifestations of fibrous dysplasia. To some observers, in fact, they were all examples of that disease. Jaffe (1953), for instance, believed this to be the case, considering even lesions such as ivory osteoma to be the possible end result of a fibrous dysplastic process, though more recently (Jaffe, 1958) he has regarded the ossifying fibroma, which he terms fibrocementoma, as an entity to be kept apart from fibrous dysplasia. Among others who support the unitarian thesis are Berger and Jaffe (1953), Zimmerman, Dahlin and Stafne (1958) and Bernier (1959). On the other hand, Sicher and Weinmann (1954), Thoma (1956), Cooke (1957), Hamner and colleagues (1968) and Eversole, Sabes and Rovin (1972) are among many others who distinguish between fibro-osseous lesions that are dysplastic and those that they consider to be neoplasms.

Clinical Features

The clinical features of ossifying fibroma are in general similar to those of fibrous dysplasia, though in some cases at least growth appears to be progressive. The condition occurs in children and in adults and presents as a localised hard swelling of the jaw, painless and not tender. Growth is generally slow, with gradually increasing facial deformity. Either jaw may be affected, the mandible more often than the maxilla, and more than one lesion may be present. Radiologically, a lesion that is mainly fibrous appears as a well defined radiolucent area, often with a thin osteo-sclerotic rim, and containing small irregular radiopaque areas. Lesions that contain much calcified material present as dense radiopaque areas, though they are still well circumscribed on the whole. However, the delimitation of the lesion is not always sharp in all areas, for at some points the radiopacity of the lesion may gradually merge with the normal pattern of the surrounding bone (Fig. 137).

Pathology

Since the lesion is well circumscribed it can often be shelled out. Relatively small lesions are often excised complete with some surrounding normal bone. The consistency of the lesion varies with the amount of calcification. The cut surface is whitish-yellow. Microscopically, the lesion consists of cellular fibrous tissue with the fibroblasts often arranged in a whorled pattern. The calcified tissue takes the form of trabeculae of bone as in fibrous dysplasia, and the microscopic appearances are indistinguishable from that condition. Differentiation is dependent on the nature of the delimitation of the lesion, those that are circumscribed, well delimited and generally tumour-like in appearance being considered as ossifying fibromas and those that are more diffuse, with ill-defined edges, being classified as fibrous dysplasia (Fig. 137).

In some lesions, numerous foci of calcified material are scattered throughout the fibrous tissue, varying in size from minute spherical deposits to larger masses. These calcifications are similar to those seen in fibrous dysplasia, but have been more frequently seen in lesions diagnosed as ossifying fibroma (Eversole and colleagues, 1972). The smaller foci are quite homogeneous and acellular, and stain deeply with haematoxylin. Slightly larger foci are still often spherical though elongated forms also occur. These larger foci are again homogeneous centrally, though at the periphery they may have a striated appearance, resulting from the calcification occurring in small globules that are arranged in a radiating manner. As the calcified foci increase in size they tend to fuse to form large irregular masses that are still strongly haematoxyphil, homogeneous and acellular and contain numerous deeply stained resting lines. The process of calcification takes place in a collagenous matrix that can be seen as a rim of eosinophilic material surrounding some of the calcified masses, though some deposits appear to be metastatic.

Nature

The circumscribed nature of this lesion helps to differentiate it from fibrous dysplasia. However, as already mentioned, the histological appearances in lesions that are described either as

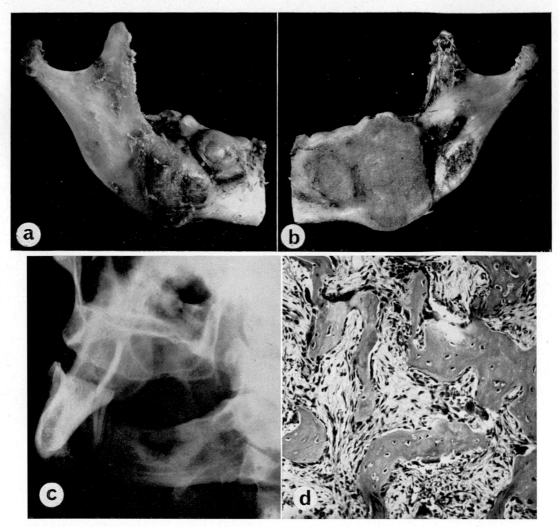

Fig. 137. **a,b,** ossifying fibroma of the mandible in a woman of 32 years. There was a history of a swelling of the mandible that had been diagnosed as a cyst and removed, 7 years previously. A year ago the swelling had recurred and had been enlarging since. Resection was now carried out. The specimen shows a circumscribed tumour in the body and angle of the mandible, with an irregularly bosselated outer surface. The cut surface of the lesion was greyish-yellow and generally firm, but harder areas were scattered throughout it. It is clearly demarcated from the surrounding normal tissue. **c,** ossifying fibroma in a woman of 46 years, showing the localised and circumscribed radiographic appearance. **d,** microscopic appearance, showing trabeculae of woven bone in a moderately cellular matrix. × 120.

ossifying fibroma or as fibrous dysplasia by different observers can be identical, and in an exhaustive survey of the literature, Eversole, Sabes and Rovin (1972) have shown that the whole range of the various histological features of these fibro-osseous lesions, including lamellar bone, woven bone, rimming of bony trabeculae by osteoblasts and the presence of spheroidal calcifications, can be found in both ossifying fibroma and fibrous dysplasia.

When spheroidal deposits of calcified material are present, they resemble the small deposits of cementum, or cementicles, that are not infrequently seen in the periodontal ligament of normal teeth. A number of workers have therefore believed that the calcified material of the lesion is also cementum, and have accordingly designated the lesion as fibrocementoma or cementoma (Bernier and Thompson, 1946; Pindborg, 1951). Thoma and Goldman (1960) use the term odontogenic fibroma, on the grounds that the cementicles indicate the origin of the lesion from odontogenic fibrous tissue. However, Geschickter and Copeland (1949) point out that the calcified spherules are typical of ossifying tumours of any membrane bones and Jaffe (1953), Weinmann and Sicher (1955), Dahlin (1967) and Waldron (1970) also note that these structures are not confined to jaw tumours. They may even be found in fibrous dysplasia lesions of cartilage bones, for example the rib. Thus, if the conventional definition of cementum as a modified type of bone covering the roots of the teeth be accepted, there are difficulties in describing as cementum the calcified spherules seen not only in certain fibro-osseous lesions of the jaws but also in similar lesions of cranial bones. Accordingly, for those who regard the lesion as a neoplasm but do not regard the calcifying material as cementum, the term ossifying fibroma has seemed the most appropriate designation. It is used in this sense by Weinmann and Sicher (1955) and others.

Many clinicians and pathologists would agree that the distinction between fibrous dysplasia and ossifying fibroma is clinical rather than histopathological. This distinction derives its validity from symptomatology and behaviour, although even on these grounds it is occasionally difficult to differentiate between the lesions. In general, the lesions diagnosed as ossifying fibroma have a thin bony shell and a distinct boundary as seen in the radiograph, whereas the lesions of fibrous dysplasia are often more diffuse and tend to extend, in membrane bones, up to suture lines. In this respect, therefore, ossifying fibroma behaves more like a neoplasm, but on the other hand some lesions of fibrous dysplasia can also appear as distinct foci, and they can also on occasion behave aggressively. Cases of this type have been reported by Williams and Faccini (1973) and Schofield (1974). When the ossifying fibroma type of lesion appears in children, it often ceases to enlarge with skeletal maturity. In Scarff's (1947) case, a lesion first seen in a young boy was subsequently observed to have remained quiescent over a period of 20 years. In adults, however, there is sometimes a history of slow though continuous growth to large dimensions. In Champion, Moule and Wilkinson's (1949) case, for example, the patient was a woman aged 54, with a mandibular tumour weighing nearly one pound and extending almost to the clavicle, which had not been noted on oral examination five years previously. Slaughter, Roeser and Smejkal (1949) also emphasise the persistent growth often exhibited by these lesions.

In most cases enucleation of the lesion results in cure, but recurrence is possible. However, even partial removal is not necessarily followed by further growth.

To summarise, it may be said that, in general, lesions diagnosed as ossifying fibroma show the characteristics of a developmental abnormality rather than a neoplasm. In favour of this are the frequent incidence in children and the younger age groups, the occasional multiplicity and the growth pattern. On the other hand, the neoplasm-like characteristics that are seen in some cases, such as clear demarcation of the lesion radiologically and pathologically, growth to large dimensions and recurrence, can all be shown at times by fibrous dysplastic lesions in extra-cranial bones.

The lesion is regarded here as in all probability a dysplastic condition of membrane bone. Fundamentally it may well be related to fibrous dysplasia but its distinctive features make it desirable to recognise it, at present, as an entity.

REFERENCES

Albright, F., Butler, A. M., Hampton, A. O., and Smith, P. (1937) Syndrome characterized by osteitis fibrosa disseminata, areas of pigmentation and endocrine dysfunction, with precocious puberty in females. Report of five cases. *New Engl. J. Med.*, **216,** 727.

Bell, W. H., and Hinds, E. C. (1967) Fibrosarcoma complicating polyostotic fibrous dysplasia. *Oral Surg.*, **23,** 299.

Berger, A., and Jaffe, H. L. (1953) Fibrous (fibro-osseous) dysplasia of jaw bones. *J. oral Surg.*, **11,** 3.

Bernier, J. L. (1959) *The Management of Oral Disease.* 2nd Edition. New York. C. V. Mosby Co.

Bernier, J. L., and Thompson, H. C. (1946) The histogenesis of the cementoma. *Amer. J. Orthodont.* (*Oral Surg. Sect.*), **32,** 543.

Bowerman, J. E. (1969) Polyostotic fibrous dysplasia with oral melanotic pigmentation. *Brit. J. oral Surg.*, **6,** 188.

Cahan, W. G., Woodward, H. Q., Higinbotham, N. L., Stewart, F. W., and Coley, B. L. (1948) Sarcoma arising in irradiated bone; report of eleven cases. *Cancer*, **1,** 3.

Champion, A. H. R., Moule, A. W., and Wilkinson, F. C. (1949) Case report of an endosteal fibroma of the mandible. *Brit. dent. J.*, **86,** 3.

Changus, G. W. (1957) Osteoblastic hyperplasia of bone. A histochemical appraisal of fibrous dysplasia of bone. *Cancer*, **10,** 1157.

Coley, B. L., and Stewart, F. W. (1945) Bone sarcoma in polyostotic fibrous dysplasia. *Ann. Surg.*, **121,** 872.

Cooke, B. E. D. (1957) Benign fibro-osseous enlargements of the jaws. *Brit. dent. J.*, **102,** 1, 49.

Dahlgren, S. E., Lind, P. O., Lindbon, Å., and Mårtensson, G. (1969) Fibrous dysplasia of jaw bones. A clinical, roentgenographic and histopathologic study. *Acta Otolaryngol.*, **68,** 257.

Dahlin, D. C. (1967) *Bone Tumors.* 2nd Edition. Springfield, Ill. Charles C. Thomas.

Dockerty, M. B., Ghormley, R. K., Kennedy, R. L. J., and Pugh, D. G. (1945) Albright's syndrome (polyostotic fibrous dysplasia with cutaneous pigmentation in both sexes and gonadal dysfunction in females). *Arch. intern. Med.*, **75,** 357.

Dustin, P., and Ley, R. A. (1950) Contribution à l'étude des dysplasies osseuse: description anatomo-clinique d'un cas d'osteosarcome polymorphe chez un enfant atteint de fibro-xanthomatose osseuse avec prematuration sexuelle. *Rev. belge path. et méd. exper.*, **20,** 52.

Eden, K. C. (1939) The benign fibro-osseous tumours of the skull and facial bones. *Brit. J. Surg.*, **27,** 323.

Eversole, L. R., Sabes, W. R., and Rovin, S. (1972) Fibrous dysplasia: a nosologic problem in the diagnosis of fibro-osseous lesions of the jaws. *J. oral Path.*, **1,** 189.

Fairbank, H. A. T. (1950) Fibrocystic disease of bone. *J. Bone Jt. Surg.*, **32B,** 403

Falconer, M. A., Cope, C. L., and Robb-Smith, A. H. T. (1942) Fibrous dysplasia of bone with endocrine disorders and cutaneous pigmentation (Albright's disease). *Quart. J. Med.*, **11,** 121.

Geschickter, C. F., and Copeland, M. H. (1949) *Tumors of Bone.* 3rd Edition. Philadelphia. J. B. Lippincott Company.

Gibson, M. J., and Middlemiss, J. H. (1971) Fibrous dysplasia of bone. *Brit. J. Radiol.*, **44,** 1.

Gorlin, R. J., and Chaudhry, A. P. (1957) Oral melanotic pigmentation in polyostotic fibrous dysplasia—Albright's syndrome. *Oral Surg.*, **10,** 857.

Hamner, J. E., Scofield, H. H., and Cornyn, J. (1968) Benign fibro-osseous jaw lesions of periodontal membrane origin. An analysis of 249 cases. *Cancer*, **22,** 861.

Harris, W. H., Dudley, H., and Barry, R. J. (1962) Natural history of fibrous dysplasia. An orthopedic, pathological, and roentgenographic study. *J. Bone Jt. Surg.*, **44A,** 207.

Henry, A. (1969) Monostotic fibrous dysplasia. *J. Bone Jt. Surg.*, **51B,** 300.

Hunter, D., and Turnbull, H. M. (1931) Hyperparathyroidism: generalized osteitis fibrosa. With observations upon the bones, the parathyroid tumours, and normal parathyroid glands. *Brit. J. Surg.*, **19,** 203.

Jaffe, H. L. (1945) Fibrous dysplasia of bone. A disease entity and specifically not an expression of neuro-fibromatosis. *J. Mt. Sinai Hosp.*, **12,** 364.

Jaffe, H. L. (1953) Giant-cell reparative granuloma, traumatic bone cyst, and fibrous (fibro-osseous) dysplasia of the jawbones. *Oral Surg.*, **6,** 159.

Jaffe, H. L. (1958) *Tumors and Tumorous Conditions of the Bones and Joints.* London. Henry Kimpton.

Kiehn, C. L., DesPrez, J. D., and Harris, A. H. (1961) Fibrous dysplasia of the facial bones. *Amer. J. Surg.*, **102,** 835.

Lichtenstein, L. (1938) Polyostotic fibrous dysplasia. *Arch. Surg.*, **36,** 874.

Lichtenstein, L., and Jaffe, H. L. (1942) Fibrous dysplasia of bone. A condition affecting one, several or many bones, the graver cases of which may present abnormal pigmentation of skin, premature sexual development, hyperthyroidism or still other extraskeletal abnormalities. *Arch. Path.*, **33,** 777.

McCune, D. J., and Bruch, H. (1937) Osteodystrophia fibrosa. Report of a case in which the condition was combined with precocious puberty, pathologic pigmentation of the skin and hyperthyroidism, with a review of the literature. *Amer. J. Dis. Child.*, **54,** 806.

Mandl, F. (1926) Therapeutischer Versuch bei einem Falle von Ostitis fibrosa generalisata mittels Exstirpation eines Epithelkörperchentumors. *Zentralb. f. Chir.*, **53,** 260.

Montgomery, A. H. (1927) Ossifying fibromas of the jaw. *Arch. Surg.*, **15,** 30.

Obwegeser, H. L., Freihofer, H. P. M., and Horejs, J. (1973) Variations of fibrous dysplasia in the jaws. *J. max. -fac. Surg.*, **1,** 161.

Perkinson, N. G., and Higinbotham, N. L. (1955) Osteogenic sarcoma arising in polyostotic fibrous dysplasia. Report of a case. *Cancer*, **8,** 396.

Phemister, D. B., and Grimson, K. S. (1937) Fibrous osteoma of the jaws. *Ann. Surg.*, **105,** 564.

Pindborg, J. J. (1951) Cémentoblastomes-cémentomes. *Rev. Stomat.*, **52,** 745.

Reed, R. J. (1963) Fibrous dysplasia of bone. *Arch. Path.*, **75,** 480.

Reed, R. J., and Hagy, D. M. (1965) Benign non-odontogenic fibro-osseous lesions of the skull. *Oral Surg.*, **19,** 214.

Riddell, D. M. (1964) Malignant change in fibrous dysplasia. *J. Bone Jt. Surg.*, **46B,** 251.

Sabanas, A. O., Dahlin, D. C., Childs, D. S., and Ivins, J. C. (1956) Postradiation sarcoma of bone. *Cancer*, **9,** 528.

Scarff, R. W. (1947) Primary malignant tumours of bone. *Brit. J. Radiol.*, **20,** 19.

Scarff, R. W., and Walker, D. G. (1948) Unilateral bony swelling of maxilla. *Proc. roy. Soc. Med.*, **41,** 485.

Schlumberger, H. G. (1946) Fibrous dysplasia (ossifying fibroma) of the maxilla and mandible. *Amer. J. Orthodont. (Oral Surg. Sect.)*, **32,** 579.

Schofield, I. D. F. (1974) An aggressive fibrous dysplasia. *Oral Surg.*, **38,** 29.

Schwartz, D. T., and Alpert, M. (1964) Malignant transformation of fibrous dysplasia. *Amer. J. med. Sci.*, **247,** 1.

Sherman, R. S., and Glauser, O. J. (1958) Radiological identification of fibrous dysplasia of the jaws. *Radiology*, **71,** 553.

Sicher, H., and Weinmann, J. P. (1954) Bone pathology: (1) fibrous dysplasia of bone; (2) cementomas. *Int. dent. J.*, **4,** 684.

Slaughter, D. P., Roeser, E. H., and Smejkal, W. F. (1949) Excision of the mandible for neoplastic disease. Indications and techniques. *Surgery*, **26,** 507.

Slow, I. N., Stern, D., and Friedman, E. W. (1971) Osteogenic sarcoma in a pre-existing fibrous dysplasia: report of case. *J. oral Surg.*, **29,** 126.

Smith, A. R., and Belcher, D. (1969) Malignant change in fibrous dysplasia. A case report. *Ohio med. J.*, **65,** 826.

Snapper, I. (1949) *Medical Clinics on Bone Diseases.* 2nd Edition. New York. Interscience Publishers, Inc.

Sutro, C. J. (1951) Osteogenic sarcoma of the tibia in a limb affected with fibrous dysplasia. *Bull. Hosp. Jt. Dis.*, **12,** 217.

Tanner, H. C., Dahlin, D. C., and Childs, D. S. (1961) Sarcoma complicating fibrous dysplasia. Probable role of radiation therapy. *Oral Surg.*, **14,** 837.

Thannhauser, S. J. (1944) Neurofibromatosis (von Recklinghausen) and osteitis fibrosa cystica localisata et disseminata (von Recklinghausen). A study of a common pathogenesis of both diseases. Differentiation between "hyperparathyroidism with generalized decalcification and fibrocystic changes of the skeleton and osteitis fibrosa cystica disseminata." *Medicine*, **23,** 105.

Thoma, K. H. (1956) Differential diagnosis of fibrous dysplasia and fibro-osseous neoplastic lesions of the jaws and their treatment. *J. oral Surg.*, **14,** 185.

Thoma, K. H., and Goldman, H. M. (1960) *Oral Pathology.* 5th Edition. St. Louis. The C. V. Mosby Company.

Valls, J., Polak, M., and Schajowicz, F. (1950) Fibrous dysplasia of bone. *J. Bone Jt. Surg.*, **32A,** 311.

Von Recklinghausen, F. (1891) Die fibrose oder deformiende Osteite. Festschrift Rudolf Virchow zu seinem 71 Geburtstage. Berlin.

Waldron, C. A. (1970) Fibro-osseous lesions of the jaws. *J. oral Surg.*, **28,** 58.

Waldron, C. A., and Giansanti, J. S. (1973) Benign fibro-osseous lesions of the jaws: a clinical–radiologic–histologic review of sixty-five cases. *Oral Surg.*, **35,** 190; 340.

Weil. (1922) 9 Jähriges Mädchen mit pubertas praecox und Knochenbrüchigkeit. *Klin. Wschr.*, **1,** 2114.

Weinmann, J. P., and Sicher, H. (1955) *Bone and Bones*. 2nd Edition. London. Henry Kimpton.

Williams, J. L. and Faccini, J. M. (1973) Fibrous dysplastic lesions of the jaws in Nigerians. *Brit. J. oral Surg.*, **11,** 118.

Windholz, F. (1947) Cranial manifestations of fibrous dysplasia of bone. Their relation to leontiasis ossea and to simple bone cysts of the vault. *Amer. J. Roentgenol.*, **58,** 51.

Zimmerman, D. C., Dahlin, D. C., and Stafne, E. C. (1958) Fibrous dysplasia of the maxilla and mandible. *Oral Surg.*, **11,** 55.

33. Cherubism

This condition was first described by Jones (1933, 1938) as familial cystic multilocular disease of the jaws, but it has subsequently been known under a variety of other designations, including "cherubism," a term introduced by the same author.

Clinical Features

Children affected by this disease appear to be normal at birth, without any clinical or radiological evidence of the lesions that will later appear in the jaws. Males are affected about twice as frequently as females. The swellings in the jaws appear between the ages of 2 and 4 years, or sometimes a little earlier, the mandible always being affected and very often also the maxilla. The mandibular lesions are practically always bilateral and the maxillary ones usually are, though unilateral lesions can occur. The lesions increase in size quite rapidly up to the age of about 7 years and then enter into a static phase, or progress only slowly, up to puberty. Thereafter, there occurs an improvement in the facial appearance though the radiological appearances still remain abnormal.

The facial deformity resulting from the lesions is the chief complaint. There is a characteristic fullness of the cheeks and jaws and often also the eyes appear to be slightly upturned, with a rim of sclera visible beneath the iris. The exposure of the sclera has been attributed to involvement of the floor of the orbit causing upward displacement of the eyeball and loss of support for the lower eyelid. Stretching of the skin over the maxillary lesions may also contribute by retracting the lower eyelids (Caffey and Williams, 1951), and this may also be the cause of the lateral spreading of the nostrils seen in some cases. The upturned eyes and full cheeks give the cherubic appearance. Marked enlargement of the submandibular lymph nodes is generally present, producing fullness in the submandibular space. The cervical nodes may also be enlarged.

The lesions consist of fibrous replacement of large areas of bone, resulting in gross expansion and irregularity. The jaws thus appear to have hard irregular masses bulging outwards from the surface. These masses are not tender or painful. In the mandible, the alveolar process may be expanded, as well as the body of the bone, and this may lead to elevation of the tongue and defective speech. In the maxilla, the lesion is often confined to the tuberosities. If it is extensive and bilateral the palate may be V-shaped and the antrum may be obliterated. The cortex of the bone may be perforated and the lesion may then grow into or intermingle with the soft tissue of the cheek, or it may appear as a localised tumour on the gum. However, epulides appear to occur occasionally as separate lesions on the gum, unconnected with the intraosseous lesion.

The dentition shows many abnormalities. The deciduous teeth are irregularly spaced and some may be absent. These teeth are lost prematurely. The permanent teeth are also abnormal, being widely separated in the expanded bone and some may be imperfectly developed. Some permanent teeth remain in the jaws unerupted and others are absent, owing to non-development of the tooth-germ. These anomalies occur constantly in the affected area of the mandible. Though they may occur in the maxilla the dentition can be normal here, even though the bone is grossly affected.

Radiologically, the mandible shows considerable expansion by a multiloculated radiolucency. The loculi are sharply defined and traversed by a few bony septa. The cortex is thinned and much expanded, and may be absent in some areas. There is no excessive periosteal new bone formation. The lesion appears to begin in the region of the angle, spreading often to affect the bone from the molar region to the coronoid notch. The incisor region may be involved, but is sometimes spared. The condyle is never affected. In the maxilla, the lesions are less well defined than those in the mandible. There is generally a diffuse rarefaction and the margins of the bone are poorly demarcated. The maxillary sinus is obscured or obliterated (Fig. 138).

The blood chemistry is normal, though the alkaline phosphatase level may be slightly raised during the period of most active lesional growth. The general health is good and no other symptoms are present.

Extraoral lesions. McClendon, Anderson and Cornelius (1962) noted a large café au lait patch of the skin in one of their cases, and a cystic area was also present in the neck of the femur. In their second case, areas of expansion and rarefaction were present in four ribs. Thompson (1962) and Bloom, Chacker and Thoma (1962) and others have also reported cases in which lesions were found in other bones in addition to the jaws, though the jaw lesions in these cases were compatible clinically, radiologically and histologically with the generally accepted picture of cherubism. Microscopic examination of extraoral lesions has not yet been made in any case. For the present, therefore, the exact nature of these lesions remains uncertain.

Familial incidence. The familial incidence of the condition is one of its characteristic features. Jones's original patients were two brothers and a sister, and other records have also made clear the inherited nature of the condition. In another case reported by Jones (1938) members of five generations of the same family were affected. Seward and Hankey (1957) suggest that a single dominant gene is responsible for the condition, since one affected parent can transmit it to a proportion of the children, but all descendants of those children who are not affected remain free of the disease. However, Anderson and McClendon (1962), who have studied very fully the reported cases in the literature, consider that a dominant gene is responsible but that its expressivity varies. This would account for the fact that fewer females than males show the overt disease and for the apparent skipping of a generation, as in Abbey and Reece's (1961) cases, and for seemingly sporadic cases (McDonald and Shafer, 1955; Dukart and colleagues, 1974). Also, unilateral mandibular lesions have been present in relatives of patients with cherubism.

Pathology

The tissue that replaces the normal bone in the lesions is soft, fibrous or friable and mottled reddish-brown or greyish-brown. Microscopically, the main constituent of the lesion is fibrous tissue, arranged in a whorled pattern. Giant cells are generally a prominent feature (Fig. 138). These cells are similar to the giant cells found in giant cell tumours and in giant cell granuloma and tend to be arranged in groups, the intervening stromal cells being plump and spindle-shaped. The lesion is vascular, numerous thin-walled blood vessels being present, and these often show perivascular cuffs of eosinophilic material which has been shown to be collagen (Hamner, 1969; Hamner and Ketcham, 1969). The giant cells are often particularly concentrated around the blood vessels and in some areas may even appear themselves to line vascular spaces. Haemosiderin is generally present. Metaplastic bone formation is occasionally seen, but this is not a prominent feature of the lesion.

Fig. 138. Cherubism in a boy of 7 years. Facial deformity had become apparent about a year previously. The mother had been similarly affected as a child. **a,** the radiograph shows bilateral expanding pseudocystic lesions of the body of the mandible extending upwards into the two rami. There is almost complete absence of the mandibular permanent teeth. **b,** microscopically, the appearances are similar to those in giant cell granuloma—numerous giant cells irregularly distributed in a vascular fibrocellular matrix. × 80. **c,** higher magnification, showing the osteoclast-like giant cells and microcysts in the matrix. × 200. **d,** giant cells are often arranged around capillaries and vascular spaces, and may partially line them. × 200.

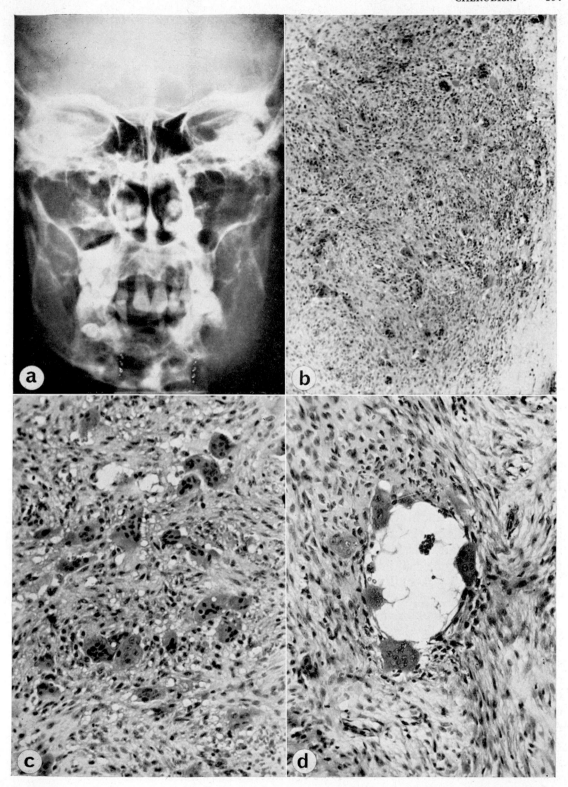

The gingival tumours that have occurred in some cases appear to be of variable structure. In Jones's (1938) cases they consisted of inflammatory tissue, but in others they have shown a similar structure to the intraosseous lesions (Small and Young, 1958).

The enlarged lymph nodes show chronic reactive changes and may contain much haemosiderin.

Histogenesis

The cause of cherubism is unknown. Though Jones (1933, 1938) first considered the lesion to represent cystic degeneration of abnormal tooth germs, this opinion was based on the clinical and radiological features only. Later, when pathological material became available in the original cases (Jones, Gerrie and Pritchard, 1950) and in those reported by subsequent authors, it was apparent that the lesion was not in fact cystic. Jones (1965) still considers that basically the condition is an anomaly of dental development, since the lesions occur only in tooth-bearing areas and dental abnormalities are regularly present. His co-workers, however, believe that the dental abnormalities are secondary to changes in the bone, and that the condition is primarily a bone dysplasia. Riley, Stuteville and Brown (1956) have also supported the idea of a fundamentally dental origin of the lesions. They point out that the onset of the condition appears to occur with the onset of the normal resorption of the roots of the deciduous teeth, and suggest that the lesion may represent an overaction of the normal resorptive processes. The decrease in progress of the lesion during adolescence corresponds in time with the natural decrease in tooth root resorption and the end of the deciduous tooth period.

Most subsequent authors have regarded the condition as a bone dysplasia, but of uncertain nature. Some have regarded it as a type of fibrous dysplasia (McDonald and Shafer, 1955; McClendon, Anderson and Cornelius, 1962), while others prefer for the time being a non-committal designation such as familial osseous dysplasia or familial fibrous swellings of the jaws (Caffey and Williams, 1951; Bruce, Bruwer and Kennedy, 1953; Riley, Stuteville and Brown, 1956; Small and Young, 1958).

Histological Diagnosis

It is not possible to make the diagnosis of cherubism solely on microscopic examination. When giant cells are plentiful in the lesion there are resemblances to giant cell tumour of bone, and some cases have been described as such (Waldron, 1951; Brannin and Christensen, 1954). However, apart from the histological differences between true giant cell neoplasm and other lesions in which giant cells may be present, the characteristic features of cherubism—familial incidence, multiple lesions and cherubic facies, typical age of onset and growth pattern—are sufficient to distinguish the two conditions. If any confusion were to arise, it would be much more likely in connection with giant cell granuloma. The microscopic appearances in cherubism may be very similar to those in giant cell granuloma, but again the clinical features of the former condition are so distinctive that confusion is unlikely. The possibility that one might be dealing with a very early or incompletely developed case of cherubism must, however, be considered.

When giant cells are present in relatively small numbers the histological appearances may suggest a lesion of fibrous dysplasia in which the replacement tissue is mainly fibrous rather than osseous. However, the absence of metaplastic bone in other than minimal amounts is a distinguishing feature, particularly in the jaws where fibrous dysplasia lesions tend to be heavily ossified rather than the reverse. Similar remarks may be made with regard to ossifying fibroma. Again, the clinical features are of great importance, for though multiple lesions of fibrous dysplasia and ossifying fibroma may occur in the jaws, these are not familial conditions and their growth pattern is different to that of cherubism.

Hyperparathyroidism must of course be considered in any lesion of the jaws in which giant cells are a feature. It is excluded by the normal biochemistry. A good discussion of the differential diagnosis of cherubism is given by Seward and Hankey (1957) and in the symposium in Oral Surg. Suppt 2 (1962).

Behaviour

As noted, the lesions show their greatest activity in the years immediately following their appearance, with subsequently a period of much slower growth up to puberty. Thereafter there is a tendency to regression. The maxillary lesions are the first to show signs of change after puberty, though the mandibular lesions may still be enlarging slowly, and may continue to do so up to about the age of 20. Then these lesions, too, regress and by middle life the facial appearance may have returned almost to normal. The lymph node enlargement subsides completely during adolescence.

The progressive improvement in facial appearance is accompanied by radiographic changes. At about puberty fine trabeculae of bone are laid down in the radiolucent areas and new cortical bone is deposited. The septa increase in number and density until by adult life the translucent spaces of the lesion have been largely filled up, to show a dense bony pattern, though a few small radiolucent spaces may still remain.

The condition is benign. Surgical intervention is often required for cosmetic reasons, as where disfigurement is severe it is hardly possible to await natural regression of the lesions. When this is undertaken, no ill-effects follow from curettage or from paring-down procedures.

Radiotherapy has been tried in a few cases. It appears to be ineffective.

REFERENCES

Abbey, F. S., and Reece, C. H. (1961) Cherubism: report of three cases. *J. oral Surg.*, **19,** 63.

Anderson, D. E., and McClendon, J. L. (1962) Cherubism—hereditary fibrous dysplasia of the jaws. I. Genetic considerations. *Oral Surg.*, **15,** *Suppl.* **2,** 5.

Bloom, J., Chacker, F. M., and Thoma, K. H. (1962) Multiple giant-cell lesions of bone. Report of a case. *Oral Surg.*, **15,** *Suppl.* **2,** 74.

Brannin, D. E., and Christensen, R. O. (1954) Bilateral giant cell tumors of the mandible in siblings: report of cases. *J. oral Surg.*, **12,** 247.

Bruce, K. W., Bruwer, A., and Kennedy, R. L. J. (1953) Familial intraosseous fibrous swellings of the jaws ("cherubism"). *Oral Surg.*, **6,** 995.

Caffey, J., and Williams, J. L. (1951) Familial fibrous swelling of the jaws. *Radiol.*, **56,** 1.

Dukart, R. C., Kolodny, S. C., Polte, H. W., and Hooker, S. P. (1974) Cherubism: report of case. *J. oral Surg.*, **32,** 782.

Hamner, J. E. (1969) The demonstration of perivascular collagen deposition in cherubism. *Oral Surg.*, **27,** 129.

Hamner, J. E., and Ketcham, A. S. (1969) Cherubism: an analysis of treatment. *Cancer*, **23,** 1133.

Jones, W. A. (1933) Familial multilocular cystic disease of the jaws. *Amer. J. Cancer*, **17,** 946.

Jones, W. A. (1938) Further observations regarding familial multilocular cystic disease of the jaws. *Brit. J. Radiol.*, **11,** 227.

Jones, W. A. (1965) Cherubism. A thumbnail sketch of its diagnosis and a conservative method of treatment. *Oral Surg.*, **20,** 648.

Jones, W. A., Gerrie, J., and Pritchard, J. (1950) Cherubism—a familial fibrous dysplasia of the jaws. *J. Bone Jt. Surg.*, **32B,** 334.

McClendon, J. L., Anderson, D. E., and Cornelius, E. A. (1962) Cherubism—hereditary fibrous dysplasia of the jaws. II. Pathologic considerations. *Oral Surg.*, **15,** Suppl. **2,** 17.

McDonald, R. E., and Shafer, W. G. (1955) Disseminated juvenile fibrous dysplasia of the jaws. *Amer. J. Dis. Child.*, **89,** 354.

Riley, P., Stuteville, O., and Brown, R. C. (1956) Familial fibrous swelling of the jaw. *Radiology*, **67,** 742.

Seward, G. R., and Hankey, G. T. (1957) Cherubism. *Oral Surg.*, **10,** 952.

Small, I. A., and Young, M. C. (1958) Familial osseous dysplasia of the jaws. *J. oral Surg.*, **16,** 35.

Thompson, E. R. (1962) Multiple giant-cell tumors. Report of a case. *Oral Surg.*, **15,** Suppl. **2,** 69.

Waldron, C. A. (1951) Familial incidence of bilateral giant-cell tumors of the jaw. *Oral Surg.*, **4,** 198.

34. Paget's Disease of Bone

The lesions of Paget's disease of bone may occur in the maxilla or the mandible, though affection of these bones is less common than of other parts of the skeleton.

Incidence

When Jaffe reviewed Paget's disease of bone in 1933, he estimated that only some 500 cases of the classical polyostotic form of the disease had been recorded since Paget's (1877) description. However, Schmorl (1932) had shown that the true incidence is in the region of 3 per cent of all persons over 40 years of age, if systematic search be made at autopsy, for in this way monostotic and subclinical lesions which would otherwise escape notice are revealed, and this estimate has been confirmed by the more recent autopsy survey of Collins (1956) and radiological survey of Pygott (1957). There are striking differences in geographical incidence, as Berry (1969) has shown in his exhaustive monograph. The disease is fairly common in the United Kingdom, France and Germany, but quite rare in Scandinavia, Spain, Italy, Central Europe, Russia and Asia. It is much less common in North and South America than in the United Kingdom. This distribution seems to be due to the fact that the disease is particularly common in people of Anglo-Saxon stock.

The lesions of Paget's disease are commonest in the vertebral column, particularly the sacrum. The lumbar vertebrae are next most often affected, then the thoracic and then the cervical vertebrae. This localisation has been attributed to the effects of mechanical stress, those parts bearing the most weight being the most often affected. After the vertebral column the skull is next most frequently involved and this again may be due to functional stress, the continued pulsation of the brain, traction of the neck muscles and the stresses of mastication having been given as determining factors.

Lesions in the jaws have been known to occur since Moore's (1923) report of a case in which there was a bony tumour of the maxilla associated with osteoporosis circumscripta of the frontal region. Osteoporosis circumscripta has been identified with an early phase of Paget's disease by Sosman (1927) and others, and subsequently a number of cases were described in which there was a co-existing lesion in the maxilla (Kasabach and Gutman, 1937; Elkeles, 1947; Rushton, 1948).

Often the patient's symptoms arise from lesions other than those in the jaws, with the result that the jaw lesions come to light in the ensuing examination. In some cases, however, the symptoms arising from the lesions in the jaws may be the first of which the patient complains, and thus lead to the subsequent detection of lesions in other parts of the skull or in other bones. Cases of this type have been reported by Novak and Burket (1944) and Jacobs (1945). Occasionally, the jaw lesions may be the only ones present (Thoma, Howe and Wenig, 1945).

The maxilla is much more often affected than the mandible. In Stafne and Austin's (1938) series, the mandible was affected in 3 cases and the maxilla in 20 cases. These 23 cases of jaw involvement were found in 138 cases in which skull lesions were present. This gives some idea of the incidence of jaw lesions.

The teeth are often affected in association with the surrounding bone, the principal abnormality being hypercementosis.

Clinical Features

An early symptom is often intermittent pain of neuralgic type, which may be very severe, and may be experienced before there is any obvious enlargement of the jaws. Bony enlargement gives rise to facial deformity and the expansion of the alveolar ridges results in dentures ceasing to fit properly. Their pressure on the gum and bone may lead to necrosis. The progressive increase in size of the dental arch causes spacing of the teeth, which also tend to erupt because of the new bone formation. The overgrowth of cementum on the roots of the teeth may lead to difficulty in extraction, or severe inflammation may follow extractions as the dense avascular areas of bone that form in the osteosclerotic phase of the disease appear to be particularly prone to infection. Excessive bleeding on extraction may occur, since the marrow is often very vascular.

Other clinical features, relating to involvement of the skull such as deafness and the characteristic disproportion between the size of the cranium and the lower face, and to involvement of the vertebral column and the limb bones, are well known and need not be repeated here.

Radiologically, the skull shows changes in most cases. There is thickening of the outer table of the vault with loss of distinction between the tables and the diploë, and irregular areas of radiolucency and sclerosis that give the characteristic cotton wool effect. The appearances characterised as osteoporosis circumscripta may be noted—well defined map-like confluent radiolucent areas with sharp irregular edges, but with no bony thickening, occupying the frontal, occipital or parietal zones. In the jaws, the earliest change is osteoporosis around the teeth (Cooke, 1956). This is followed by osteosclerosis, with the formation of dense areas of bone with ill-defined outlines that tend to merge with the hypercementosis that affects the teeth (Fig. 139). These sclerosed areas produce the appearance of cotton wool patches similar to those seen in the skull. Occasionally they may be so dense as to be mistaken for odontomes or embedded teeth. Cook notes that in some cases of maxillary disease there may be a uniform increase in density, without any cotton wool patches, giving a ground glass appearance.

Pathology

Bone. Microscopic examination of bone from the jaws shows the characteristic changes of Paget's disease as seen in other parts of the skeleton. These are due, as Weinmann and Sicher (1955) express it, to a combination of destruction and repair occurring without relation to the statics or dynamics of the affected bone.

According to Schmorl, the earliest changes occur in the haversian canals, and consist of osteoclastic resorption. As the removal of bone proceeds, the canals gradually enlarge and ultimately adjacent spaces coalesce. The marrow in these spaces then comes to contain numerous connective tissue cells and new bone is laid down, in trabeculae in the marrow and on the walls of the enlarged spaces. This initial phase is followed by continued resorption of the old bone, and of the newly deposited bone, together with further deposition of more new bone. These two processes, deposition and resorption, then continue, sometimes more or less side by side, sometimes in an alternating manner, so that ultimately the bone becomes extensively remodelled. As this occurs without any apparent reference to the functional requirements of the part of the skeleton in which the process is taking place, the bony pattern comes to present a quite irregular appearance, consisting of fragments juxtaposed like the pieces of a jigsaw puzzle. The cement lines between these pieces, often broad and markedly haematoxyphilic, give rise to the characteristic curvilinear markings of Knaggs (1925) or mosaic pattern (Fig. 140). The rate of turnover of the bone is rapid, as has been shown by the isotope studies of Bauer and Wenderberg (1959) and Macdonald (1960). Lee (1967) has similarly demonstrated a high turnover rate by using tetracycline markers.

The deposition of new bone frequently occurs in the form of small acellular spheroidal masses

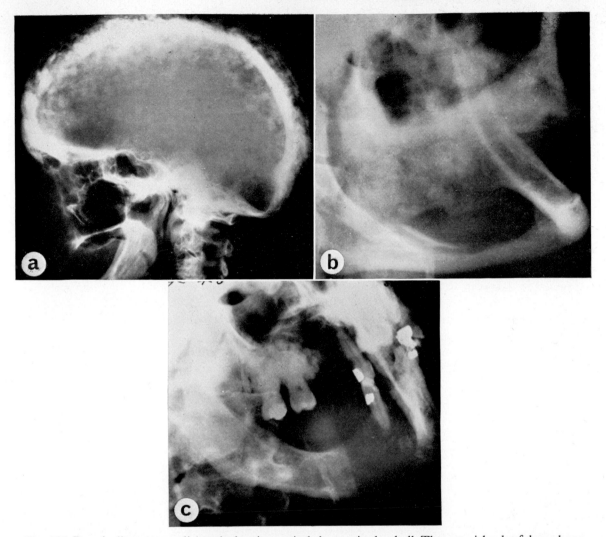

Fig. 139. Paget's disease. **a,** radiograph showing typical changes in the skull. There are islands of dense bone on the inner and outer surfaces with thickening of the vault. The variations in radiodensity give rise to the "cotton-wool" appearance. **b,** Paget's disease affecting the maxilla. There is diffuse enlargement of the pre-molar and molar regions, with thickening of the alveolar ridge. The maxillary sinus is encroached upon and reduced in size. The mandible is not involved. **c.** hypercementosis is a characteristic feature of Paget's disease of the jaws. In this woman of 60 years there is an irregular opaque mass around the upper right second and third molar teeth, due to the deposition of much cementum. The specimen is shown in Fig. 139 **a.**

that gradually enlarge and fuse to form larger areas of dense sclerotic bone. In turn, there is fusion between this dense bone and the hyperplastic cementum covering the roots of the teeth. In this way ankylosis of the teeth occurs.

The Teeth. Involvement of the teeth in Paget's disease was first described by Fox (1933), who reported a case in which the maxilla was affected and the roots of all the maxillary teeth showed radiographically the presence of knob-like irregularities, due to excessive deposition of cementum. Later, Stafne and Austin (1938) showed that hypercementosis is a characteristic of Paget's disease and many other authors have reported similar findings. However, it is to be noted that the cemental proliferation occurs only after the bony changes in the jaws are well established, and in a relatively early case this feature may be lacking.

An extracted tooth with hypercementosis shows a mass of hard tissue around the root or roots (Fig. 140). The excessive cementum may be diffusely deposited over the whole of the root, or it may be confined mainly to the apical portion, forming a roughly globular mass. Rushton (1938) pointed out that the excessive cementum may be deposited in the same manner as is the abnormal bone in Paget's disease—in successive irregular increments, with intervening phases of resorption. Hence the characteristic mosaic appearance is seen also in the cementum as well as in the bone. Even in cases where the cementosis is of lesser extent this appearance may also be detected (Lucas, 1955).

In some cases resorption of the roots of the teeth may take place, rather than hypercementosis —there may occur, in fact, cementosis of one root with resorption of another, in the same tooth. Thoma and Goldman (1960) have pointed out that the resorbed cementum and dentine may be repaired by the ingrowth of Paget bone.

Histological Diagnosis

Since in most cases of Paget's disease of the jaws the skull is also affected, and often also other bones, the diagnosis is generally made on clinical and radiological grounds, together with the results of biochemical examination. The pathologist may then receive portions of bone for confirmatory examination, or bone may become available for examination when removed from the enlarged maxilla or mandible for prosthetic reasons.

In cases where the jaws alone are affected the clinical and radiological diagnosis may be difficult, particularly in early cases. The appearances may be interpreted as those of chronic osteomyelitis but histological examination of bone or teeth leads to the correct diagnosis or, where the histology is suggestive but not conclusive, to the performance of biochemical tests and adequate follow-up of the patient. It should be noted, however, as Cahn (1948) and Snapper (1949) have pointed out, that the serum alkaline phosphatase level may not be raised in cases where the disease is localised to one small area.

With regard to the histological picture itself, chronic osteomyelitis and fibrous dysplasia are the principal conditions requiring differentiation. Jaffe has noted that the bone of the jaws contains more cement lines than does bone from other parts of the skeleton, and that these are often irregularly disposed. No doubt this is due to the very active turnover of bone that occurs in the jaws as a result of the stresses of mastication. He also mentions healing infective periostitis with excessive bone formation as a possible cause of numerous cement lines, and generalised osteitis fibrosa cystica as a cause of chaotic bony architecture. However, a definite mosaic appearance is diagnostic of Paget's disease. When mosaics appear in other conditions, their extent is limited and the cement lines tend to be more regular.

Though ossifying fibroma generally occurs in younger patients it may also be seen in the age range at which Paget's disease occurs. Histologically, the osteoblastic phase of Paget's disease, characterised by the formation of dense acellular masses of bone, may resemble ossifying fibroma. However, a definite mosaic pattern is not seen in the latter condition, though the thick, deeply staining cement lines may be vaguely suggestive.

Fig. 140.   Paget's disease. **a,** the excised teeth shown in Fig. 139 **c.** They are surrounded by a dense mass of cementum. × 2. **b,** section of one of the teeth, showing the hypercementosis. × 3.5. **c,** alveolar bone, showing the characteristic mosaic pattern. × 150. **d,** heavily staining incremental lines in the cementum. × 80. **e,** at some distance from the teeth there is deposition of new calcified tissue in the form of small acellular masses. × 150.

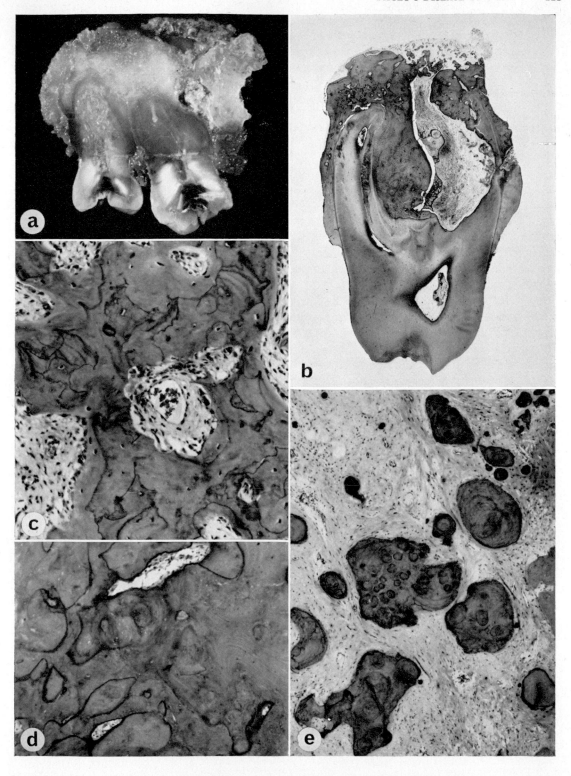

When teeth alone are available for examination it is still possible to make a histological diagnosis of Paget's disease if there is well marked hypercementosis showing the mosaic pattern. However, as has been seen, hypercementosis is not always present, but in such cases any resorption of the roots may be repaired by bone showing Paget characteristics.

Neoplasia in Paget's Disease

The incidence of neoplasia in Paget's disease is quite high in those cases in which there is involvement of many bones, being in the region of 10 per cent. Where only one or a small number of bones are affected the incidence is much lower, and Jaffe (1958) gives the overall figure as 2 to 3 per cent. Over one half of the neoplasms are osteosarcomas and a quarter are fibrosarcomas. Chondrosarcoma and giant cell tumour have also been reported, and although neoplasms may occur in any bone, the femur and the humerus are the commonest sites. Jaw tumours are rare, but it is of interest that McKenna and colleagues' (1964) survey of the literature showed that of the 12 benign giant cell tumours that have been reported, 3 occurred in the jaws. A fourth jaw tumour was malignant. A giant cell tumour of the maxilla has also been reported by Shklar and Meyer (1958). Malignant giant cell tumours have also been reported in Paget's disease, but it may well be that some at least of such tumours were basically osteosarcomas. Brooke (1970) reviews the literature.

Reports of osteosarcoma are scanty. In Karpawich's (1958) case the patient had Paget lesions in the skull and jaws and in the pelvis, and developed osteosarcomas in the maxilla and ilium. Foote (1961) reports one maxillary and one mandibular case, and in Berry's (1969) review of 116 patients with neoplasms, there was one mandibular and one maxillary case. There is one mandibular case in McKenna and colleagues' (1964) series; Tillman (1962), Rosenmertz and Schare (1969) also report cases and mention others. Taylor and Shklar (1964) have reported squamous cell carcinoma of the maxillary antrum in a patient with Paget's disease in the skull and jaws.

REFERENCES

Bauer, G. C. H., and Wenderberg, B. (1959) External counting of ^{47}Ca and ^{85}Sr in studies of localised skeletal lesions in man. *J. Bone Jt. Surg.*, **41B**, 558.

Berry, H. C. (1969) *Paget's Disease of Bone*. Edinburgh & London. E. & S. Livingstone Ltd.

Brooke, R. I. (1970) Giant-cell tumor in patients with Paget's disease. *Oral Surg.*, **30**, 230.

Cahn, L. (1948) Bone pathology as it relates to some phases of oral surgery. *Oral Surg.*, **1**, 917.

Collins, D. H. (1956) Paget's disease of bone. Incidence and subclinical forms. *Lancet*, **2**, 51.

Cooke, B. E. D. (1956) Paget's disease of the jaws: fifteen cases. *Ann. roy. Coll. Surg. Engl.*, **19**, 223.

Elkeles, A. (1947) Osteoporosis circumscripta and leontiasis ossea faciei associated with Paget's disease. *Proc. roy. Soc. Med.*, **40**, 466.

Foote, F. W. (1961) In Foote, F. W., and Horn, R. C. Seminar on diseases of maxillo-facial region including salivary gland. Proceedings of the Twenty-sixth Seminar of the American Society of Clinical Pathologists. 1960.

Fox, L. (1933) Paget's disease (osteitis deformans) and its effect on maxillary bones and teeth. *J. Amer. dent. Ass.*, **20**, 1823.

Jacobs, M. H. (1945) The jaws in Paget's disease (osteitis deformans): with special reference to osteoporosis circumscripta cranii. *Amer. J. Orthodont. (Oral Surg. Sect.)*, **31**, 104.

Jaffe, H. L. (1933) Paget's disease of bone. *Arch. Path.*, **15**, 83.

Jaffe, H. L. (1958) *Tumors and Tumorous Conditions of the Bones and Joints*. London. Henry Kimpton.

Karpawich, A. J. (1958) Paget's disease with osteogenic sarcoma of maxilla. *Oral Surg.*, **11**, 827.

Kasabach, H. H., and Gutman, A. B. (1937) Osteoporosis circumscripta of the skull and Paget's disease. Fifteen new cases and a review of the literature. *Amer. J. Roentgenol.*, **37**, 577.

Knaggs, R. L. (1925) On osteitis deformans (Paget's disease) and its relation to osteitis fibrosa and osteo-malacia. *Brit. J. Surg.*, **13,** 206.

Lee, W. R. (1967) Bone formation in Paget's disease. A quantitative microscopic study using tetracycline marks. *J. Bone Jt. Surg.*, **49B,** 146.

Lucas, R. B. (1955) The jaws and teeth in Paget's disease of bone. *J. clin. Path.*, **8,** 195.

Macdonald, N. S. (1960) The radioisotope osteogramkinetic studies of skeletal disorders in humans. *Clin. Orthop.*, **17,** 154.

McKenna, R. J., Schwinn, C. P., Soong, K. Y., and Higinbotham, N. L. (1964) Osteogenic sarcoma arising in Paget's disease. *Cancer*, **17,** 42.

Moore, S. (1923) Observations on osteitis deformans. *Amer. J. Roentgenol.*, **10,** 507.

Novak, A. J., and Burket, L. W. (1944) Oral aspects of Paget's disease, including case reports and necropsy findings. *Amer. J. Orthodont. (Oral Surg. Sect.)*, **30,** 544.

Paget, J. (1877) On a form of chronic inflammation of bones (osteitis deformans). *Trans. roy. med. chir. Soc. Lond.*, **60,** 37.

Pygott, F. (1957) Paget's disease of bone. The radiological incidence. *Lancet*, **1,** 1170.

Rosenmertz, S. K., and Schare, H. J. (1969) Osteogenic sarcoma arising in Paget's disease of the mandible. Review of the literature and report of a case. *Oral Surg.*, **28,** 304.

Rushton, M. A. (1938) The dental tissues in osteitis deformans. *Guy's Hosp. Rep.*, **88,** 163.

Rushton, M. A. (1948) Osteitis deformans affecting the upper jaw and osteoporosis circumscripta of the skull. *Brit. dent. J.*, **84,** 189.

Schmorl, G. (1932) Über Ostitis deformans Paget. *Virchows Arch.*, **283,** 694.

Shklar, G., and Meyer, I. (1958) A giant-cell tumor of the maxilla in an area of osteitis deformans (Paget's disease of bone). *Oral Surg.*, **11,** 835.

Snapper, I. (1949) *Medical Clinics on Bone Diseases.* 2nd Edition. New York. Interscience Publishers, Inc.

Sosman, M. C. (1927) Radiology as an aid in the diagnosis of skull and intracranial lesions. *Radiology*, **9,** 396.

Stafne, E. C., and Austin, L. T. (1938) A study of dental roentgenograms in cases of Paget's disease (osteitis deformans), osteitis fibrosa cystica and osteoma. *J. amer. dent. Ass.*, **25,** 1202.

Taylor, R., and Shklar, G. (1964) Carcinoma of the maxillary antrum in a patient with osteitis deformans (Paget's disease of bone). Report of case. *J. oral Surg.*, **22,** 428.

Thoma, K. H., Howe, H. D., and Wenig, M. (1945) Paget's disease of the mandible. *Amer. J. Orthodont. (Oral Surg. Sect.)*, **31,** 265.

Thoma, K. H., and Goldman, H. M. (1960) *Oral Pathology.* 5th Edition. London. Henry Kimpton.

Tillman, H. H. (1962) Paget's disease of bone. A clinical, radiographic, and histopathologic study of twenty-four cases involving the jaws. *Oral Surg.*, **15,** 1225.

Weinmann, J. P., and Sicher, H. (1955) *Bone and Bones.* 2nd Edition. London. Henry Kimpton.

Index